THE SAVVY WOMAN'S GUIDE TO MENOPAUSE

A JOHNS HOPKINS PRESS HEALTH BOOK

The Savvy Woman's Guide to Menopause

BEFORE, DURING, AND BEYOND

Julia Schlam Edelman
MD, FACOG, MSCP

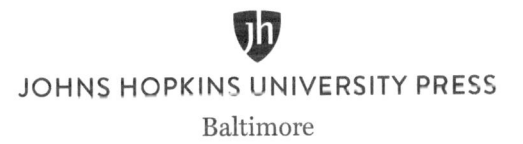

JOHNS HOPKINS UNIVERSITY PRESS
Baltimore

Note to the reader: This book is not intended as a substitute for the medical or healthcare advice of physicians or other licensed professionals. Readers should consult healthcare providers in matters relating to their health, particularly with respect to any symptoms that may require diagnosis or medical attention.

© 2025 Julia Schlam Edelman
All rights reserved. Published 2025
Printed in the United States of America on acid-free paper
9 8 7 6 5 4 3 2 1

Johns Hopkins University Press
2715 North Charles Street
Baltimore, Maryland 21218
www.press.jhu.edu

Library of Congress Cataloging-in-Publication Data is available.

ISBN 978-1-4214-5296-8 (hardcover)
ISBN 978-1-4214-5297-5 (paperback)
ISBN 978-1-4214-5298-2 (ebook)

A catalog record for this book is available from the British Library.

Special discounts are available for bulk purchases of this book. For more information, please contact Special Sales at specialsales@jh.edu.

EU GPSR Authorized Representative
LOGOS EUROPE, 9 rue Nicolas Poussin, 17000, La Rochelle, France
E-mail: Contact@logoseurope.eu

To every woman who wants to take charge of her health—whether preparing for menopause, navigating its changes, or embracing life beyond it—may this book be a trusted companion, empowering you with knowledge and confidence.

To the clinicians dedicated to guiding women through these transitions, your commitment to compassionate, evidence-based care is invaluable. May this book support you in helping your patients thrive.

And to the spouses, partners, family members, and friends who stand beside the women in their lives, offering understanding and support—thank you. Your encouragement makes all the difference.

CONTENTS

Preface ix

1. Successful Health Strategies for Women: Before, During, and Beyond Menopause *1*
2. Handling Hot Flashes Without Hormones *32*
3. Taking Hormones in Menopause *66*
4. Heart Disease: The Risk of Doing Nothing *105*
5. Understanding Unexpected Bleeding *133*
6. Common Concerns *176*
7. Smoother Sex *203*
8. Compatible Contraception *249*
9. Moods, Memory, and Mental Health *269*
10. Successful Sleep *320*
11. Better Bones *345*
12. Lifestyle Choices for Living Longer *390*
13. Curbing Your Risk of Cancer *436*
14. Conclusion: Going Forward *480*

Acknowledgments 483
References 485
Glossary 499
Index 505

PREFACE

Are you noticing changes in your body and wondering what they mean? Or perhaps you feel great and want to stay that way for years to come. Wherever you are in your journey, whether in your 30s, 40s, 50s, 60s, or beyond—this book is for you.

Menopause isn't just a single moment in time; it's a transition with lasting effects on your health. Yet many women assume it doesn't apply to them until they have symptoms or have already gone through "the change." The truth is the years before and after menopause present crucial opportunities to make choices that will shape your long-term well-being.

This book is a comprehensive guide to women's health, covering far more than hot flashes and hormone therapy. In these pages, you'll find expert guidance on:

- Optimizing your heart health, metabolism, and brain function at every stage of life
- Preventing osteoporosis, cancer, and other chronic conditions
- Managing sleep, stress, and lifestyle factors to support overall well-being
- Navigating changes in sexual health and intimacy with confidence
- Understanding hormone therapy and natural alternatives, what doesn't work, and what's right for you

As a gynecologist and certified menopause clinician, I have spent decades helping women take charge of their health. Since publishing *Menopause Matters* in 2009, I've continued to learn from my patients, reading and teaching, and my own experiences. The result is this book—a practical, science-based, and easy-to-use resource designed to help you live a vibrant and healthy life, no matter where you are on the timeline of menopause.

For clinicians reading this book, you'll find peer-reviewed references and resources to guide your patients through every stage of menopause: before, during, and beyond.

If you've ever thought menopause is something to worry about "later," think again. The choices you make in your 30s, 40s, 50s, and 60s will shape the quality of your life in your 70s and beyond. *The Savvy Woman's Guide to Menopause* is here to help you take control of your health today so you can enjoy every decade to its fullest.

CHAPTER 1

SUCCESSFUL HEALTH STRATEGIES FOR WOMEN

Before, During, and Beyond Menopause

INTRODUCTION

It's a time of change. It's a new phase of your life. You're not alone and your doctor can help.

If there's one certainty about a woman's aging, it's this: If you were born with ovaries, you will become postmenopausal at some point. If your ovaries are not surgically removed or impacted by chemotherapy or radiation, you will also experience years of menopause transition or perimenopause. While each of us experiences these changes differently, there are many aspects that all women share. In this chapter, I'll provide historical context for societal views of menopause and address some of the most common questions I receive from patients about menopause. These include the following:

- What exactly is menopause?
- What factors affect the timing of menopause?
- What stage of menopause am I in, and why does it matter?
- How long does each phase of menopause last?
- How will my hormone levels change during perimenopause, menopause, and post menopause?
- How can my doctor help me before, during, and beyond menopause?

SOCIETAL VIEWS OF MENOPAUSE

Just 40 years ago, there was little medical research on women including minimal research on menopause. Researchers studied men because it was more straightforward: no risk of pregnancy, no concerns about the influence of the menstrual cycle on the results, and no influence of menopause and changing hormones. Medically, women were regarded as physically smaller versions of men, meaning they had the same medical needs but on a smaller scale. This translated into occasionally lowering doses of a given medication for women. Over time, the medical community learned that there were more differences than size between men and women. Researchers have shown that women metabolize certain medications differently than men. There are also ongoing studies to sort out how the menopause transition and menopause affect women's health apart from aging. Researchers are becoming more adept at studying the differences in how women's brains and bodies function.

Over the past three decades, advances in gender-based medicine and research have led to a paradigm shift in medical thinking and practice. Fundamentally, the philosophy of medical care—particularly medical care for aging women—has changed. Consider the example of a broken arm due to osteoporosis. Decades ago, if you broke your arm, you underwent surgery, or had a cast put on. Now, if you are a midlife woman, the goal is to prevent your first fracture from ever occurring. The medical community also seeks to prevent your first heart attack or stroke. Further, there are strategies to lower your chances of getting certain cancers based on your personal and family history. You and your clinician can determine your risk of heart disease, stroke, diabetes, and osteoporosis. In some cancers, you may also consider preventive strategies to avoid the risk altogether. While you are not obliged to act on any of this information, you will likely benefit from considering it.

EVOLVING SOCIETAL VIEWS OF MENOPAUSE

Before I discuss the specifics of perimenopause and post menopause, I would like to provide historical context. In the past 70 years, societal views of menopause in the United States have gone from one extreme to another. More than half a century ago, society viewed menopause as a sign of aging to be hidden—something that should not acknowledged or discussed. Women were expected to "deal with it" on their own. Society didn't acknowledge menopause as a natural transition. Instead, it was viewed only as an unwelcome sign of aging.

During other decades, estrogen replacement was touted as the antidote to aging. Physicians and others recommended estrogen to preserve youth, femininity, and mental acuity while lowering the risk of heart disease and osteoporosis. Today, with additional research and understanding, we know that neither of these extreme views serves women well.

In the past, if you suffered from debilitating hot flashes, society made you feel like an outlier and not psychologically robust if you were unable to weather this natural process with ease. When hormone replacement therapy (HRT) came onto the scene, it was touted as the fountain of youth and an antiaging strategy. If you declined to take estrogen, you were viewed as not taking pride in your appearance or sex life. During this time in history, society viewed menopause as a medical condition to be treated. Physicians wrote prescriptions to "cure" it. Today, I still encounter colleagues and patients who embrace one of these perspectives to the exclusion of others. The first group continues to regard HRT as something to avoid at all costs. The second group continues to medicalize menopause and insist that all women should be taking bioidentical hormones for their health.

I have safely prescribed low-dose hormones to patients my entire career that spans more than 35 years. However, I do not completely agree with either group. I strongly recommend each of you consider menopause as a natural condition that does not necessarily require medication. Most of you will not need to take estrogen to feel well or stay healthy as you age. Some of you may wish to take low-dose estrogen for a short time to maintain your well-being because your hot flashes or night sweats are debilitating. Or, you may benefit from low-dose vaginal estrogen to prevent recurrent urine infections or stop discomfort with intercourse.

I am writing this book to clarify the current state of research and medical knowledge about menopause. While there are still significant knowledge gaps in the medical community, there have also been significant advances with ongoing progress. Each year, the medical research community and menopause clinicians enhance their understanding of menopause. This allows doctors to offer patients more options to weather bothersome symptoms. In some cases, these options include hormones as well as other types of medications and strategies such as lifestyle modifications or nonhormonal medications.

DEFINING PERIMENOPAUSE, MENOPAUSE, AND POST MENOPAUSE

Before diving into this chapter, it's important to acknowledge the three phases of change:

- Perimenopause: The 7 to 12 years prior to the final menstrual period
- Menopause: Can refer to peri- or post menopause or both
- Post menopause: This phase occurs when you experience 12 consecutive months of no bleeding without any underlying medical explanation.

You will also come across the term "premenopause." Premenopause refers to the reproductive years prior to any changes associated with menopause. Typically, these years encompass individuals in their twenties and early to mid-thirties.

EXPLORING THE TIMING OF MENOPAUSE

When researchers studied menopause patterns of more than 234,000 women in seven different countries, they found the median age to achieve post menopause was 50. However, this is only the median. The actual age at which you experience post menopause will vary, depending on your unique scenario and any underlying medical conditions. For example, if your ovaries permanently stop releasing eggs and estrogen before age 40, you have premature ovarian insufficiency. This occurs in 1.9 percent of women.[2]

If your final menstrual period occurs between ages 40 and 45, you underwent early menopause. Since the median life expectancy for a woman living in the United States is 81, many of us will spend 30 percent or more of our lives in post menopause.

Researchers have used the Stages of Reproductive Aging Workshop (STRAW) framework to divide the phases leading up to the final menstrual period.[1] The STRAW framework improves our understanding of perimenopause by allowing researchers to evaluate lab values such as follicle-stimulating hormone (FSH), anti-Müllerian hormone (AMH), and the number of antral follicles in the ovary. Clinically, it also includes monitoring the presence or absence of hot flashes or night sweats as well as menstrual periods over time. So far, no reliable blood test can predict when your last menstrual period will occur. FSH is too volatile, and AMH is too unreliable. Clinically, if you have 90 consecutive days of no bleeding, your menstrual periods are likely to stop permanently within three years.[1] Not exactly the accuracy of a crystal ball.

WHAT INFLUENCES THE NATURAL TIMING OF MENOPAUSE?

A host of factors influence the natural timing of menopause. I provide several below.[2]

Ethnicity

Ethnicity is one of several important factors. For example, Japanese American women may experience post menopause later than Caucasian American women. Hispanic, Native American, Hawaiian, and Black women may experience post menopause at a relatively earlier age. Studies are ongoing to learn more about ethnic influence.

Age of First Menstrual Period 11 Years or Younger

Women who started menstruating at age 11 or younger have an 80 percent increased risk of entering menopause before age 40 (primary ovarian insufficiency, POI). They also have a 32 percent risk of early menopause or having a final menstrual period between ages 40 and 45. The risk of early menopause or POI is double in women who do not give birth.

> **DID YOU KNOW?**
>
> Women who start menstruating at age 11 or younger have an 80 percent increased risk of premature menopause and a 32 percent risk of early menopause. This risk is double in women who do not give birth.

Body Mass Index

Body mass index (BMI) is another factor. If you have a higher BMI in premenopause and a higher waist-to-hip ratio (i.e., greater than 1:2), you may experience natural menopause at a later age. If you are underweight or have a low BMI in your early or mid-adult years, you have a greater chance of having an earlier final menstrual period. Genetic variations may also play a role.

Timing of the Final Menstrual Period

Recently, researchers have identified a connection between women's premenopausal heart health and the timing of their final menstrual period. Data from the Framingham Heart Study indicates that premenopausal women who have a less favorable heart health profile in premenopause (i.e., a profile that includes higher total cholesterol, higher systolic and diastolic blood pressure, and other worrisome cardiovascular risk factors) may anticipate entering post menopause at an earlier age.

Physical Activity
Physical activity also influences the timing of natural menopause. More specifically, activity is associated with lower concentrations of reproductive hormones in the blood and less frequent ovulation. Therefore, physical activity is likely associated with a later age at natural menopause; however, this is not yet definitive.

Smoking
For more than 15 years, more than 100 studies have confirmed that cigarette smoking leads to natural menopause at an earlier age. Seventeen studies of more than 220,000 women across seven countries found that the younger a woman is when she starts smoking—and the more cigarettes she smokes per day—the more likely she is to experience early and premature menopause. This is true for both current and former smokers.

Genetic Patterns
Genetic patterns are also influential. Mother–daughter trends and similarities among sisters in the timing of the final menstrual period have been found. Having a final menstrual period at age 45 years or younger in a mother, sister, aunt, or grandmother is associated with a sixfold increase of early menopause after adjusting for smoking and childbearing and body mass index.[3] There is a stronger risk of early menopause if a woman has a sister or multiple relatives with early menopause (9–12 times increased risk) and if there is a history of POI/premature menopause at age 40 or under (eightfold increased risk).

Twins and Premature or Early Menopause
Registries of twins in the United Kingdom and Australia show that twins are more likely to experience POI or premature menopause. Also, if you are a child of a multiple pregnancy (birth parent is a twin

or one of a multiple pregnancy), you have a 50 percent greater chance of early menopause.[2] This finding is not related to birth weight.

Early Menopause and Heart Disease

New correlations have emerged linking age at natural menopause and risk of cardiovascular disease. In 2016, researchers grouped 32 different studies of more than 310,000 women. They found that the women who had early onset of their final menstrual period (i.e., before age 45) had a higher risk of coronary heart disease (CHD), fatal CHD, and heart failure than other women in menopause who had a final menstrual period between ages 45 and 50. These different studies are leading researchers to conclude that early menopause influences heart health and aging, but poor heart health may also contribute to early or premature menopause.

In addition, individuals who have both of their ovaries surgically removed before natural post menopause or before age 45 will have a higher risk of CHD. This is true regardless of whether the uterus is removed as well.

WHAT TO EXPECT FROM THIS BOOK

Why devote a book to the medical strategies for women before, during, and beyond menopause? In my community-based gynecology practice, I have had the privilege and opportunity to follow individual women over years and, in some cases, even decades. Like each woman I see in my office, each of you has different medical needs and priorities. These needs and priorities often change over time. Your needs will likely differ as you encounter the menopause transition and then enter post menopause for the rest of your adult life. While you may not have any menopausal symptoms at one point, you may at another. While you may not be interested in lifestyle modifications or medical treatment at one point, you may change your mind and explore your options to feel and function well at another time. Your friends, family members, or coworkers may become debilitated by changes during midlife that range from worse moods to hot flashes to fitful sleep, painful sex, lost libido, worsening memory, or broken bones. Most likely, your priorities will change over time as you experience mental and physical changes. During your journey, you may hear comments such as, "Menopause is a natural process. I see no reason to medicate or 'medicalize' it." Another perspective is to view menopause as reversing the hormonal changes of adolescence. We don't medicate adolescents during their teen years while their reproductive systems mature.

It's true that during adolescence, the hormones shift to prepare for the reproductive years. During perimenopause, these hormone systems wind down for 7 to 12 years until the final menstrual period, when there are no longer any cyclic hormone patterns. However, the process of dismantling the hormone patterns of the reproductive years can be more disruptive than adolescence and may last more than twice as long.

THE COLLECTIVE EXPERIENCE: YOU'RE NOT ALONE

Even though everyone experiences menopause differently, many commonalities can help empower women to seek the help they need. The following are some of the statements my patients have made about menopause:

"Who hijacked my body?"
"I have brain fog, fatigue, and poor-quality sleep."
"I can no longer multitask."
"I have debilitating hot flashes and night sweats."
"I have erratic mood changes and get angrier at small things."
"I have difficulty functioning well at work and at home."
"I have no libido."
"Sex is painful."
"It is overwhelming to be caring for elderly parents who need my
    help as well as teenagers and grandchildren."
"Since the pandemic, work demands have escalated. Some remote
    workers never came back. I'm expected to do three people's jobs."

Whether you are managing well and notice few or no disruptive changes or are looking for options to feel better, it is helpful to understand what body changes are taking place. This book is dedicated to discussing the mental and physical changes that women may experience as well as options to manage the changes to optimize your health and well-being at this often-challenging time.

VISIBLE AND INVISIBLE CHANGES THAT MAY OCCUR

Even when you feel well and have no concerns during menopause, your body is changing. The most common visible/noticeable changes women report in menopause include:[4]

- Anxiety
- Brain fog
- Breast tenderness
- Depressed mood or major depression
- Hair loss
- Heavy, irregular, prolonged, or infrequent menstrual periods (80 percent of women experience this)
- Hot flashes and/or night sweats (80 percent of women experience this)
- Low libido
- Pain with sex
- Trouble sleeping
- Vaginal dryness
- Worse premenstrual syndrome (PMS)

There are also invisible/less noticeable changes that take place. These include:

- Higher cholesterol
- Higher risk of dementia or Alzheimer's disease
- Higher risk of diabetes, metabolic syndrome, or both
- Higher risk of heart attack or heart disease
- Higher risk of stroke

- Thin bones, low bone mass, or osteoporosis in the spine or hips
- Vaginal dryness that you don't yet feel

SORTING THROUGH INFORMATION OVERLOAD

In the past, information wasn't as easily accessible as it is today. Now, you and I are bombarded with facts and advertisements from Facebook, the Internet, Instagram, Pinterest, television, YouTube, Twitter, and TikTok. We may also be inundated with unsolicited recommendations from friends, family, and coworkers. Despite this abundance of information, not everything we see or hear is accurate, and some of the information we receive is presented out of context. For example, a well-intentioned friend might encourage you to take supplements that have a poor or nonexistent safety profile and that may not produce the desired/promised effect.

> **DID YOU KNOW?**
> The average age for a North American woman to have her last menstrual period and become postmenopausal is 51 years. This age has remained constant since the Roman Empire. However, post menopause is more significant now than even 100 years ago. That's because of the dramatic increase in longevity. An American woman is now likely to spend 30 years or more in post menopause.

While more comfortable, our modern lifestyle puts us at greater risk of osteoporosis, obesity, diabetes, and heart disease, as well as breast, ovarian, and uterine cancer. Today, many women live into their eighties and beyond, but this increase in life expectancy does not come with a warranty ensuring a good quality of life. The choices you make now set the stage for your health and well-being during the last third of your adult life. There are many options to consider in the areas of nutrition, dietary supplements, exercise, stress management, and screening for hidden medical problems. Even if you are over 65, you can still benefit from making better-informed choices.

Visiting your doctor and taking preventive measures will save you time, expense, and hassle. In the long run, you will make fewer trips to the doctor and spend less time waiting in reception areas for visits to treat high blood pressure, diabetes, osteoporosis, and advanced cancer. Embracing preventive care will lighten your financial burden as well. You will avoid paying for expensive medications and make fewer visits to doctors to monitor your more fragile state of health.

Women who reject preventive care strategies miss opportunities to be proactive about their health. They can expect to have more numerous and severe health problems. The most devastating consequence of this adverse medical status can be the loss of independence.

"BUT I FEEL FINE! WHY DO I NEED TO TALK WITH MY DOCTOR?"

Many women entering menopause have told me: "I feel well, so I must be healthy. I don't want to have expensive tests when I feel fine!" Some of these women dislike the time, expense, and experience of the tests themselves, and some dislike the notion of taking medications because they are concerned about side effects. The hazards of taking hormones and the perils of other prescription medications have been overemphasized in the media. Many women have simply concluded it is safest to tough out the perimenopause transition without a doctor's input and to "let nature take its course" during post menopause.

Our entire lives, most of us have relied on doctors to treat acute problems. I find that people are very accepting of "fix-it" medicine. If they develop a urinary tract infection, for example, they are willing to take antibiotics. If they break a hip, they are willing to have surgery to repair or replace it. You may have the mindset, "I won't fix it if it isn't broken." However, good medical care today *must* include good preventive care as well.

Neglecting your health is never a good idea, and as you get older, the consequences can become grave. It can be difficult for a woman to care for herself during perimenopause and beyond because she is often juggling the demands of elderly parents as well as her own partner, children, and grandchildren. I know what it is like to be a member of the "sandwich generation," caring for family members who are both older and younger, with different needs, at the same time. The caregiver, often a midlife woman, is in the middle of the sandwich trying to meet the needs of more than one generation. My advice: Even if you have a very busy life—and even if you feel fine— please take the time to meet with your doctor and have a checkup. You may have invisible health problems that require attention, and the sooner you identify and deal with them, the better. On the other hand, if you get a clean bill of health, you can take comfort knowing you are on the right track. Find the time now to see your doctor, and consider your medical options based on your age and menopause status. The adage is still true: "An ounce of prevention is worth a pound of cure!" Consider Lenore's story.

Lenore's Story
"I'M THROUGH WITH MENOPAUSE!"

At age 60, I assumed I was done with menopause. I felt fine and had no bleeding or hot flashes, so I decided I no longer needed to keep going to the doctor on a regular basis.

One day, while I was gardening, I was bitten by a tick. Several days later, I developed a fever and muscle aches. When I went to my family doctor, he ordered a blood test to check for evidence of Lyme disease. Since I was overdue for a complete physical examination, he ordered additional blood work as well.

When the lab results came back, it was clear I not only had Lyme disease but also very high cholesterol. My doctor explained to me that high cholesterol dramatically increases my risk of heart attack and stroke. My doctor prescribed antibiotics for Lyme disease and talked to me about exercising and modifying my diet. He told me that if these lifestyle changes did not have a great enough effect, he would recommend a type of medication called a statin to further lower my cholesterol and reduce my risk of heart attack and stroke. Although I weathered the storms of perimenopause, I had not continued to take care of my health. My Lyme disease turned out to be a blessing in disguise because it ultimately led me to take control of my cholesterol.

HIDDEN THREATS YOUR DOCTOR CAN EVALUATE

Women who have hot flashes, urinary problems, vaginal dryness, or other concerns are more likely to find their way to a doctor's office because they are looking for relief. However, even women with none of these physical discomforts still need medical care. The body's hidden needs do not correlate with hot flashes, night sweats, or menstrual irregularities. Relying on these symptoms to gauge whether you need care can be misleading. One goal of this book is to familiarize you with the hidden health threats you may not be monitoring. These hidden threats include:

- *Cardiovascular disease*, including heart attack and stroke. Your risk of heart disease rises after you enter post menopause. This is especially true after age 50. Cardiovascular disease is women's largest silent killer. In the United States, one out of every two women over age 50 will die of heart disease. This exceeds the combined death rate of women from all types of cancer.
- *Weight gain.* As you age, your metabolism slows, making weight gain an issue even as early as age 35 or 40. Excess weight strains your heart, increases your risk of cancer, stresses your joints, and puts you at risk of developing diabetes.
- *Diabetes.* Obesity and diabetes are rapidly growing concerns. More than 60 percent of the U.S. population is now overweight, and the incidence of diabetes has reached

epidemic proportions. The onset of type 2 diabetes is linked to obesity and is a huge factor in heart disease and heart attack, among other serious conditions.
- *Osteoporosis.* Rapid bone thinning occurs early in post menopause when estrogen levels plummet. Thin bones put you at risk for fracture. In addition, serious fractures, such as fractures of the hip, put you at risk for pneumonia and other complications of being bed-bound.
- *Cancer.* It looms large in nearly every woman's mind. Your risk of breast cancer continues to increase every year of your life until you reach roughly 80 years old. For men and women, the incidence of colon cancer, which you can easily avoid by following preventive measures, increases at age 50 and beyond.

These hidden threats are more common and more threatening to your well-being during menopause than they were when you were younger. The good news is that treatments are available that may preserve your lifestyle and independence. Some may even save your life. Working with a doctor to prevent problems and catch disease early means you will enjoy better health than if you wait until a hidden problem, normally amenable to medical treatment, becomes obvious but difficult to treat.

PARTNERING WITH YOUR GYNECOLOGIST

At this stage, your gynecologist or menopause specialist plays a key role in helping you maintain or achieve all-around good health. That's because so many aspects of your health are linked to your hormone levels. If you experience hot flashes, night sweats, and irregular periods during perimenopause, you may assume this is all part of aging. However, I encourage you to avoid the temptation of self-diagnosing menopause and assuming these symptoms are always benign. Self-diagnosis may result in overlooking health problems that you and your doctor must address. For example, thyroid abnormalities can cause many of the symptoms associated with perimenopause and post menopause. In these instances, diagnosing and treating the underlying thyroid imbalance can put an end to the symptoms.[4]

Similarly, it is not safe to assume that if you are a postmenopausal woman who doesn't have sex, you do not need gynecologic exams. Regardless of whether you are currently sexually active, it is still important to have regular gynecologic exams to stay healthy.

Rupa's Story
A SLUGGISH THYROID

I'm 46 years old and am struggling with the fact that I recently gained 15 pounds and started experiencing hot flashes. My nails stopped growing, and my hair was falling out in clumps when I washed it. I missed six menstrual cycles in seven months; however, based on the experiences of my friends with similar issues, I thought it was just part of perimenopause. When I discussed my symptoms with my doctor, he wanted to see whether my thyroid gland was functioning normally.

A blood test revealed that my thyroid was underactive. My doctor said its function was sluggish and that my metabolism went into "slow motion." He prescribed a thyroid medication that I now take orally once a day. Eight weeks after I started taking it, my hot flashes were gone. Six months after I started it, my hair had stopped falling out and my nails began to grow back. My menstrual cycles also became more predictable, and I was finally able to shed the excess weight I had gained.

WHAT STAGE OF MENOPAUSE ARE YOU IN—AND WHY DOES IT MATTER?

It's important not to assume you are postmenopausal when you are still in perimenopause. Post menopause is a permanent phase that follows perimenopause. Post menopause also marks the end of your fertile years. Once you enter the postmenopausal phase, you remain in it for the rest of your life. These two distinct phases affect your health differently. For example, postmenopausal women cannot conceive. Perimenopausal women can and do. The ability to conceive is just one example of the differences between them.

Treatment options also differ by phase of menopause. The risks, benefits, and safety profiles of a given hormone, medication, supplement, or surgical procedure may be drastically different for a postmenopausal woman than they are for one who is perimenopausal. Measures that maintain or restore health in one phase can be detrimental in another. For example, a perimenopausal nonsmoker who experiences severe hot flashes may benefit from taking a low-dose birth control pill. The hormones in the pill might relieve her symptoms. On the other hand, even a low-dose birth control pill is not suitable for a postmenopausal woman over 50. The hormone levels are too high for her system. Moreover, the pill delivers hormones in a cyclic pattern that does not match a postmenopausal woman's biology. Since she no longer has a menstrual cycle, her hormones stay constant.

Even if your body seemingly behaves the same way in post menopause as it did in perimenopause, there are significant differences to note. For example, if you are perimenopausal, bleeding is expected. If you are postmenopausal, even a small amount of bleeding is a warning sign. It can signal that there is a problem in the uterus. While 9 out of 10 times that problem is not due to cancer, this means that 1 out of 10 times, the postmenopausal bleeding *is* due to cancer. In post menopause, a single episode of bleeding may be a woman's only warning sign.

DID YOU KNOW?

For postmenopausal women, even a small amount of bleeding is a warning sign.

The term "menopausal" can be misleading because it means different things to each of us. For example, if you say, "I am menopausal," that indicates to me you are no longer menstruating and that you are technically postmenopausal. However, if your next sentence is, "I have drastic mood swings!" I conclude that you are more likely experiencing mood swings associated with perimenopause. This language mix-up is problematic. Perimenopause and post menopause are not the same thing, and the terms are not interchangeable. It is important to know which phase of menopause you are in. Your doctor can help you find out.

CHANGING HORMONE LEVELS

The role of the ovary changes over time from birth to the postmenopausal years. When puberty arrives, the ovaries become the conductor of the childbearing orchestra. They produce key female hormones (i.e., estrogen and progesterone) and are responsible for releasing eggs. Throughout life, the ovaries also produce the male hormone (i.e., testosterone) that contributes to a healthy woman's sex drive. Even in post menopause, the ovaries continue to produce small amounts of testosterone. In post menopause, the ovary no longer makes estradiol and no longer releases eggs. Spontaneous conception is no longer possible in post menopause.

The ovaries in a female fetus can contain up to two million follicles, tiny cysts that may develop into eggs. Some follicles dissolve before a baby girl is born, but most follicles remain in a woman's body. At birth, a female infant begins releasing eggs from her ovaries. However, she cannot conceive until her body goes through puberty and is primed for her first menstrual period. This happens somewhere between ages 9 and 16. Puberty marks the beginning of her reproductive years when her biology is geared toward conceiving children. After menstruation is established, follicles release eggs during ovulation. Eggs released during ovulation are available for fertilization by male sperm. Eggs that are not fertilized by sperm dissolve in the pelvis.

While the ovaries play an important role in releasing eggs and manufacturing hormones, they do not act alone. Other organs, such as the hypothalamus in the brain, also influence their performance.

The most regular menstrual cycles occur in a woman's twenties and early thirties with a recurring pattern each month that includes mid-cycle ovulation when the ovary releases an egg. During each cycle, the ovaries make predictable amounts of estrogen and progesterone in a set sequence. These levels rise and fall in a natural rhythm that repeats itself about every 28 days, and women know what to expect. After ovulation, progesterone is responsible for shedding the uterine lining. This usually happens two weeks later with the menstrual period.

HORMONES IN PERIMENOPAUSE: UNPREDICTABLE FLUCTUATIONS

Wider fluctuations in estrogen and progesterone levels occur during the menstrual cycles of women in their late thirties, forties, or fifties. By the time a woman is 40, her ovaries are starting to shrink, and they have fewer follicles to release. They continue to shrink in size over the next 20 years or so. As the ovaries begin to show signs of age, hormones no longer rise and fall in a smooth, predictable pattern over a four-week cycle. Ovulation still occurs, but it is less frequent and more erratic. During perimenopause, ovary hormones fluctuate wildly and move away from the regular, predictable patterns established in the childbearing years. Irregular menstrual cycles are common, and changes in your body's level of estrogen and progesterone can be difficult to endure.

> DID YOU KNOW?
>
> Estrogen levels are erratic in perimenopause. It is a common misconception that the discomforts of perimenopause are all caused by a lack of sufficient amounts of estrogen. Ironically, during perimenopause, estrogen levels often are too high. Some of the hallmarks of perimenopause, such as heavy bleeding, are a result of excess estrogen.

Your body makes different types of estrogen. Your ovaries make a type of estrogen (i.e., estradiol) during the reproductive and perimenopausal years. If your estradiol levels are high, taking extra estrogen during this time may make you feel worse. During the reproductive years, estrogen levels rise and fall smoothly like gentle hills and valleys. During the perimenopausal years, the pattern becomes erratic. The graph of perimenopausal hormones looks like throwing spaghetti against the wall. The erratic peaks and valleys of estrogen levels include rapid, unexpected shifts from very high to very low estrogen levels. This erratic pattern creates a rocky time for many perimenopausal women.[4] After rising too high, estrogen levels can plummet and sink too low. Periodically, estradiol levels sink so low that they trigger a hot flash or night sweat. Unpredictable and erratic estrogen levels can also wreak havoc in the form of mood changes and abnormal bleeding.

Women usually spend anywhere from 2 to 10 years in perimenopause. For some women, this is a trying time. The erratic hormone shifts may produce debilitating hot flashes and night sweats, irregular menstrual periods, disturbing mood changes, and poor sleep quality. For other women, these changes are mild and barely noticeable. For a fortunate minority, the transition is invisible. Twenty percent of women do not experience any hot flashes or night sweats.

During perimenopause, levels of progesterone, the other female hormone made in the ovaries, are also erratic and often too low. They may be too low to effectively counterbalance the high estrogen levels. Bloating, irritability, and breast tenderness may result. Some women with erratic hormone fluctuations benefit from additional progesterone—not estrogen—to balance their estrogen peaks (you can read more about this in chapter 3). Imbalances of estrogen, progesterone, or both are characteristic of the perimenopausal years. When there is no ovulation for a cycle, little or no progesterone is released. As a result, the monthly shedding of the lining does not take place, often resulting in a missed period.

HORMONES IN POST MENOPAUSE: LOW AND STEADY

Steady, low estrogen levels do not appear until post menopause. Once they are established, a woman maintains them for the rest of her life. This can be a relief to women who suffered with the erratic peaks and valleys of perimenopause.

Estradiol is no longer the dominant estrogen in your body in post menopause. Another type of estrogen plays an even more important role in post menopause: estrone, a weaker form of estrogen. Estrone becomes the dominant form of estrogen in your body during post menopause; it is not made in your ovaries. Your body's fatty tissues, also called adipose tissue, manufacture estrone. There is a reason for the extra belly fat that none of us can seem to avoid at this age. It is helpful to have a modest amount of extra fat during post menopause to maintain your supply of estrone. Estrone helps maintain bone strength. However, as in life, too much of a good thing isn't always better. Women with a great deal of adipose tissue produce excess amounts of estrone that may cause abnormal bleeding and increase the risk of breast and uterine cancer.

FERTILITY AND PERIMENOPAUSE

Perimenopause represents the transition a woman's body undergoes when it changes from childbearing status to non-childbearing status. Fertility gradually declines for women in their thirties and continues to diminish until their fifties, depending on their personal biological schedule. Many women think that the signs of perimenopause mean they are no longer fertile. In reality, fertility persists until post menopause. Women in their forties have unplanned pregnancies at a rate second only to that of teenagers. Postmenopausal women cannot become pregnant. Perimenopausal women can and *do*.

Daniella's Story
PREGNANT AT 46

I began to have hot flashes when I turned 45 and then missed four menstrual periods in a row. I assumed I was in post menopause and told my husband to cancel his appointment for a vasectomy. We had decided on a vasectomy for him because we had recently sent our youngest child off to college and did not want to risk an unplanned pregnancy.

I was actually perimenopausal and had missed menstrual periods because I was pregnant. Subsequently, I miscarried. After we weathered the stress of the unplanned pregnancy and miscarriage, my husband rescheduled his appointment to have a vasectomy. I continued to have irregular menstrual periods. It wasn't until I was 55 that I had 12 consecutive months with no bleeding. At that time, my doctor confirmed I had entered post menopause and was no longer fertile.

MENSTRUAL BLEEDING AND PERIMENOPAUSE

Irregular menstrual periods are the most frequent sign of perimenopause. Eighty percent of women experience changes in their menstrual cycle for 7 to 12 years preceding post menopause. Menstrual cycles in perimenopause often disappear only to reappear without warning. I have heard horror stories about the sudden, unexpected return of a menstrual period that can involve bleeding through clothes in a public setting. If this happens to you, rest assured: you are not alone!

During perimenopause, your menstrual flow may become lighter or heavier. You may bleed for longer or shorter periods of time. You may miss periods or bleed more often. Even though each woman's experience is unique, doctors use specific medical guidelines to determine whether something is wrong. The more information you can share with your doctor about your experience, the easier it is for them to recognize anything abnormal. I ask all my patients to keep a record of their bleeding patterns so I can see at a glance when something changes.

HOW LONG DOES PERIMENOPAUSE LAST?

"When will this end?" is a question my patients ask me daily. You have a right to know, but neither you nor your doctor has a way to tell until after the fact. Determining the end of perimenopause is a retrospective process. Doctors look back after the fact to see if you have experienced 12 consecutive months without any menstrual bleeding. Once this occurs, you and your doctor can typically assume you're in post menopause.

When my patients pose this question, I can't help but think about how ironic it is that we live in a world where we can send an astronaut to the moon but still can't pinpoint when perimenopause begins, how long it will last, and when it will end.

Perimenopause can last as long as 7 to 12 years and even longer in some cases. Unfortunately, there is currently no blood test to confirm that you are in perimenopause or a test that accurately predicts when your perimenopause will end. New testing is in the works, but it is not yet available, reliable or accurate. Currently, perimenopause is usually established by taking a careful medical history.

In my experience, the most frequently requested test for perimenopause is a blood test for follicle-stimulating hormone (FSH). FSH is reputed to tell you whether you are perimenopausal and when you can expect to enter post menopause. In fact, FSH usually *cannot easily* give you this information. Here's why.

If you are in perimenopause, your levels of FSH fluctuate widely. So, a single blood test result showing elevated FSH could represent just one part of a given menstrual cycle. I will tell you what I tell my perimenopausal patients: You can have your blood drawn one day and get an FSH result that is incredibly low, indicating premenopause or perimenopause. Yet on another day that same week, you could get a result that is incredibly high, indicating that you are in post menopause. These erratic results may reflect your perimenopausal status, but they do not predict whether post menopause is imminent. In post menopause, FSH is consistently elevated. However, this rise does not begin until one year after your final menstrual period. We need a better test.

Recently, researchers discovered that a woman who missed three menstrual periods in a row could expect to enter post menopause within the next three years.[4] Typically, post menopause was farther away for women who only skipped one menstrual period at a time or continued to have regular cycles.

Your doctor can order blood tests of certain hormones. You can also contact mail-order companies that offer saliva tests to measure estrogen, progesterone, and testosterone. They offer kits to allow you to perform your own saliva testing and then get the results by phone, email, or a mailed report. This may appeal to you for several reasons. First, you avoid the unpleasant experience of having your blood drawn. Second, you can perform the saliva test yourself in the privacy of your home without a doctor's visit. Third, you can take charge of your own care. Unfortunately, the accuracy of these saliva tests is not established. Hormone levels in saliva are not biologically meaningful. It is not possible to test for the concentration of free unbound hormone in the saliva. Free unbound hormone is not attached to a carrier molecule and not free to circulate in the blood. Further, there is no biological relationship between salivary sex steroid hormone concentration and the amount of free hormone in the blood. Researchers don't understand the large differences in salivary hormone concentrations between individual women. In addition, there is variability for individual women at different times during their menstrual cycle and during different phases of menopause. Salivary hormone levels also vary with diet, the time of day of testing, and the specific hormone being tested. In the future, there will, no doubt, be better tests. Testing levels of inhibin, a hormone that plays a role in the timing of post menopause, shows promise. Levels of inhibin are elevated in post menopause but not in perimenopause. The timing and accuracy of this blood test are still being investigated: it is not yet available for clinical use.

DIAGNOSING POST MENOPAUSE

Post menopause begins when a woman has had 12 consecutive months with no menstrual bleeding. In post menopause, menstrual cycles are no longer possible, and fertility ends. The ovaries have released their last follicles, and no eggs remain. Post menopause is a permanent state.

Each woman is born with a certain number of eggs and uses them up at her own rate. Women who have had two full-term pregnancies enter post menopause later than those who do not. During full-term pregnancies, ovulation is suspended, so eggs are not used up as quickly. You also have a break from ovulation during the time you spend nursing your infant.

The average age for post menopause in North America is 51 years, although women commonly reach this milestone seven years before or after this age. So, the normal age range for entering post menopause is 44 to 58 years old.

> DID YOU KNOW?
>
> Perimenopause usually precedes post menopause; however, post menopause can occur rapidly when the ovaries are surgically removed or are inactivated by infection, radiation, chemotherapy, or severe stress while an individual is still perimenopausal.

Although postmenopausal ovaries have retired from childbearing, they still have other functions. A common misconception is that the ovaries stop making hormones in post menopause. In fact, ovaries continue to make testosterone. Postmenopausal ovaries also continue to make estradiol; however, they just make it in drastically reduced amounts, and they release it slowly and steadily. This is a stabilizing, tranquil time for many women after they have weathered the storms of perimenopause.

Sometimes it can be hard to tell whether you are postmenopausal or just experiencing a longer gap between menstrual cycles in perimenopause. If you suspect you are postmenopausal, ask your doctor to confirm it. They will perform a physical exam, update your personal medical history, and perhaps order lab work to confirm whether you are truly in post menopause.

Once you establish steady, low levels of estrogen and progesterone in post menopause, you will maintain steady, low levels of these hormones for the rest of your life. They will not fluctuate each month. This means that monthly mood changes are a thing of the past. If your moods vary, you and your doctor should look for other causes, such as depression, stress, anxiety, sleep issues, thyroid imbalances, or another metabolic disorder such as thyroid disease.

Post menopause may be associated with discomforts such as vaginal dryness or pain with sexual intercourse. Another medical issue that can arise is unexpected urine loss. Hot flashes may persist in the postmenopausal years, but they are less likely to begin then.

EARLY POST MENOPAUSE

While the average woman in North America becomes postmenopausal at age 51, younger women may be postmenopausal for many different reasons. Women who become postmenopausal in their early forties (i.e., between ages 40 and 44) are referred to as having early post menopause.

Several factors influence the timing of premature menopause and post menopause:

- *Premature menopause.* Premature menopause refers to the cessation of menstrual periods and the end of fertility before the age of 40. This can occur naturally or after radiation or chemotherapy. Survivors of childhood cancer are more likely to experience premature menopause.

- *Surgical menopause.* Surgical menopause occurs when a woman's ovaries are surgically removed before she has made the transition into post menopause on her own. (Note: If the ovaries are surgically removed after age 55, for example, and a woman is already postmenopausal, she has not experienced a surgical menopause.)
- *Cigarette smoke.* Smoking is toxic to the ovaries, and it nearly doubles the chances of premature menopause. It is also associated with an earlier arrival of post menopause by up to two years.
- *Early onset of menstruation.* A woman whose first menstrual period occurs at age 9 or younger is more likely to have premature menopause or early post menopause.
- *The pill.* Using oral contraceptives or birth control pills lowers the risk of early menopause. This is probably related to the fact that ovulation is suppressed while a woman is on oral contraceptives. This conserves follicles for later release.

Surgical menopause is a cloudy concept because the term "hysterectomy" is loosely used to describe several different operations. In my experience, the most common misconception is that a "total hysterectomy" results in instant menopause. However, in surgical terms, a total hysterectomy represents the surgical removal of the uterus and the cervix. It does not indicate the status of the ovaries, which is what determines postmenopausal status. The surgical procedure that produces post menopause is a *bilateral oophorectomy*, or the removal of both ovaries. You could have a total hysterectomy at age 42, but if you have healthy ovaries that are not surgically removed, you will not become postmenopausal at that time. The ovaries will continue to make normal amounts of estrogen and progesterone, and they will continue to release follicles that are absorbed into the abdominal cavity. If you have even one functional ovary remaining, you are still perimenopausal. The remaining ovary will take over and continue to manufacture hormones, including estrogen, progesterone, and testosterone.

In this case, you cannot determine your menopausal stage by your menstrual periods because you will not have any periods after your uterus is surgically removed.

Petra's Story
TOTAL HYSTERECTOMY WITHOUT OOPHORECTOMY
(OVARIES CONSERVED)

I was 43 years old when I found out that I had a large uterine fibroid. The size was comparable to a four-month pregnancy. I had been experiencing pelvic pressure and abdominal bloating. I also had heavy menstrual bleeding and clots and had become anemic. My doctors recommended a hysterectomy, and told me they planned to conserve both of my ovaries if they appeared normal at the time of surgery. They expected the ovaries to continue to function normally, providing me with adequate levels of hormones. If my ovaries were abnormal, they said they would remove them and prescribe estrogen so I wouldn't experience sudden "surgical menopause." Fortunately, my ovaries were normal and were left in place. I had a total hysterectomy with conservation of my ovaries and removal of my uterus and cervix and both fallopian tubes. I didn't notice any hormonal shifts or mood changes that were different from what I was experiencing before surgery. My doctor explained that I was perimenopausal at the time of surgery and still am. My ovaries are still functioning. Since the operation, I really have only two significant changes: I can no longer become pregnant, and I no longer have any menstrual bleeding.

HOW YOUR DOCTOR CAN HELP YOU

Your doctor does not have a crystal ball to see your future, and neither do I. However, we are well equipped to identify your risk factors for cardiovascular disease, osteoporosis, and diabetes. Extensive research has shown us what to look for when we analyze your personal medical history and family history. We know what to check during your physical examination, which tests to order, and how to interpret the results.

To customize prevention strategies that suit your needs and preferences, your doctor needs your input. An effective prevention strategy meets two criteria: It helps you stay healthy, and it includes recommendations that you are willing to follow.

Many people become motivated to get more exercise, improve their nutrition, or take preventive medication only after their first heart attack or stroke, after they have been diagnosed with diabetes, or after fracturing their backbone or hip. Others will be proactive and embrace preventive measures before they have a medical crisis.

Even if you feel fine, don't let a hidden problem catch you by surprise. By the time it comes to your attention, it will be much harder to correct. Every year, fine-tune your prevention and treatment regimens with your doctor. They can help you decide if your current approach is best or if it is time to incorporate the results of a new medical breakthrough or newly available natural remedy.

Your doctor wants to partner with you to help you be healthy. While some illnesses cannot be prevented, many can. It is sad to see women as patients whose lives become limited by preventable illnesses. It is heartening to see active, energetic, and motivated women as patients who take control of their health and future.

IMPORTANT TAKEAWAYS

In summary:

- While there are still significant knowledge gaps about menopause in the medical community, there have also been significant advances and ongoing progress.
- The actual age at which you experience post menopause will vary, depending on your unique scenario and any underlying medical conditions.

- Even though everyone experiences menopause differently, many commonalities can empower women to seek the help they need.
- Treatment options for symptoms of menopause vary by phase. Measures that maintain or restore health in one phase can be detrimental in another.
- Avoid the temptation to self-diagnose menopause. Also don't assume that menopause-related symptoms are always benign.
- To customize prevention strategies that suit your needs and preferences, your doctor needs your input.

PREPARING FOR YOUR DOCTOR'S APPOINTMENT

During your appointment, consider asking your doctor questions such as these:

1. I am 50 years old and have missed six consecutive menstrual periods. I assume I am in post menopause and plan to stop using contraception. Am I correct? Should I get blood tests?
2. I had an endometrial ablation to correct heavy bleeding at age 46 and no longer have menstrual periods. I don't have hot flashes or night sweats. How will I know when I am in post menopause, and why does it matter?
3. I have been on a low-dose birth control pill and get a short light menstrual period. I only get one or two mild hot flashes during the pill-free week. Will the pill hide when I go into post menopause? And how long should I continue to take the pill?
4. I had no menstrual bleeding for 11 consecutive months, and then I bled again. Isn't that just one last period? It was short and light. Isn't it common? What does it mean?
5. I have never experienced hot flashes or night sweats and am now 53 years old. My last menstrual period was more than

12 months ago. Am I postmenopausal or perimenopausal? And what supplements should I consider at this time?

6. A close friend ordered mail-away saliva tests to check her levels of estrogen and testosterone and suggested I do the same. Should I consider this? And what should I do if I have low levels of testosterone or estrogen?

RESOURCES

Menopause Guidebook 10th edition, December, 2024. Published by The Menopause Society, this manual is an overview of all aspects of menopause, including perimenopause and early menopause. It can be ordered and viewed online (www.menopause.org/edumaterials/guidebook) or obtained in print.

www.ACOG.org: The American College of Obstetricians and Gynecologists. See Patient tab for topics such as Menopause, Healthy Aging, Menstrual Health, Heart Health, and Vulvovaginal Health.

CHAPTER 2

HANDLING HOT FLASHES WITHOUT HORMONES

"Hot flash," "power surge," "furnace blaster." Whatever you call it, it can be one of the most noticeable and uncomfortable parts of menopause. But there are ways to move through it.

HOT FLASHES ARE THE MOST common symptom of menopause. Hot flashes are also the most likely reason you may seek the help of a doctor during the menopausal transition or during post menopause. What's going on, and what can be done?

In this chapter, I'll answer some of the most common questions women have about hot flashes and what they can do about them.

- What can I do to help cope with hot flashes?
- I don't like taking medications. Are there any natural supplements that work for hot flashes?
- What about taking something from the drugstore?
- When should I go to the doctor? What questions would be helpful for me to ask?
- Can any medications potentially help me?

EVOLVING VIEWS ON MENOPAUSE

For more than half a century, medical experts thought that women's menopausal hot flashes were something to be tolerated (when mild) or treated (when severe or disrupted) and were otherwise not medically significant. Researchers are now finding that vasomotor symptoms (i.e., hot flashes and night sweats) may be associated with blood vessel changes in the heart and brain, providing a window into other potential health outcomes over time. This gives women an opportunity to manage their health more proactively. For example, they can treat their already existing high blood pressure to prevent severe hypertension.

While some of you may never experience a hot flash or night sweat, most of you will. If you are among the 80 percent of women who do experience hot flashes and night sweats, you may have found that there are three categories of so-called vasomotor symptoms:

1. Mild vasomotor symptoms: You get a warm surge with no associated sweating.
2. Moderate vasomotor symptoms: You get a warm feeling day or night associated with sweating, but the vasomotor symptoms are not disruptive.
3. Severe vasomotor symptoms: You get an intensely warm feeling followed by sweating that is disruptive and stops you from continuing with your current activity.

If your vasomotor symptoms are mild, you may never seek the help of a medical practitioner. Lifestyle modifications, described in more detail later in this chapter, may be all you need to weather these symptoms. If your symptoms are moderate or severe, however, lifestyle modifications may not suffice. Instead, you may find your work, mental health, sleep, ability to focus, and home life disrupted.

> WHAT IS A HOT FLASH?
>
> As its name suggests, a hot flash is sudden, temporary warmth, with flushing and perspiring. In other words, you become hot, red-faced, and sweaty, sometimes at the worst of times like during a Zoom meeting.

HOT FLASHES AND PHYSICAL CHANGES

What exactly happens to your body during a hot flash?

- First, the body's core temperature goes down, producing central cooling.
- Then heat is lost through the skin. Skin temperature measurements show that the skin becomes several degrees warmer as a hot flash takes place.
- Perspiring and evaporation cause additional rapid heat loss. A chill may follow the hot flash.

WHO GETS HOT FLASHES?

One hundred years ago, women spent less time in post menopause. Their life expectancy was decades shorter, and hot flashes were not a major issue. Today, about 80 percent of women experience hot flashes—and about 20 percent do not.

Scientific research has consistently shown that you can make two lifestyle choices to help alleviate symptoms: diet and exercise.

Vegetable-based diets are associated with less frequent, milder hot flashes. Vegetarians in the United States as well as those in other parts of the world report fewer hot flashes.

In Japan, women eat mostly vegetables, have a more active lifestyle, and are seldom overweight. Fewer than 25 percent of Japanese women have hot flashes. In fact, the Japanese language does not include a word for hot flashes. Women in certain African tribes also meet these criteria and, similarly, have fewer hot flashes.

In addition, those who exercise regularly or are physically active have fewer, less intense hot flashes. Women who walk daily report fewer hot flashes.

Diet and exercise, however, may only partially explain why women in other cultures enjoy a smoother midlife transition with fewer medical concerns. Middle-aged women in Japan, the Mayan culture, and some Arabic and African nations are more highly regarded during midlife and beyond. Their status in society increases with their seniority. They gain more respect from society and their families as they age. These women welcome the end of childbearing responsibilities. For them, this time of life is associated with attaining the highest status possible. I suspect this is a positive incentive to weather the changes of perimenopause and post menopause, and it may decrease the stress levels of women living in these societies.

Contrast this experience with that of North American women who live in a youth-centered culture. Many of these women mourn the end of their childbearing years and the loss of their youth. A quick glance at the magazines on any newsstand illustrates the message clearly: Look young, banish wrinkles, and attain a thinner, more youthful body at any cost. Do whatever it takes—creams, Botox, liposuction, plastic surgery—or, in Madonna's case, a grueling exercise routine reported to exceed six hours a day. The price is never too high.

The first general menopause book I read was Gail Sheehy's *Silent Passage*, published decades ago. The author laments aging in a youth-centered culture. Despite her insights, our society's view of adult female citizens has not matured. In a room full of older women, before the pandemic of 2020, few had gray or white hair, and many perimenopausal and postmenopausal women are still reluctant to reveal their age.

HOW YOU CAN REFRAME HOT FLASHES

It can help to see how your roles change in interesting ways as you leave the childbearing years. The "empty nest" involves more than the departure of offspring—it brings a different perspective on life. When it coincides with post menopause, it is also relief from the relentless biology of reproduction and a quieting of the hormone storms of perimenopause. As our hormones shift, our "wiring" also shifts, and we end up with a different emotional perspective on the world when we cross the threshold into post menopause. How would we feel if we were given increased respect and consideration as we aged? What if we were encouraged to share our life experience rather than our repertoire of techniques to look younger?

HOT FLASHES VARY FROM WOMAN TO WOMAN

The intensity and frequency of hot flashes vary dramatically between individual women. Hot flashes also vary over time for each woman as she progresses from perimenopause to post menopause.

- Your hot flashes may come and go over days, weeks, or months.
- You may experience hot flashes briefly before the flashes disappear for good.
- You may have hot flashes or night sweats while you still have menstrual periods, or you may get vasomotor symptoms when your menstrual periods are infrequent or after they have stopped.
- And although it is less common, you may find yourself in the small group of women who report troublesome hot flashes that linger for decades.

LET'S TALK ABOUT NIGHT SWEATS

You may be comfortable during the day but awaken every hour or two during the night with night sweats. Night sweats are identical to hot flashes except for their timing. It is possible to have only daytime hot flashes, only night sweats, or both. It is not clear why hot flashes or night sweats plague some women and not others; however, new DNA research is emerging that shows a genetic mutation in a gene in the thermoregulatory zone—the thermostat in the brain's hypothalamus region.

TREATING HOT FLASHES AND NIGHT SWEATS—YES OR NO?

It's a big myth that women must treat their hot flashes. You don't need to treat mild or infrequent hot flashes at all. Hot flashes are harmless unless they compromise your ability to function in daily life. Frequent or severe night sweats can disrupt sleep, causing sleep deprivation, irritability, and memory loss. They are life-threatening if they make you sleepy enough to risk falling asleep at the wheel of your car. If this is the case, talk to your doctor!

> DID YOU KNOW?
> Contrary to popular belief, hot flashes do not predict when perimenopause ends or when post menopause begins. Hot flashes can come and go, without warning, over days, months, or years. They may resolve spontaneously without any intervention, or you or someone you know may only find relief with treatment.

YOUR HOT FLASHES AND NIGHT SWEATS MAY CHANGE OVER TIME

Hot flashes and night sweats may be easily tolerated or debilitating. At one point, your hot flashes may be mild or infrequent, causing little or no disruption in your routine. At another time, you may suffer from intense hot flashes that recur every hour or are severe enough to compromise your ability to function effectively at home or work. If your hot flashes are not incapacitating, they may or may not stay mild and tolerable. Or, over time, they could become debilitating.

HOT FLASHES AND NIGHT SWEATS THAT COME AND GO

A postmenopausal woman whose hot flashes have completely resolved for more than a year without medication can expect them not to return. If they do return, work with your doctor and find out why. Some other causes for hot flashes that are unrelated to post menopause include the following:

- Certain prescription medications (e.g., niacin to reduce cholesterol, Lupron to shrink fibroids or control endometriosis, or Evista to build bones)
- Some over-the-counter supplements
- Common medical conditions, including thyroid disease, high blood pressure, and hepatitis
- Unusual medical conditions, including tuberculosis and sarcoid

With a medical history, exam, and lab tests, your doctor can identify why you are experiencing hot flashes.

> **DID YOU KNOW?**
> Hot flashes have nothing to do with willpower. In the past, women were told, "Hot flashes are all in your head." This suggested you could control or suppress your hot flashes using willpower. Some of my patients have the idea that they should be able to banish their symptoms of menopause—that is, conquer them through sheer will. Hot flashes may be triggered by anxiety, and they are often made worse by stress. This does not mean they are imaginary. Many women in previous generations were told to "Just tough it out, the hot flashes will go away on their own." Now we know this is not always possible. While it's true that you may never have night sweats or hot flashes, this is not due to your willpower. Your body may not have a vulnerable thermostat based on your genetic makeup, lifestyle, or both.

HOT FLASHES DUE TO THYROID PROBLEMS

The thyroid is a soft, butterfly-shaped gland in front of the trachea (windpipe) in the neck. The thyroid gland regulates metabolism, telling your body how fast to move and process food and waste.

Thyroid function affects hair health, including breakage, texture, and rate of growth and loss. It affects nail health and growth. It also affects your reflexes and the quality of your sleep.

You may not know this, but thyroid disease is the most common cause of hot flashes other than menopause. Sometimes a combination of thyroid disease and perimenopause can cause hot flashes. An underactive thyroid may cause hot flashes as well as night sweats, weight gain, and irregular menstrual periods. When the thyroid condition is treated, these symptoms may vanish. That's why it's important to check with your doctor, who can assess your thyroid function with a blood test. If your thyroid function is sluggish or overactive, either can be associated with vasomotor symptoms. It is also possible to have a thyroid imbalance and vasomotor symptoms from perimenopause simultaneously. While hot flashes due to perimenopause may be simply watched, thyroid disease must be identified and treated to avoid serious complications affecting the rest of the body.

Thyroid disease is very common, especially in women. For every man with a thyroid problem, there are 10 women with thyroid disease. Thyroid disease also is more common with increasing age. Although thyroid disease runs in families, it is often present in women with no family history of thyroid disease. Thyroid disease shows up in two different ways:

- Hyperthyroidism, or an overactive thyroid, is associated with racing thoughts, unintended weight loss, poor sleep, and a rapid heart rate, as well as increased sweating.
- Hypothyroidism, or an underactive thyroid, may cause sluggishness of thought and motion, depression, and unplanned weight gain without any changes in eating or exercise.

Both types of thyroid disease can cause hot flashes and irregular menstrual periods.

It is possible to experience hot flashes caused by thyroid disease before, during, or after perimenopause. Thyroid disease can be detected by a careful medical history and then confirmed with a blood test. Sometimes you may have troublesome symptoms, but your thyroid blood tests are only mildly abnormal. This could represent subclinical hypothyroidism. Additional specialized blood tests could show that your thyroid gland function has been disturbed. In the past, individuals with subclinical thyroid problems have not always received medication to treat the imbalance. In England, a group of patients was so upset about not being treated for subclinical hypothyroidism that they formed a patient advocate group that petitioned the medical community to be more aggressive about diagnosing and treating subtle thyroid disorders.

Rarely, thyroid disease can be present with normal laboratory results. This requires specialized blood work or an ultrasound of the thyroid to check for nodules that may disrupt metabolism.

It is less common to develop hot flashes for the first time if you have spent more than 18 months in post menopause. If you do, ask your doctor about getting tested for thyroid disease.

Divjot's Story
HOT FLASHES DUE TO A THYROID PROBLEM

Nine years ago, when I was 55, I had a total hysterectomy with the removal of both ovaries. I began using a hormone patch after the surgery and was free of hot flashes. However, after extensive media coverage of the negative effects of hormones in July 2002, I became concerned about the risks of estrogen and stopped using the patch. I felt well for six months, but then the hot flashes—severe and frequent—returned. My doctor suspected a thyroid problem because the hot flashes had already been resolved when I was off estrogen. They said that because I was in a stable postmenopausal state, my estrogen levels should not be fluctuating. The thyroid blood test showed that I had become hypothyroid. My sluggish thyroid was causing the hot flashes. My doctor prescribed thyroid medication and, after three months, my hot flashes are now gone.

HANDLING HOT FLASHES WITH PACED RESPIRATION

Smaller early studies published 10–15 years ago showed that slow, deep diaphragmatic breathing, known as paced respiration, could decrease hot flashes by 80 percent. At that time, I advised my patients to try paced respiration, and many found it to help stop hot flashes. More recently, however, larger studies have shown that paced respiration does not help as many women as was initially thought, and it is no longer advised as an evidence-based strategy by The Menopause Society. Paced respiration, however, does help treat high blood pressure naturally, in some cases lowering it into the normal range. With paced respiration, you breathe only five to seven times per minute—much slower than the normal breathing rate that averages more than 12 breaths a minute.[2]

REMEDIES, LIFESTYLE STRATEGIES, NONHORMONAL PRESCRIPTIONS, AND SUPPLEMENTS

HANDLING HOT FLASHES WITH LIFESTYLE MODIFICATIONS

Hot flashes can arrive hourly, daily, weekly, or monthly. Although hot flashes may occur in a cyclic pattern, they don't always appear on cue.

Medical researchers are starting to better understand why vasomotor symptoms occur. Common established triggers (i.e., behaviors, circumstances, or substances) commonly induce hot flashes. Caffeine and alcohol, for example, frequently trigger hot flashes or night sweats. An upcoming menstrual period can also be a trigger.

Avoiding your triggers reduces the number and severity of hot flashes. At times, avoiding or eliminating triggers may even erase the need for other lifestyle modifications, natural remedies, or prescription medication.

Neal Barnard, MD, a physician, researcher, and expert in the benefits of a vegan diet, has performed research demonstrating that ½ cup of soybeans or edamame daily may ease vasomotor symptoms. To benefit, you may eat the ½ cup of soybeans or edamame on its own, or you can add it to soup or salad.[1]

HOW TO REDUCE YOUR STRESS

Stress is a trigger for many women, although it is not clear why. There are a variety of strategies to reduce stress and help you cope with it. Decreasing the number of stressful situations you face each day at home and/or at work may decrease the number of hot flashes you have. To reduce your stress, ask yourself these questions:

- Can I delegate tasks to others?
- Can I reduce my commitments?
- Can I change my priorities?
- Can I shorten my work hours?
- Can I eliminate a long or stressful commute?
- Can I change to a different type of work that is less stressful?

WHAT TECHNIQUES DO YOU FIND HELPFUL TO LOWER YOUR STRESS?

Stress reduction techniques are taught by psychologists, social workers, and other mental health professionals. (See chapter 9 in this book about the role of cognitive behavioral therapy vs. interpersonal therapy and how both can help.) Your strategies may also include relaxation tapes, meditation, or other approaches.

CONSIDER COGNITIVE BEHAVIORAL THERAPY

Cognitive behavioral therapy (CBT) has been shown to help hot flashes and night sweats. Many therapists are trained in cognitive behavioral therapy (see Chapter 9 for more information). This form of talk therapy provides insight and does not require an individual to delve into their past. In addition to alleviating hot flashes and night sweats, CBT has also proven helpful in easing the extra anxiety that many women experience during perimenopause.[4,5,6]

AVOID ALCOHOL

Whether it is consumed in the form of beer, wine, hard liquor, or a mixed drink, alcohol is almost certain to bring on hot flashes or night sweats. Alcohol also disturbs the quality of your sleep. Although it is typically easier to fall asleep after a drink or two, doing so compromises the deepest, most restful part of sleep, otherwise known as rapid eye movement sleep. Decreasing the amount of alcohol you consume improves the quality of your sleep. It also reduces the frequency and severity of hot flashes and night sweats.

Carmen's Story
HOT FLASHES AND RED WINE

I was going through perimenopause smoothly. I had been experiencing hot flashes, but they resolved after I cut down my daily coffee from an extra-large coffee (24 ounces) to an 8-ounce coffee a day. One February, my hot flashes returned, so I went to see my doctor. As we chatted, I mentioned that my brother was staying with me for a month. He is a wine connoisseur, and his way of repaying my generosity was to bring home different wines for us to have with dinner every night. This was not my usual routine. My doctor thought the wine was causing the hot flashes and suggested that I try eliminating it. As soon as I did, my hot flashes were once again under control.

CUT BACK ON COFFEE

Coffee is a very common trigger. It's also a beverage that is more popular than ever. The number of specialty coffee shops is multiplying, and the coffee cups are getting larger. An extra-large Dunkin' Donuts cup of hot coffee is 24 ounces. A "venti" at Starbucks is

20 ounces. The more coffee you drink, the longer it takes to eliminate the caffeine from your body. Half the caffeine in a cup of coffee consumed by a healthy, nonpregnant adult is eliminated in six hours. If you drink a large cup of coffee (which may have 200 milligrams of caffeine) at 4:00 P.M., 100 milligrams of caffeine will be eliminated from your body by 10:00 P.M., leaving another 100 milligrams in your body that evening. This will disrupt your normal sleep pattern and promote night sweats. For some women, the caffeine in chocolate, tea, or soda also induces hot flashes.

> DID YOU KNOW?
> Most hot flash/night sweat sufferers are relieved to hear that it is not necessary to give up coffee entirely. Even a modest decrease in coffee consumption may banish the hot flashes and night sweats.

Abruptly eliminating coffee from your routine, however, is not advised, as doing this may trigger headaches. To taper off your regular java, decrease the amount by just two ounces the first week. Pour off two ounces every day before taking your first sip. If you still have severe hot flashes the second week, pour off two more ounces of coffee. Now you'll be at four fewer ounces per day. Continue the process until the hot flashes are bearable or gone. After two or three months with no hot flashes or night sweats, it's often possible to add back some coffee slowly in small increments without the hot flashes returning.

KEEP COOL

Hot weather triggers hot flashes, as does a warm room. Sometimes even slight increases in your body's core temperature can trigger a hot flash. Here are some suggestions for keeping cool:

- Set the thermostat at a lower temperature.
- Open a window.

- If you're feeling hot, sip a cold drink.
- Wear layers of light clothing. A sleeveless cotton shell under a shirt, sweater, or jacket works well. The outer layer can be peeled off, then replaced if a chill follows.
- Choose loose-fitting cotton clothing that breathes and is more comfortable.
- Try using a personal fan, either electric or handheld.
- Be Kool Strips® are another option. The small strips adhere to the skin and provide local cooling for about eight hours. They may be purchased over the counter at a pharmacy.

NEWER COOLING OPTIONS: TEMPERATURE CONTROL DEVICES

Women battling hot flashes now have a newer option as well: a personal thermostat. Researchers have validated these devices to varying degrees, and none of them have been subject to rigorous medical research trials in which large numbers of women are observed and compared to a control group (i.e., one that uses a sham device).

That said, some women find relief with these devices. I will list a few of the readily available temperature control devices here:

1. EMBR (www.EMBRlabs.com). Developed by engineers at MIT, this device can make you warmer by touching a red area on the device and cooler by touching a blue area on the device. The nerves in your wrist (i.e., peripheral nerves) where the device is worn perceive the local change in temperature from the device and send a message to the brain that warming up or cooling down is required. This device also has settings to promote sleep and lessen carsickness/motion sickness. Some of my patients who tried it found it helpful.

2. KULKUF (https://kulkuf.com/benefits/). This tech firm, based in Brooklyn, New York, developed a battery-operated

Velcro wristband that is a cooling device only. It assists with heat dissipation and ensures less sweating in addition to temperature comfort. It was initially designed for pro-athletes and gymgoers to reduce muscle soreness from heat exhaustion and increase stamina. They tweaked the design for menopausal women and discovered that 9 out of 10 women stated their hot flashes were eliminated in under 10 seconds. They report that those men and women with hot flashes from other medical conditions, such as multiple sclerosis and thyroid problems, as well as tuberculosis, HIV, and stress, may also benefit from using KULKUF.

3. MENOPOD (www.uncommongoods.com/product/meno pod). The MENOPOD is a small electronic cooling device that looks like a computer mouse and fits in your palm. You may charge it from a USB or an outlet. After pressing a button, you hold the device over the back of your neck for one minute. It blends into the workplace as it is indistinguishable from a wireless mouse. This device is designed in Canada and made in China.

4. REON POCKET (www.sony.com.hk). REON POCKET, developed in Hong Kong, is a wearable heating and cooling device worn on the back of the neck that can be tucked under your collar. REON POCKET Version 3 does not have to operate from your phone.

At the time of this writing, prices for all four of the devices above range from 150 to 199 US dollars. The American Congress of Obstetricians and Gynecologists reports that 27 million women (20 percent of the American workforce) experience menopause each year. As you read earlier, 80 percent are symptomatic. In addition to the devices above, there are chilling pillows and even a bed with a cooling system built in. None of these have undergone side-to-side comparisons.

EAT MORE VEGETABLE-BASED MEALS

Eating more vegetable-based meals helps reduce hot flashes. The good news is that it isn't necessary to become a vegetarian to get the benefit. Decreasing the size of each meat portion and serving meat less frequently may lessen hot flashes. Recently, another research study showed that those whose daily intake includes 30 grams of fiber had fewer hot flashes than those who did not. Vegetable-based meals, in addition to consumption of soy foods, may be responsible for the dramatically lower rate of hot flashes in Asian women.[1]

THE POTENTIAL ROLE OF SOY FOODS

Some plants, including soy, contain compounds called phytoestrogens that are plant-derived, estrogen-like substances. Phytoestrogens are biologically active compounds like the estrogens in a woman's body; however, they are not identical. They do not act the same way in the body, and they are weaker.

There are different types of phytoestrogens. Isoflavones are the type used most often to relieve menopausal symptoms. The two most prominent isoflavones in soy are genistein and daidzein. Isoflavones attach to receptors in the human body but do not behave the same way a woman's own estrogen would. Some behave similarly to estrogen but with less effect. Others are anti-estrogens and behave in a way opposite to estrogen.[7]

No doubt you have read at least one article promoting the role of soy foods and phytoestrogens as a method of handling hot flashes. But to date, there is no definitive data about their effectiveness. Studies about eating soy have produced contradictory findings. Soy foods have been shown to decrease the frequency and severity of hot flashes in some studies but not in others. And there are a few concerns. The safety of soy supplements has not been established. Soy foods are preferable. One concern about soy that has not been resolved is its effect on women who have had breast cancer. Currently, women who have had breast cancer are advised not to take soy supplements. Consuming one or two servings of food that contains soy on a regular basis is not thought to be harmful, but more data is needed. Asian women consume more soy foods than North American women and have a lower rate of breast cancer.

The second area of complexity that may contribute to the contradictory findings about soy is that phytoestrogens possess both estrogen-like properties and anti-estrogen properties. In some ways, these phytoestrogens may act like estrogen, alleviating hot flashes, and in other ways, they may act as estrogen antagonists and behave exactly opposite to the way estrogen would behave. For many years, women, regardless of their health history, were cautioned to avoid taking soy supplements. Although some women prefer the ease of taking a soy supplement as a pill or tablet, it may be detrimental—and there is no evidence that it is beneficial. In addition, the additives used to manufacture the supplements may not be healthy. Further, some supplements may contain too much of a particular type of soy—even more than the body can use or eliminate.

There are two promising exceptions to the general tenet that whole soy foods (e.g., soybeans, edamame, tofu, and tempeh) are healthier and more beneficial than soy supplements.

One exception is Equelle, which contains the active ingredient, S-Equol.[10] S-Equol is produced in small amounts in the female gut. Most inactive soy supplements need to be converted to the active S-Equol. Many women in the United States, however, don't have the gut bacteria to readily convert these supplements to the active ingredient. For them, soy products are not usually effective. A preparation that includes the active form of soy S-Equol, however, overcomes this disadvantage of individuals who cannot convert a supplement with daidzein and/or genistein to the active S-Equol. Only 25 to 35 percent of Western adults can produce Equol from daidzein. In contrast, 50 to 65 percent of Asian populations have gut bacteria that readily convert daidzein to the active S-Equol. Over decades of use, Equelle has not been associated with any hormone changes, changes in thyroid function, or changes in the risk of breast or uterine cancer in women who take Equelle. If forthcoming larger studies show Equelle use is safe and effective, it will be a wonderful nonhormonal option for women to consider if they have moderate or severe hot flashes. That's because the S-Equol acts on the estrogen beta-receptor and enhances estrogen activity in the brain without increasing the risk of breast cancer, uterine bleeding, or blood clots.

Another study looking at S-Equol used phytoSERM to evaluate an estrogen receptor B-selective phytoestrogenic formulation in perimenopausal and postmenopausal women.[8] This retrospective study was designed to evaluate the ability of PhytoSERM to manage vasomotor symptoms and cognitive decline. The researchers identified women who were both vulnerable to dementia and who had the APOE genotype. They found that women who took 50 mg daily of PhytoSERM for 12 weeks had fewer hot flashes per day than at baseline. They also had improvements in verbal learning and executive functioning, indicating preservation of cognitive functioning. These small, exploratory studies are encouraging, and they open the door for larger studies that can prove true efficacy.[9]

Soy supplements deserve larger, more rigorous trials to determine whether they will help you or someone you know and exactly what they will do for you. More specifically, research can provide whether they can potentially relieve vasomotor symptoms and/or promote improved cognition. Existing studies have small numbers of women, a high placebo response, and poor study design. These small studies, however, tell us that larger studies are worth the time and effort because they may provide crucial information to improve cognition and vasomotor symptoms using an estrogen-like compound with none of the drawbacks of estrogen itself.

Lastly, researchers have shown that extracting and processing soy affects the amount of isoflavone that remains in the product. Sometimes, removing the fat, taste, or color of natural soy to turn it into a supplement product removes the beneficial isoflavones. If the beneficial isoflavones are removed, the soy supplement may not provide the benefits found in foods such as tofu, soybeans, soymilk or soy cheese, and other types of beans.

GET REGULAR EXERCISE

Regular exercise decreases the frequency and severity of hot flashes. Exercise can also reset the body's thermostat and reduce stress. It can be as simple as walking or dancing, or it can be an exercise class or a class with a specific relaxation component such as yoga or tai chi (for more information on the role of exercise on your overall health, see chapter 12). A few small studies show that yoga effectively decreases vasomotor symptoms; however, other studies have not confirmed this finding. There is no definitive proof to support recommending yoga as a strategy to substantially decrease vasomotor symptoms. Larger studies are needed, and when they are designed, I hope they evaluate the role of different types of yoga and how each one affects vasomotor symptoms. A large well-designed study may even be able to tell us whether specific individuals can rely on certain types of yoga to decrease bothersome vasomotor symptoms.[3]

OVER-THE-COUNTER REMEDIES AND SUPPLEMENTS

DO SUPPLEMENTS WORK?

My patients often ask me about using supplements to help with their hot flashes. I always tell them to be careful because there is no one-size-fits-all approach. For women who do not get adequate relief from hot flashes using the lifestyle strategies mentioned so far, there are other options to consider. These various remedies, however, merit a discussion with your doctor, as they may affect your health in other ways. There is not sufficient space here to discuss every natural remedy being touted as beneficial for hot flashes or other menopausal symptoms. What follows are the handful that tend to attract the most interest from women seeking relief without hormones. That's because they typically receive the most attention in the media or have been included in studies to determine efficacy.

Before I jump onto the list, keep in mind that the Food and Drug Administration (FDA) does not review supplements before their release. This means no rigorous testing and data on potential interactions with other medications exist. As a result, these remedies may have unpredictable interactions with other medications or supplements you take. In addition, they may not be advisable if you have certain medical conditions.

I would like to tell you that natural remedies are safer and better for you, but proof of safety and effectiveness is lacking for most of the over-the-counter options that are currently available. Some remedies, however, such as flaxseed, look more promising than others. In fact, others have a wide range of quality standards between different brands or methods of preparation.

As a group, these remedies have not been studied rigorously, so they may also have side effects that are not well known or understood. That is why it is important to tell your doctor about all the supplements you take, as well as your prescription medications, before you try these remedies.

The testing and review process in place for FDA-approved prescription medicines is designed to test for safety and effectiveness and to determine whether the medication will help the person who takes it with the fewest possible side effects. The process determines whether manufacturing is reliable and uniform and whether pills or capsules are made to a precise standard. Without this type of safety check, a given pill or capsule may have no active ingredient in it. Or there can be too much of an active ingredient, which could cause harmful side effects. The FDA checks that the side effects of a medication are studied and disclosed so you don't take it with something else that is not compatible. Medication manufacturers must include this information when they advertise and sell the product. Although the FDA process is not foolproof, it is rigorous.

Unfortunately, natural preparations and nutritional supplements in the United States have none of these safety precautions in place. As a result, one can purchase a remedy that contains too much of an ingredient in one dose and too little of an active ingredient in another dose. They also are not required to list side effects or warnings about use or possible interactions with other products or prescriptions. This leads to the false impression that they are safer.

Further, if there is a precaution, such as sun sensitivity, the manufacturer of an over-the-counter remedy is not required to disclose it on the packaging.

If a natural remedy has no precautions written on the package, it does not mean there are no safety considerations. For example, St. John's wort is an over-the-counter remedy that relieves mild depression. Studies have shown that it is effective, but it can also cause abnormal bleeding, and you should stop it before surgery or anesthesia. Also, it may weaken the effectiveness of your low-dose oral contraceptive (i.e., birth control pill). Lastly, St. John's wort is not safe to take at the same time as a prescription antidepressant medication such as Prozac or Paxil.

Before I review some of the most requested over-the-counter remedies and the results of studies on their effectiveness, I would like to review one of the most challenging aspects of interpreting studies on vasomotor symptoms in menopause. Different researchers use a variety of criteria in choosing the women they study and how they measure the symptoms and report them. Over the past 75 years, there has been no standardization, making it difficult to compare different treatments. It's also difficult to apply various conclusions from different studies to clinical practice.

In 2021, The Menopause Society published a critical study from Australia that outlined standards for designing studies of vasomotor symptoms worldwide. Sarah Lensen, PhD, also published an original study titled "A Core Outcome Set for Vasomotor Symptoms Associated with Menopause: The COMMA (Core Outcomes in Menopause Global Initiative)." In this study, researchers standardized the outcome measures after looking at various randomized controlled trials of treatments for vasomotor symptoms in postmenopausal women from November 2019 to March 2020. To refine the results, they held international consensus meetings with clinicians, researchers, and women who experience these symptoms. Once this standard is implemented, we can better understand what approaches work when addressing vasomotor symptoms for certain women.[13] Based on the standardized outcomes, the following information will be reported in all future randomized trials evaluating interventions for women with vasomotor symptoms:

1. Frequency of vasomotor symptoms
2. Severity of vasomotor symptoms
3. Distress, bother, or interference of vasomotor symptoms
4. Impact on sleep
5. Satisfaction with treatment
6. Side effects of treatment

Manufacturers of over-the-counter remedies are not required to prove that the remedy produces the desired effect. While a prescription medication must include the percentage of individuals who can expect to benefit, the over-the-counter remedy does not demonstrate it works, how often it works, or for whom it works best. In addition, manufacturers do not need to specify who should avoid these remedies. When you read the material included with a natural remedy, you may be reading the equivalent of a television commercial.

In addition, the length of time that it is safe to take natural remedies is not well established with sound research. Aside from safety issues, there is no proof that some natural remedies work. Also important: There's no requirement to prove effectiveness prior to selling a natural remedy unless that remedy is classified as a drug.

Note that some natural remedies are both safe and effective. One example is B vitamin folate, which lowers the risk of birth defects. Solid research is still needed to learn which natural remedies are best suited to which individuals, in what quantity, and for what duration. As this information becomes available, women can use natural remedies more safely and with more confidence.[14]

RESVERATROL

The Resveratrol for Healthy Ageing in Women study evaluated women taking resveratrol and compared them to women taking inert pills (placebo-controlled with crossover for 24 months). The women were randomized: neither the women nor the researchers knew who took the active resveratrol (75 mg) and who took the placebo. The study, which relied on questionnaires, evaluated resveratrol's effect on pain perception, mood and depressive symptoms, menopausal symptoms, sleep quality, and quality of life. These researchers showed that resveratrol supplements reduced chronic pain in age-related osteoarthritis and improved menopause-related quality of life in postmenopausal women. I look forward to future larger studies evaluating resveratrol since many of my patients request estrogen hormone replacement for their achiness and joint discomfort. Not all patients can take estrogen. If it lives up to its promise, resveratrol would be a welcome alternative.[12]

WILD YAM CREAM

Wild yam cream is sold as a natural remedy to help reduce hot flashes. How does it work? By supplying natural progesterone to the body. Although it is true that progesterone is helpful in reducing hot flashes, yam cream is not effective because humans do not have the enzyme necessary to convert its plant compound into active progesterone in the body. The manufacturer is not required to disclose this information. To date, research data indicates that short-term treatment with topical wild yam cream does not reduce hot flashes.

Verdict: Don't bother trying wild yam cream because there's no proof it works.

BLACK COHOSH

Black cohosh is made from the underground stems of *Cimicifuga racemose*, a plant that is native to North America and has been used by Native Americans for hundreds of years. Europeans have been using it for more than 50 years, and in 1989, the German Kommission E, a federal institute, approved the use of black cohosh for menopause-related symptoms.

Studies of black cohosh have evaluated only its short-term use (i.e., for six months or less). The mechanism of action is not known. In addition, many different preparations of black cohosh are available, and they are not interchangeable. One preparation may be less effective than another, and side effects may differ. This can be attributed to the unique processing and dosing of each preparation, as well as the different types of ingredients from the various sources being used for each product. Even Remifemin, a popular formulation of black cohosh in this country, is prepared differently than it was 40 years ago when the initial study of the plant's effectiveness was performed. At that time, a study showed the original preparation was effective.

Black cohosh should not be taken at the same time as other hormone preparations, such as oral contraceptives or hormone prescriptions.

Verdict: It's OK to try the Remifemin preparation of black cohosh due to the high standard of manufacturing and supporting studies. Avoid taking black cohosh with oral contraceptives.[11]

RELIZEN

Relizen is a hormone-free, over-the-counter preparation to relieve hot flashes and night sweats. One of the main ingredients is bee pollen. It has been used by European women for more than 15 years. You take two tablets a day by mouth with or without food. In a small study of 64 women with 5.4 hot flashes a day, Relizen decreased the number and severity of vasomotor symptoms by 65 percent. A survey of more than 3,500 women showed Relizen reduces hot flash frequency and intensity while improving quality of sleep and quality of life. There is no specific data on which individuals benefit from Relizen and which do not. Relizen will not affect your hormone levels. Relizen does not act like estrogen and will not change your bleeding pattern. As long as you are not allergic to bees, there is no harm in trying Relizen; however, you may need to wait two months or more to see whether it works for you.[3,14]

Verdict: It is worth trying for mild to moderate vasomotor symptoms.

DONG QUAI

The root of this plant, which is a member of the celery family, has been used in Eastern medicine for thousands of years. It has not been well studied in the West, but one research study indicates that using dong quai alone does not relieve hot flashes any better than a placebo. Practitioners of complementary medicine advise that you can use dong quai with other herbs. These preparations have not been formally studied, so more data is needed. A known side effect of dong quai is sunlight sensitivity. If you take this remedy, wearing sunglasses, sunscreen, and a hat or visor is important. Dong quai can trigger heavy uterine bleeding, so women with fibroids should not try it. In addition, women on blood thinners should also avoid it, as should women with bleeding problems or other blood clotting problems.

Verdict: Dong quai is no better than a placebo, so it makes sense to avoid it.

RED CLOVER

Red clover is another source of isoflavones. Six different studies looking at two different preparations of red clover concluded that it did not help to reduce hot flashes. Because there is no evidence that it has a significant effect on hot flashes, and because it contains processed isoflavones that do not have a track record for being safe or effective, I do not recommend red clover.

Verdict: Avoid it due to potential safety problems.

FLAXSEED

A small study by the Mayo Clinic indicates that flaxseed may be effective in treating hot flashes. In the study, women who had at least

14 hot flashes a week added four tablespoons of crushed flaxseed a day to their diet for six consecutive weeks. The result? Flaxseed halved their number of daily hot flashes. In addition, the intensity of their hot flashes dropped by 57 percent. The women in the study also reported improved mood. While some consider it premature to strongly recommend flaxseed, this option looks promising, and so far, no adverse effects have been reported. Flaxseed also contains healthy omega-3 fatty acids, giving it heart-health benefits as well. It is easily added to cereal, juice, yogurt, or fruit dishes, so most women do not find it difficult to introduce it into their daily meals.[15]

Verdict: Looks promising, but larger studies are needed to assess efficacy.

VITAMIN B6 SUPPLEMENTS

Vitamin B6 may provide some relief from hot flashes when taken in doses of 50 milligrams by mouth once a day. It is important not to exceed the recommended dosage. Taking more than 100 milligrams of vitamin B6 daily may cause irreversible nerve damage. Be sure to check the label of the multivitamin supplement that you take, as well as the labels of other vitamins, such as B-complex, that may contain additional vitamin B6. The goal is to not exceed the recommended dose in your combined supplements.

Verdict: OK to try, especially if your blood level is low. Do not take high doses as high doses are associated with nerve damage.

VITAMIN E SUPPLEMENTS

While some studies suggest that vitamin E may help relieve hot flashes, other studies indicate just the opposite. Trying up to 400 international units of vitamin E per day is safe for most women. Women on blood thinners such as coumadin or aspirin (including low-dose aspirin), nonsteroidal anti-inflammatory drugs such as ibuprofen or naproxen, dong quai, evening of primrose oil, garlic or ginger supplements, or ginkgo biloba should avoid taking extra vitamin E because it may prolong bleeding. It interferes with platelet function and impairs normal clotting. Women who have active bleeding with ulcers, brain hemorrhage, heavy vaginal or uterine bleeding, rectal bleeding, or a history of a bleeding disorder should also avoid vitamin E.

Verdict: There's no definitive proof that vitamin E supplements work to relieve hot flashes. Be particularly cautious if you are on blood thinners as you may experience excess bleeding if you take both vitamin E and blood thinners.

ACUPUNCTURE

Acupuncture has not been shown to reduce the number of hot flashes a woman experiences. Some small studies point to the success of acupuncture in relieving vasomotor symptoms. Other studies show no benefit. Larger well-designed studies would be helpful. Although all studies do not agree that acupuncture is effective, it is reasonable to try it for hot flashes or night sweats if it is performed by a licensed practitioner and the needles are sterile.[20]

Verdict: Research studies do not prove acupuncture works for hot flashes and night sweats in most women.

CANNABIS

One study I found queried women on their use of cannabis for menopause symptoms, including hot flashes and night sweats. At this time, the study established that women are trying different forms of cannabis, whether edible or smoked, to quell vasomotor symptoms. Further studies are needed to determine the effectiveness of this approach.[16]

Verdict: There's no data yet on the efficacy of cannabis to treat hot flashes.

WHAT PRESCRIPTION MEDICATIONS CAN HELP WITH HOT FLASHES?

If you continue to have troublesome hot flashes despite making lifestyle and dietary modifications, you may benefit from a non-hormone-based prescription medication. A variety of options may provide relief. Some medications, commonly prescribed for other medical conditions such as high blood pressure, depression, or nerve pain, have been shown to diminish hot flashes and night sweats.

Not all medications in a particular category of medications will help hot flashes. For example, many antidepressants and most medications available to treat high blood pressure do not affect hot flashes.

The advantage of using these types of medications is that they are not hormones, so they do not increase the individual's risk of blood clots, stroke, heart disease, breast cancer, or uterine cancer. Discuss these options with your doctor and consider these medications if:

- You choose not to take hormones, but you need relief from hot flashes and have already tried the lifestyle modifications described in this chapter.
- You are a breast cancer survivor or the survivor of a stroke or heart attack.
- You need to stop hormone therapy.
- You have both hot flashes and another medical condition that requires one of these types of medications.
- You are taking a low dose of hormones, but you have not obtained complete relief from your hot flashes or night sweats, and you want additional relief without taking a higher dose of hormones.
- You are older than 60 or more than 10 years from your last menstrual period.

ANTIDEPRESSANTS

Low doses of certain antidepressants, such as Paxil, Prozac, Effexor, or Lexapro, can be used to decrease hot flashes. In some cases, the dose is lower than the dose used to treat depression. Antidepressants are not associated with a risk of breast cancer or uterine cancer.

Do not stop taking antidepressants suddenly. As the hot flashes become more manageable or subside completely, taper off the medication under your doctor's supervision to avoid unnecessary side effects.[6,14,21]

Each antidepressant medication will affect individuals differently. If one antidepressant is associated with unacceptable or unpleasant side effects (for example, weight gain or sexual problems), a sister antidepressant medication may provide relief from hot flashes without the same difficulties. You may end up trying several different medications before you find the one that is best for you.

Shoshana's Story
HOT FLASHES AND ANTIDEPRESSANT MEDICATION

I'm a 52-year-old postmenopausal woman who has been on hormones for a year. This includes two prescription hormones that I take daily: Prometrium, a plant-based FDA-approved progesterone, and Estradiol, a plant-based FDA-approved estrogen. My doctor explained that taking estrogen alone, without progesterone, could lead to uterine cancer. Unfortunately, I had a suspicious finding on a routine mammogram, and subsequently, the breast biopsy showed cancer. My doctor did not attribute the breast cancer to hormone use because I had used the hormones for only one year. However, they did tell me to stop taking hormones. After I stopped taking hormones, I developed severe night sweats. My gynecologist suggested a low dose of Effexor, an antidepressant that works through the nervous system to reduce hot flashes. They also cautioned me not to take any synthetic soy preparations, such as soy powders, pills, or supplements, as the effect on breast cancer is still unknown. Thankfully, I've gotten dramatic relief on Effexor. And my gynecologist has assured me that I can taper off this medication over time once the hot flashes have subsided.

BLOOD PRESSURE MEDICATION

Clonidine (or Catapress) is a medication that helps lower high blood pressure by working through the central nervous system. It also helps decrease hot flashes and night sweats. In some cases, a woman's primary care physician, internist, or family doctor may be able to prescribe clonidine to control high blood pressure and simultaneously reduce hot flashes.

Some women need more than one type of medicine to control high blood pressure, and clonidine may be selected as one of the prescriptions. An individual on clonidine would then benefit from its dual effects in reducing her hot flashes and lowering their blood pressure.

Zhang's Story
FLASHES AND HIGH BLOOD PRESSURE

At age 49, I didn't expect to be diagnosed with high blood pressure. After all, as a school nurse, I know a lot about health. But I had to admit I was overweight, and I know that contributes to hypertension. At the same time, I shared with my doctor that my hot flashes have never subsided. My doctor put me on clonidine, a blood pressure medication that also helps hot flashes. It really helped. After I was able to start exercising, I also modified the way I ate and lost the extra weight I'd gained over the past few years. When my blood pressure remained at a healthy level, I was able to stop the clonidine, and my hot flashes did not return.

NERVE ADJUSTMENT MEDICATION

Neurontin (gabapentin) is a medication prescribed to decrease nerve pain. Recent research shows that it also reduces hot flashes at night or night sweats even in the absence of nerve pain. Neurontin may be a good choice to decrease hot flashes or night sweats and may be prescribed "off label" (it is off label because it is designed and approved to treat a different medical condition, but studies show it is effective for this additional reason). You'll want to discuss this with your doctor, however, to determine whether it might be a good choice for you. It is usually prescribed to be taken at bedtime. At first, the doctor may prescribe a lower dose and then increase it every few weeks until you get relief from your hot flashes. It can also help you sleep better.[22]

Candela's Story
HOT FLASHES AND NEURONTIN (GABAPENTIN)

I'm 68 and have been postmenopausal for 12 years. I stopped taking hormones in August 2002 after the media coverage of the Women's Health Initiative. Now I have hot flashes that are annoying and inconvenient. Night sweats interrupt my sleep, and I feel tired during the day. I don't want to restart hormones and my gynecologist agrees with me. We discussed my options. They recommended I try a low dose of gabapentin before bed. This reduced the frequency and severity of my night sweats enough for me to get a good night's sleep.

OVERACTIVE BLADDER MEDICINE

Oxybutynin is a medication taken by mouth that works through the nerves in the bladder to lessen frequent urgent bladder contractions that promote urge urinary incontinence (UUI). With UUI, you can leak on the way to the bathroom, or you may need to urinate frequently or suddenly. Off-label, 5 mg of oxybutynin taken daily may ease vasomotor symptoms. Long-term safety is not yet assured, however. The good news is that relief for months or one to two years can be helpful for some women who have bothersome hot flashes or night sweats (or both) and also have urinary urgency.[17]

NEW CLASS OF MEDICATION

For more than half a century, doctors and researchers had only a crude understanding of the physiology of vasomotor symptoms. Now, we know the body's thermostat is in the hypothalamus, an area of the brain that contains specific receptors to regulate temperature. Estrogen influences the behavior of three critical receptors in this region: kisspeptin, neurokinin B, and Dynorphin. Together, these receptors are called the KNDy neurons. When the estrogen levels fall in menopause, neurokinin B becomes overactive, and the temperature range you can tolerate comfortably becomes extremely narrow. Even a one- or two-degree rise in temperature can set off a hot flash or night sweat. With genetic studies and more sophisticated mapping of neurons and receptors, researchers have isolated the neurokinin B receptors and made an antagonist that blocks the excess firing of neurokinin B just as estrogen would. The result? Temperature regulation is restored. Studies are continuing to show that that Fezolinetant and other neurokinin B antagonists help more than 85 percent of women who take it within a few days of starting it. Larger studies are needed to determine whether there are hidden side effects. In addition, other similar medications are in development to block the KnDY neurons. [18]

Clinicians and researchers are beginning to ask whether hot flashes are only a symptom of menopause or if they are a signal that the nerve regulation in an individual's body is altered. More research is needed to explore this possibility.[19]

IMPORTANT TAKEAWAYS

In summary:

- Certain women are more prone to hot flashes than others.
- The intensity and frequency of hot flashes and night sweats may change over time.

- Hot flashes and night sweats could be due to an underlying health condition.
- There are many ways to reduce hot flashes, such as lifestyle modifications, , stress reduction, and more.
- Diet and exercise play a critical role in reducing hot flashes and night sweats.
- Before taking a supplement for your hot flashes and night sweats, be sure to speak with your doctor.
- You may benefit from a non-hormone-based prescription medication, but only a conversation with your doctor can determine that.

QUESTIONS FOR YOUR DOCTOR

1. My hot flashes are mild. Do I need to treat them? What lifestyle options should I consider?
2. My night sweats are debilitating, and I was given a sleeping pill but want other treatment options. What should I consider?
3. I have estrogen receptor—positive breast cancer. What options do I have for severe hot flashes and night sweats?
4. I am a BRCA carrier. What options do I have for my moderate to severe hot flashes and night sweats?

Also be prepared to answer these questions your doctor may ask you:

5. How often do you bleed?
6. Have you had 12 consecutive months with no bleeding?
7. If you had a final menstrual period, when was it, and how old were you?
8. Are your hot flashes associated with sweating? If so, do they prevent you from continuing with your current activity? Do you have night sweats? Do you wake up tired even after a full night's sleep?

RESOURCES

American Academy of Family Physicians (www.familydoctor.org). This professional organization has excellent resources for medical professionals and the public about menopause and more general health topics.

American College of Obstetricians and Gynecologists (www.acog.org). This site has Patient Education Pamphlets for the major topics in women's health and preventive care.

Mayo Clinic (www.mayoclinic.com). This is a world-class medical center with resources for the public on its website. They also publish a newsletter about general health topics of interest to men and women.

Menopause Flashes® E-Newsletter. This is a free monthly email newsletter for consumers containing information about all aspects of menopause and available therapies, both traditional and complementary, to ease symptoms and preserve long-term health. You may preview an issue and subscribe at www.menopause.org/newsletter.aspx.

The Menopause Society (formerly the North American Menopause Society) (www.menopause.org). In addition to the newsletter available online, there are print brochures on special aspects of menopause, including early menopause (*The Early Menopause Guidebook*). They also publish *Pause*, a print journal available quarterly through your gynecologist's office. Book reviews and other resources are also featured.

National Center for Complementary and Alternative Medicine (http://nccam.nih.gov/). This site has objective reviews of studies showing the benefits and risks of complementary and alternative strategies. It is also helpful to look at what has not been studied completely and what is not known.

CHAPTER 3

TAKING HORMONES IN MENOPAUSE

Taking hormones during menopause is a very personal decision. Here's how to know what may be right for you.

ALTHOUGH HORMONE THERAPY IS highly effective for certain symptoms of menopause, the decision to take them is unique to you based on your age, personal health risks, and stage of menopause. There is no universal answer, which is why it's important to explore your options before deciding. In this chapter, I'll answer several questions about taking hormones in menopause such as:

- Will I benefit from hormones, or might they increase my risk for certain diseases and cancers?
- What are bioidentical hormones, and how do they differ from synthetic ones?
- What questions should I consider as I decide whether hormones are right for me?
- What if I want to stop taking hormones? How can I do that effectively?

HORMONES: SETTING THE RECORD STRAIGHT

Menopause is a natural process that all women encounter in midlife or sooner. You may have read or heard that you should avoid taking hormones at all costs since menopause is a natural process. Or you may have read or heard that hormones help you maintain your youth. At times, the medical community has been accused of medicalizing menopause—that is, influencing you to take hormones to maintain youth and well-being, regardless of whether you need or ask for them. And there are clinicians who do just that.

While estrogen levels do stabilize at low levels in post menopause, menopause is not an estrogen-deficient state. Young girls who have not begun to menstruate are not estrogen deficient. They are young girls who have not experienced puberty yet. Women who become postmenopausal are entering a normal phase of life when they do not menstruate. This postmenopausal state does not require medication.

WHY ALL THE FUSS ABOUT HORMONES?

You may never want or need hormones. Or you or someone you know may find menopause challenging. Your symptoms may impair your ability to function well in your daily life. When this is the case and absent any medical risk factors, you may meet current safety guidelines for taking hormones. In fact, a prescription for low-dose hormones may provide much-needed relief. I encourage you to consider framing menopause as a natural passage that you will experience. You may or may not want help along the way, and that help may or may not include low-dose estrogen at some point in your journey.

HORMONES: A LOOK BACK AT HISTORY

For more than 40 years, middle-aged women were encouraged to take prescription medications containing female hormones to replace the hormones their bodies were no longer making at youthful levels. Menopausal hormone therapy (MHT) was prescribed to ease the troublesome symptoms of menopause, and it was thought to confer other benefits as well. MHT was believed to help preserve memory; maintain young-looking skin; control hot flashes and night sweats; improve sleep and moods; ease vaginal dryness; prevent weak bones, heart disease, and Alzheimer's disease; and lower the risk of colon cancer. Some of these assumptions have turned out to be incorrect, while others are still true for certain groups of women.

Now that additional research has been done, taking hormones has become increasingly controversial. A woman who is thinking about using hormones must consider multiple factors such as her age, the date of her final menstrual period, her stage of menopause, whether she has had a hysterectomy, whether she has heart disease, whether she has any history of breast cancer, and so on. Each of you is unique with your own individual profile. The information in this chapter will help you clearly understand the risks and benefits of hormone therapy so you'll be able to ask your doctor the most appropriate questions and work together to find the best approach for you.

Your personal preferences are also an integral part of the decision-making process. If you are against certain lifestyle changes or medications, hormones cannot improve your health. Even if you are certain that you would never take hormones or other prescription medications, stay informed about the risks and benefits. The benefits will increase, and the risks will diminish as newer, better medications are developed. Also, with time, your risk for age-related conditions such as osteoporosis, stroke, and heart disease will increase. Review your health history with your gynecologist regularly and be on the lookout for new treatments that may become available.

TODAY'S VIEWS ON HORMONES

Since 2002, the pendulum has swung away from hormones, and many clinicians who do not focus on menopause are reluctant to prescribe them. So, you may wonder why I am going to discuss them. Here's why: startling headlines, inaccurate and incomplete assessments of research results, and important information reduced to soundbites have not helped the discussion of what's best for women's health during perimenopause and beyond. My goal is to help you sort through the confusing barrage of information and be able to have a frank, educated discussion with your doctor about what's best for you.

HORMONES: MY RECOMMENDATIONS

I am not recommending that you take hormones, nor am I advising you to avoid them. Here is my only recommendation: that you and your doctor arrive at a safe, reasonable approach that meets your individual needs.

When you discuss hormones with your doctor or read about them on your own, you are likely to encounter the issue of bioidentical hormones as well as many ways of taking hormones other than by mouth. Each of these is discussed in detail in the pages that follow. Making the right choice begins with being informed.

In the discussion of MHT, there has been no greater influence for women today than the Women's Health Initiative (WHI). The results of this important study have been so misconstrued that until you have a clear, full understanding of what these results mean, you cannot make an informed decision about HT. That is why I begin this chapter with an examination of what the WHI has really taught us.

MAKING SENSE OF THE WOMEN'S HEALTH INITIATIVE STUDY

The federally funded WHI was the largest, most comprehensive examination of postmenopausal women's health ever undertaken. It was a pivotal study because thousands of women were included, and it was designed in the classic randomized double-blind, placebo-controlled manner that is the gold standard for scientific studies. Women were randomly assigned to receive either active hormone pills or sugar pills (placebo). Neither they nor their doctors knew which pills they were getting. The hormones studied were Premarin (synthetic estrogen, synthesized from horse urine) and Prempro (synthetic estrogen combined with synthetic progesterone).

In July 2002, however, WHI investigators stopped their research early for the Prempro group due to the increased risk to the health of the women involved. The medical community was disturbed when the WHI report stated the study was stopped because initial data showed that the women who were taking these hormones had higher rates of breast cancer, heart attacks, strokes, and blood clots than the women who were taking placebos. Although the study was supposed to run for eight years, it was halted after five years due to these alarming results.

In April 2004, the WHI also stopped its research on estrogen-only therapy because it appeared to increase the risk of strokes and blood clots without providing any added protection against heart disease.

These events had an enormous impact on women and the medical community. Many women who were taking hormones stopped abruptly, and women who were not on hormones avoided starting them. Prescriptions for hormone therapy plummeted. Findings from the WHI study are still being reanalyzed, debated, and reported.

The current interpretation of the WHI data on hormones and heart disease is in keeping with what researchers and clinicians have observed for the past 30 years: healthy women (those without established heart disease, strokes, or blood clots) between ages 50 and 59 do NOT have a higher risk of heart attack if they take estrogen or an estrogen and progesterone combination if they initiate hormone therapy less than ten years after their final menstrual period. Healthy women in this age group who have spent fewer than 10 years in post menopause may consider taking hormones to control severe hot flashes. In fact, some studies looking at hormone use in this group of healthy postmenopausal women show that their risk of heart disease is lower with hormone use.

Initially, the WHI reported the outcomes for most women in the study, all over 60 years old, as if these outcomes represented those for all women, including those ages 59 and younger. In reality, the outcomes differed depending on a woman's age. Researchers also combined outcomes of women more than 15 years out from their last menstrual period with those fewer than 10 years into post menopause. They reported their results as a global finding—as if it applied to all of the age groups studied. In fact, these early published results were very different from the experience of women in the study who were younger than 59 and closer to their last menstrual period. But the data for the women under 59 was not interpreted separately or published until 2007.

Other differences have emerged as the information gathered from the WHI study has been reexamined. For instance, more of the women who were 60 and older were also obese when compared to participants in the younger age group. The older groups of women also had established heart disease in the form of high blood pressure and high cholesterol. Their arteries had already begun to harden. Estrogen is not advised for women who already have heart disease. Estrogen may lower the risk of heart disease in a younger woman, but only when heart disease is not present. Once heart disease is established, there is no role for estrogen. In fact, it worsens heart disease.

The risk of stroke is low for certain healthy postmenopausal women with no history of stroke. This includes women who are under the age of 60 or fewer than 10 years from their final menstrual period. The risk of stroke in 50- to 59-year-old women is much lower than the risk for women in their sixties and seventies. This means if hormone prescriptions increase the risk by a small amount, few additional women ages 59 or younger are likely to experience a stroke as long as they are healthy and have no predisposition to having a stroke before filling the prescription and no history of blood clots in the legs or lungs (deep vein thrombosis or pulmonary emboli).

A more in-depth review of the WHI data confirms that starting (or restarting) hormones in certain women over age 60 (i.e., those who are more than 15 years away from their last menstrual period) is not beneficial. A very different circumstance exists for women aged 59 or younger or who have had their final menstrual period less than ten years prior. These women may need and benefit from hormones to quell severe, debilitating hot flashes. The risks and benefits for each group of women are not the same.

The influence of hormones during post menopause on breast cancer risk is being debated. It is so complicated that researchers and clinicians have not reached a consensus, but they can agree on the following:

- The risk of breast cancer increases each year until a woman turns 79. That risk remains almost as high until age 85, when it begins to decline. The risk of breast cancer increases with age, even without taking hormones.
- Obese women have a higher risk of breast cancer.[5]
- Estrogen affects breast tissue and cancer risk differently when taking an estrogen and progesterone combination (Prempro, discussed shortly) than when taking estrogen alone.
- Some types of breast cancer are affected by estrogen, and others are not. Hormones affect breast cancer risk differently, depending on the type of breast tissue involved.
- The longer a postmenopausal woman over 50 takes supplemental estrogen and progesterone, the more likely it is to increase her risk of breast cancer. This is especially true after five years of use.[5]
- The higher the dose of hormones, the higher the risk of getting breast cancer over time.
- After an individual stops taking hormones, the risk of breast cancer decreases over time until it is no longer elevated.[5]

Since more of the women aged 60 and older in the WHI study were obese than women in the younger group, they were already at higher risk of breast cancer (as well as heart disease) because of their obesity as well as their age.[1]

ARE THERE ANY DRAWBACKS OF THE WHI STUDY?

Yes. The study had some drawbacks, some of which were overlooked, that prevent the results from applying to all women. These include the following:

1. Only 10 percent of the women in the WHI study were younger than 55. The early, general conclusions drawn from the study do not apply to all perimenopausal and postmenopausal women. The results are, however, helpful in learning about women who have spent more than 10 years in post menopause. They do not predict outcomes for perimenopausal women or younger, newly postmenopausal women.
2. Seventy percent of the participants were over 60 years old. Most of the women were 15 or 20 years into post menopause. Based on professional guidelines, this is not a group of women that menopause specialists start on hormones for hot flashes or night sweats.
3. The women in WHI were not screened for heart disease at the beginning of the study. Some of them had already developed heart disease, and most of them would have had an elevated risk of heart disease and stroke because of their age and length of time in post menopause.
4. Some of the WHI participants already took estrogen before they enrolled in the study, although they were required to stop taking hormones for three months before the study. This confuses the data regarding the length of time participants took hormone therapy. The total length of time some participants took hormones is much longer than the study suggests.
5. The WHI study excluded women with severe hot flashes. Women who wanted estrogen to relieve these symptoms could not participate in the study. This is unfortunate because one of the principal reasons for prescribing hormones is to relieve debilitating hot flashes or night sweats.

WHAT HORMONES DID THE WHI STUDY?

Decades ago, researchers found that women with a uterus who take estrogen alone have an increased risk of getting uterine cancer. Adding progesterone to the estrogen prescription reduced this risk. This information was factored into the WHI study from the outset.

The women in the WHI study were divided into two groups to study both scenarios:

1. The first study started with 10,739 women who had hysterectomies. These women were divided into two groups:
   - Group A (5,310 women) took 0.625 milligrams a day of Premarin, a synthetic estrogen prepared from the urine of pregnant mares.
   - Group B (5,429 women) took a placebo.
2. The second study started with 16,608 women ages 50–79 years who all had an intact uterus.
   - Group A (8,506 women) took Prempro 2.5, which is a combination of 0.625 milligrams of Premarin and 2.5 milligrams of Provera (synthetic progesterone).
   - Group B (8,102 women) took a placebo.

WHAT WERE THE RESULTS OF THE PREMARIN STUDY?

When it became clear that the women in the WHI study taking Premarin (synthetic estrogen alone, without progesterone) had a higher risk of stroke, the study was halted. It is important to note, however, that for the duration of their participation, the women taking estrogen alone did not have a higher risk of heart attack or breast cancer than the women taking a placebo. They also had stronger bones and a lower risk of colorectal cancer than they would have had without Premarin. When the data for women ages 50 to 59 was reanalyzed, it showed that the women ages 59 and younger who took Premarin alone had a lower risk of breast cancer. In addition, the Premarin group had more than twice the risk of certain types of benign breast disease. The Premarin group experienced 155 cases of benign breast disease while the placebo group had 77 cases.

Now that the results have been reanalyzed and sorted out by age and menopause status, experts believe that the increased risk of stroke mainly affects women over age 60 and have spent more than 10 years in post menopause. Women over 60 who are more than 10 years from their final menstrual period are discouraged from starting or restarting estrogen therapy.[1]

WHAT WERE THE RESULTS OF THE PREMPRO STUDY?

Prempro, a synthetic version of estrogen and progesterone, was thought to prevent heart disease when the WHI study began. One purpose of the study was to determine whether this was true. Initially, researchers reported that Prempro worsened the risk of heart disease. As of 2007, this applies to study participants over 60 years old and were more than 10 years into post menopause. Healthy women 59 and younger who were less than 10 years from their last menstrual period did not have a higher risk of heart attack in the WHI study. In fact, women ages 59 and younger who took Prempro had a lower risk of heart disease if they were less than 10 years into post menopause.

Prempro did not prevent heart disease in the women over 60 because they already had it—it was too late for prevention. In women 59 and under who have not been postmenopausal for more than 10 years, however, estrogen does prevent heart disease. This does not mean that you should take estrogen to prevent heart disease if you are younger than 59. What it does show is that certain healthy women who choose to take estrogen to treat debilitating hot flashes will not increase their risk of heart disease. This includes women who are in the low-risk group who have been in post menopause for fewer than 10 years.

A noteworthy effect of taking combination estrogen/progestin hormones was an increase in false alarms from mammograms and more benign breast disease. The estrogen component increases the density of a breast tissue. This makes mammograms harder to read, and it leads to more false positives. Higher breast density is also an independent risk factor for breast cancer. Since hormone therapy may make it harder to detect breast cancer, women who use it will want to make sure they keep up with checkups, including annual breast exams and mammograms.

Most hormone studies have been done on the synthetic hormones Premarin, Provera, and the combination, Prempro. Other hormone preparations, whether derived from plants or bioidentical or compounded, are thought to have the same risks. In the absence of large studies that look at other hormone preparations, experts advise women and their doctors to assume that all types of hormones have the same risks regardless of the way they are taken or how they are made. This includes natural, bioidentical, or plant-derived hormones. And higher doses of hormones, such as those found in pellets and implants, have a higher risk. These are discussed in more detail at the end of this chapter.

Since menopause experts use synthetic hormones as studied in WHI as the standard for assessing the risks and benefits of hormones in general, I think it is helpful to review the safety concerns and precautions that the WHI research study showed in more detail.[1,3]

WHAT DID DOCTORS LEARN FROM THE WHI STUDY AND ITS REINTERPRETATION?

The WHI findings were splashed across headlines in a blanket fashion: "Hormones are dangerous—do not take them!" We now know this is an oversimplification and does not represent the WHI findings in an accurate way. It cheated many women of the benefits of estrogen by implying that all women on hormones are in danger. From the alarming press reports, women got the idea that all hormones are bad for all women in all settings.

HORMONE THERAPY AND THE RISK OF HEART DISEASE

In early observational studies of younger postmenopausal women, estrogen lowered the risk of heart disease. The reanalysis of the WHI study results for women under age 59 has reaffirmed this fact.

Based on data from the Nurses' Health Study, a large study where women were observed for changes in their health over decades, women who begin taking combination hormones while they are still perimenopausal have a 30 percent lower risk of heart disease than women who do not take hormones. Perimenopausal women and women in early post menopause may benefit from estrogen to prevent heart disease before their arteries have hardened and lost their flexibility.[11]

HORMONE THERAPY AND RISK OF BREAST CANCER

Initially, the WHI results showed that women did not increase their risk of breast cancer when they took Prempro (the combined hormone used in the study) for five or fewer years. Those who took Premarin alone had a lower risk of breast cancer. These results have held up in subsequent studies.

More about hormones and breast cancer. In the WHI study, a daily continuous-combined dose of conjugated estrogen and medroxyprogesterone showed a small increased risk of breast cancer with nine additional breast cancer cases for every 10,000 women per year of treatment. This is less than one additional case of breast cancer diagnosed in 1,000 users a year. This risk is slightly greater than if you drank one glass of wine a day. It is a lower risk of breast cancer than you would have if you drank two glasses of wine a day. It is like the risk you would have if you were obese with low physical activity.[1]

If you take estrogen or an estrogen/progesterone combination, commit to regular mammograms to detect early breast cancers and precancers before they can be felt on exam. Ways to decrease the risk of breast cancer are discussed in chapter 13.

STATISTICAL RESULTS

WHI STUDY, PREMPRO GROUP[3]

To clarify the study results, they are expressed in terms of the increased or decreased risk in "person years." If you were to put 10,000 women on Prempro for one year (10,000 person years), you could expect these outcomes for the higher-risk group by age and menopause status:

Increase in Absolute Risk	Increase in Relative Risk
7 more coronary heart attacks	29 percent increase in risk
8 more cases of breast cancer	26 percent increase in risk
8 more strokes	41 percent increase in risk
18 more blood clots	100 percent increase in risk

Decrease in Absolute Risk	Decrease in Relative Risk
6 fewer cases of colorectal cancer	37 percent reduction in risk
5 fewer hip fractures	37 percent reduction in risk

Remember, as of 2007, the increased risk of heart attack does not apply to women under age 59 who have spent fewer than 10 years in post menopause. These women are a lower-risk group and will not experience the higher risk of heart attack.

The increase in relative risk is often quoted as unacceptably high. Who would want to take something that increases the risk of breast cancer by 26 percent? And what doctor would write such a prescription? The answer lies in the absolute risk. The relative risk looks at the degree of increased risk that the medication adds, not the actual number of women affected. In the case of breast cancer, taking Prempro for one year adds eight more cases of breast cancer per 10,000 women taking the prescription hormone. That is less than one additional case of breast cancer per 1,000 women per year.

It is not a desirable outcome, but a healthy individual who suffers from debilitating hot flashes or night sweats may consult her doctor and accept that risk if she cannot obtain relief with other strategies.

HORMONE THERAPY AND THE RISK OF OVARIAN CANCER

In Denmark, a study of more than 900,000 postmenopausal women was done from 1995 to 2005 to assess whether taking hormones increases a woman's risk of ovarian cancer. Different types and dosages of hormones were studied, including bioidentical hormones. Women who took hormones were slightly more likely to develop ovarian cancer than those who did not take them. Two years after the hormones were stopped, there was no increase in risk. For every 8,300 women who took hormones for one year, there was one extra case of ovarian cancer. These results are similar to those of the Million Women Study.[2]

Is this risk great or small? For an individual woman, the risk is not great. Ovarian cancer is rare, so even doubling the rate would still yield a low number. But any case of ovarian cancer is devastating, and when the effect is multiplied by hundreds of thousands of women, it becomes a public health issue. This increase in ovarian cancer may be due to greater vigilance and diagnosis since women on hormones get close follow-up before refilling their prescriptions. More data are needed on the doses and types of hormones that influence these results.

HORMONE THERAPY AND ALCOHOL

Alcohol increases the risk of breast cancer even without hormones. A Danish study that included more than 5,000 women found that women who took estrogen and other hormones increased their risk of breast cancer threefold by consuming one or two drinks a day. Drinking more than two drinks daily was associated with almost five times the risk. Women who know they are going to be drinking will want to factor this into their decisions about hormone therapy. (More information in chapter 13.)

WHO SHOULD AVOID STARTING SYSTEMIC ESTROGEN?

The goal of systemic estrogen is to provide safe, low blood levels of estrogen to improve your menopause symptoms. Systemic estrogen may be taken by mouth or by applying a patch to the skin, rubbing a lotion into the skin, or spraying the skin. It can also be taken by using Femring, a ring placed in the vagina that releases enough estrogen to alleviate hot flashes as well as vaginal dryness. These forms of estrogen are meant to be absorbed into the body and raise the blood level of estrogen. Avoid starting systemic estrogen if:

- There is any possibility you are pregnant.
- You have not had a menstrual period for more than 10 years.
- You have any unusual vaginal bleeding that has not been checked by your doctor.
- You have liver disease.
- You have had a heart attack, stroke, or other heart disease.
- You have spent more than 10 years in post menopause and are over 60 years old.
- You do not have severe hot flashes or night sweats.
- You have had a deep vein clot in your leg or a pulmonary embolus (lung clot) or you have an inherited high risk of blood clots (thromboembolic disease).
- You have untreated gallbladder disease.
- You were recently diagnosed with breast cancer or have already had an estrogen-sensitive breast, ovary, or uterus cancer in the past and have not discussed estrogen with your oncologist, breast surgeon, gynecologist, and internist or primary care physician.[1,3]

HOT FLASHES THAT BEGIN AT OR AFTER AGE 60

Hot flashes, night sweats, or both that begin after age 60 warrant further evaluation. Starting hormone therapy older than 60 years and more than 10 years from menopause onset is linked to a high risk of stroke and deep vein clots of the legs and lungs.

If you develop hot flashes or night sweats more than 10 years into post menopause or after age 60, check with your doctor. Other causes may include the following:

- Carcinoid (a rare cancer that causes hot flashes)
- HIV/AIDS
- Lyme disease
- Lymphoma
- Medications such as antidepressants or hypoglycemic agents
- Obstructive sleep apnea
- Sarcoid (an uncommon lung disease)
- Thyroid imbalance
- Tuberculosis
- Withdrawal from alcohol or opioids

WHO MAY SAFELY START TAKING ESTROGEN?

If you find the quality of your life is compromised by severe, debilitating hot flashes or night sweats, you will benefit the most and incur the least risk from taking hormones. This may be true if you exhibit the following four characteristics:

1. You are under 60 years old.
2. You are perimenopausal or in early post menopause, your last normal menstrual period was fewer than 10 years ago, or you are fewer than 10 years into post menopause (medical history or lab results).
3. You have no personal history of heart disease, stroke, or estrogen-sensitive breast, uterus, or ovary cancer.
4. Your hot flashes or night sweats are not due to another medical condition such as a thyroid disorder. Your doctor may safely prescribe estrogen if you have stable, treated thyroid disease.

If you cannot get adequate relief from your symptoms by other means, you may accept the risk associated with hormone therapy. With close monitoring, you may benefit from taking low-dose hormone therapy.[1,3,10]

OTHER PRECAUTIONS WHEN CONSIDERING HORMONES

Ask your doctor about precautions for the estrogen or progesterone prescribed for you. For example, Prometrium, a plant-derived progesterone taken by mouth, is made from peanut oil, so do not take it if you are allergic to peanuts.

In general, if you are taking any type of estrogen, avoid direct sun. You will be more sun sensitive. A discoloration may develop on your skin, even on your face. Use sunscreen. Wear a hat or visor and sunglasses. While taking hormones, you may not metabolize alcohol as well. Both alcohol and estrogen taken by mouth are processed through the liver. If you drink on a regular basis, you may increase the amount of estrogen in your blood because your liver is busy processing alcohol instead of estrogen. With the alcohol load, the processing of estrogen is less efficient and effective. A consequence of this may be a higher risk of breast cancer since higher levels of alcohol are associated with a higher risk of breast cancer. Also, higher levels of estrogen are associated with higher rates of breast cancer.[5] Consider Jodelle's story.

Jodelle's Story
HOW OLD IS TOO OLD FOR HORMONE THERAPY?

I'm 57 and started taking plant-based estrogen and progesterone to control severe hot flashes and night sweats eight years ago when I was 49. At that time, I was healthy, and both my gynecologist as well as primary care physician were confident that the estrogen would also lower my risk of heart disease and keep my bones strong. I did well on the hormones but recently decided to stop taking them. While my mammograms have been normal, my doctors and I are concerned that my risk of breast cancer may increase if I stay on them. We agreed I would stop the hormones. I'm also going to decrease the amount of alcohol I drink. This decision is based on a discussion with my doctor about lowering my risk of breast cancer. I also know that alcohol can affect hot flashes, and I want to keep those under control. Since I cut back on the number of days a week that I drink and the number of drinks that I have in an evening, my hot flashes and night sweats are milder and occur less often.

HORMONES AND EARLY MENOPAUSE

A woman's body is designed to release estradiol from her ovaries until about the age of 50. As you read in the first chapter, some women go into menopause prematurely. When this occurs, hormone therapy can help postpone the effects of post menopause. The side effects of hormones for these women are low compared to the substantial benefit.

Latisha's Story
PREMATURE MENOPAUSE
(PRIMARY OVARIAN INSUFFICIENCY, POI)

I had my last menstrual period when I was 33. I never felt well on progesterone and was unable to take birth control pills because I felt poorly on progesterone. My doctor offered me a progesterone releasing intrauterine device (IUD) to protect my uterus lining and gave me a plant-based estrogen to take by mouth at age 34. I have felt well since. Now that I'm 41 and have been on estrogen for seven years, the results of the WHI study have made me very anxious. I made an appointment with my gynecologist to talk about stopping estrogen. They explained that I became estrogen-deficient prematurely and that, in general, a woman's body is meant to have estrogen until her early fifties. They also explained that because I'm much younger than the women in the WHI study, the study does not address my problem directly. They encouraged me to continue using a progesterone-releasing IUD and take estrogen by mouth or as a patch until I'm 50 to "imitate the biology of natural post menopause" as if my unusually early menopause had not interrupted it. My doctor has convinced me that the benefits of the hormones, including maintaining stronger bones and preventing heart disease, outweigh the possible risks in my case.

HORMONES AND HYSTERECTOMY

A hysterectomy is the surgical removal of the uterus, or womb. A complete hysterectomy means that the cervix was removed with the uterus. (There are separate terms for the removal of the fallopian tubes and ovaries.)

Taking estrogen alone, without progesterone, is not appropriate for a woman with an intact uterus because it is associated with an increased risk of uterine cancer. If you have undergone a hysterectomy and no longer have a uterus, however, you may take estrogen alone to relieve hot flashes or night sweats. You may take it in pill form, such as estradiol (plant based), or Premarin. Or you may use estrogen in the form of a plant-based skin patch (such as Climara, Estraderm, Estradiol, or Vivelle). Another option is to apply estrogen to the skin as a gel (Estradiol gel, Divigel) or a spray form of estrogen (Evamist).

It is possible to have a complete hysterectomy and still have fallopian tubes and ovaries. If you have had a hysterectomy and still have your ovaries, the ovaries will still produce a cyclic pattern of hormones, and you will continue to ovulate and produce estradiol. You may still experience PMS (premenstrual syndrome) if you had it before your hysterectomy. You will not get pregnant (the sperm have no way to reach the eggs), and you will not experience any more menstrual periods. Menopause will eventually occur on your body's natural schedule when your ovaries stop releasing eggs and making estrogen. You may or may not experience hot flashes at that time.

Premenopausal or perimenopausal women who have both ovaries and tubes removed at the time of a hysterectomy (described as a total abdominal hysterectomy with bilateral salpingo-oophorectomy) usually experience severe hot flashes within three days of surgery due to the sudden loss of estrogen. If you have already entered post menopause, this typically does not occur, particularly if you have already spent more than one year in post menopause.

Severe hot flashes after surgical removal of the ovaries may be avoided in most cases with the use of an estrogen patch after surgery.[10]

Sandita's Story
HYSTERECTOMY AND PREMARIN

When I was 43, I had my uterus and ovaries removed because of large, painful ovarian cysts, in addition to a large fibroid in my uterus that caused pelvic pressure and hemorrhaging. After surgery, my doctor prescribed a plant-based estrogen patch (Climara), and I felt fine. When the WHI study results were publicized, I wondered if I should continue to use the patch. My friends and coworkers were discouraging me from using the medication. But my gynecologist felt differently. First, they pointed out that since I had no uterus, I was not at risk of developing uterine cancer. Second, the data indicated I could continue taking the plant-based estrogen patch until age 51. And having surgical menopause at an early age meant I had started taking hormones while they could still lower my risk of heart disease. The hormone would also help me postpone or avoid early bone thinning. My doctor explained that while the WHI study indicated a higher risk of blood clots and stroke for the women over 60 years old who took Premarin, a synthetic pill form of estrogen, I was much younger than the women in the study and I was using an estrogen patch that has a much lower risk of blood clots. I decided to continue taking the estrogen patch for a while longer. My doctor advised me that in my case, the benefits at my age and stage of menopause outweigh the risks.

VAGINAL ESTROGEN

Vaginal estrogen was not studied in WHI. It is used to relieve vaginal dryness or pain with intercourse in perimenopausal and postmenopausal women of all ages. It can be used in the form of an estrogen cream, a tablet, or a vaginal ring that slowly releases small doses of estrogen into the vaginal walls (for more information, see chapter 7). Vaginal estrogen has not been associated with a high risk of breast cancer or heart disease and is not formulated to achieve a blood level of estrogen.

HORMONES AND ORAL CONTRACEPTIVES

Estrogen and progesterone hormones are used in birth control pills but in higher doses than the amounts for postmenopausal women. Oral contraceptives use hormones to block ovulation and thin the uterine lining to prevent pregnancy. In contrast, hormone therapy for menopause is designed to make up for an age-related decline in natural hormone levels that cause debilitating symptoms. In a young perimenopausal woman who is still menstruating and wants contraception, oral contraceptives may be helpful in relieving hot flashes. They may also help regulate irregular menstrual cycles, once a medical evaluation has shown there are no structural causes of the irregular cycles. If you are a nonsmoker who is still perimenopausal, your doctor may be able to prescribe a low-dose oral contraceptive for you (for more information, see chapter 8).[10]

Priscilla's Story
HOT FLASHES AND THE PILL

I'm 43 and still have regular periods. My husband and I divorced recently, after 22 years of marriage, and I've been under a lot of stress. I had returned to work full-time a year before the divorce. I need to work now to have my own health insurance as well as for the income. In the past I was able to manage the occasional, mild hot flashes I get the week before my period by cutting back on coffee, wearing layers of clothing, and carrying a small paper fan. For the past three months, the hot flashes have been occurring five times a day, and night sweats wake me up more than three times a night. My gynecologist explained that I'm still making estradiol, the same type of estrogen as before in my ovaries, but the levels of estradiol are erratic. Since I'm a nonsmoker without any risk factors for blood clots or stroke, they recommended a low-dose birth control pill to control the hot flashes and night sweats. They said the low doses of estrogen and progesterone in the pill will give me a steady, predictable hormone pattern and minimize or eliminate my hot flashes. Plus, I want to avoid an unplanned pregnancy when I start dating again. The birth control pill has worked well for me. I don't wake up with night sweats and I don't get embarrassing flushes and sweating at work.

HORMONES FOR HOT FLASHES

If approaches such as lifestyle modifications, over-the-counter remedies, or nonhormone prescriptions described in chapter 2 don't work for you, and your symptoms are debilitating, you and your doctor may conclude that the benefits of hormone therapy outweigh the risks.

ESTROGEN ALONE

Estrogen provides the best and most complete relief for hot flashes and night sweats. Because of the WHI study results, women are less likely to be offered a starter prescription for estrogen. Women with early (under age 45) or premature ovarian insufficiency (POI, under age 40) typically benefit from taking estrogen much longer, or until they reach 51 years old. A healthy woman who is younger than 59 years old, has had her uterus surgically removed, and has spent less than 10 years in post menopause may be a good candidate for low-dose estrogen if other options have failed to provide adequate relief. There are many types of estrogen available, as well as a range of doses and various routes of delivery. The decision about which type of estrogen is best for you should be thoroughly discussed with your gynecologist and primary care physician.[1,3,5]

PROGESTERONE ALONE

Another option to decrease hot flashes is to take progesterone alone, such as norethindrone or progesterone or progestin. Progesterone is available in different forms, including some that are plant based.

Progesterone helps with hot flashes and does not cause uterine cancer, but it is associated with other risks. The manufacturer of Provera (medroxyprogesterone) notes on its website that the drug may cause difficulty controlling blood sugar levels, and you have read about the results of the WHI study for Prempro, which includes Provera. Progesterone may be associated with irregular bleeding as well as weight gain or bloating, and in some cases (less than one in 100), it is associated with depression. The manufacturer also cautions against the use of progesterone for women who have had breast cancer.

ESTROGEN AND PROGESTERONE COMBINED IN OTHER PREPARATIONS

As you have already seen, the WHI study using Prempro (conjugated equine estrogen and medroxyprogesterone) helped clarify the risks of combination hormone therapy for postmenopausal women. There are many plant-based preparations that are approved by the US Food and Drug Administration (FDA) for safety and effectiveness. These include the following:

- Activella, an oral preparation that includes both plant-based estrogen and progesterone.
- CombiPatch, a plant-based estrogen and progesterone in a patch form (for women with a uterus) that is worn daily on the lower abdomen or buttocks and changed once or twice a

week. Note that there is a lower risk of blood clots with CombiPatch since it is not initially processed by the liver.
- Femring, a ring placed in the vagina that releases a small dose of estrogen into the vagina and the bloodstream 0.1 mg a day. Unlike Estring (designed purely for vaginal treatment), Femring provides systemic doses of bioidentical estrogen to help hot flashes as well as local estrogen for the vagina.[1] See Selena's story for more information.

Selena's Story
ESTROGEN AND PROGESTERONE FOR HOT FLASHES

I am a 51-year-old who teaches high school equivalency courses in the evening. My last menstrual period was a year ago. My classroom is not air-conditioned, and I frequently must interrupt teaching to wipe the sweat off my face and neck. During a hot flash, my face turns bright red, and I know it distracts my students from focusing on the subject matter. My best friend Janelle, who is 52, is opposed to hormone use. Her hot flashes were very mild and had already stopped. She encourages me to "tough it out" without taking hormones until the hot flashes resolve naturally. Due to the severity of my hot flashes and night sweats, my gynecologist encouraged me to try a low dose of estrogen and progesterone every evening. I was experiencing such discomfort and loss of sleep that I agreed to try it. Within three weeks, I was sleeping through the night and was comfortable teaching again. The doctor advised me that my increased risk of breast cancer is minimal if I stay on the low dose of hormones for less than five years. They also advised me to keep up with breast exams and annual mammograms.

WHEN ORAL ESTROGEN STOPS WORKING

If you take prescription estrogen by mouth for more than a year, you may find that the same dose of estrogen pills is no longer effective in relieving your hot flashes. You may get relief by changing to an estrogen skin patch, lotion, ring, or spray. When taken in pill form, estrogen is processed through the liver. As the liver metabolizes estrogen, the metabolic process itself changes how much estrogen is bound to a carrier protein and how much is free in the blood. The change in free estrogen occurs because the process of metabolizing oral estrogen in the liver increases a binding protein (sex hormone binding globulin [SHBG]) that removes the estrogen from circulation and keeps it bound rather than free. Estrogen taken in the form of a skin patch, cream, lotion, or gel avoids this step and can banish the hot flashes without the need to take a higher dose of estrogen to get relief.[10] See Kalinda's story.

Kalinda's Story
FROM ESTROGEN PILLS TO ESTROGEN PATCH

I'm 41 and work as a librarian. At 33, I was diagnosed with severe endometriosis and had my uterus and both ovaries removed. My hot flashes have been controlled with 0.625 milligrams of Premarin I take by mouth once a day. However, for the past three months, I've been waking up with terrible night sweats. During the day I have hot flashes even though the library is air-conditioned. I spoke with my gynecologist, and they advised changing to a patch form of estrogen in a comparable dose. They prescribed the estradiol patch, from which my body absorbs 0.05 milligrams of estrogen per day. Although the doses sound different, they explained that it is equivalent. I apply a new estrogen patch to my lower abdomen at the same time each Sunday and Thursday. The patch remains in place even during baths, showers, and swimming. The relief I'm getting from hot flashes now is comparable to when I first took the oral estrogen pill, Premarin. My doctor tells me I will be safely able to continue to use the patch for years.

STOPPING ESTROGEN

Many women have the misconception that if they start taking estrogen, they will never be able to get off it without suffering from severe hot flashes or night sweats all over again. In truth, most women can stop their hormones without the return of troublesome hot flashes or night sweats. That said, some women find that hot flashes or night sweats do return.

If you take hormones and have not tried any lifestyle modifications, I recommend you put the lifestyle modifications in place first, then try to stop the hormones. (Chapter 2 has tips.) For example, slowly decrease the amount of coffee and alcohol you consume. These strategies will make it more likely you will feel comfortable after tapering off hormones.

The possibilities for stopping hormones include:

- Stopping "cold turkey." While some women can do this with no ill effects, others cannot. If you miss a pill or two and do not experience hot flashes, you may be able to stop taking estrogen without tapering off.
- Tapering off by taking a slightly lower dose for weeks or months at a time. So far, studies have not shown a benefit to tapering off hormones rather than just stopping them. Many of my patients who want to stop their hormones, however, feel more comfortable slowly tapering off rather than stopping abruptly. If you feel this way, your doctor may gradually lower the dose of hormones you take by giving you a prescription for a lower dose. Alternatively, you can cut your pills or patches in half, but discuss this with your doctor first. As soon as you adjust to the new hormone dose and have no hot flashes, you can try taking an even lower dose, until you have stopped hormones completely.
- Tapering off by changing the intervals—that is, taking the same dose, but less often, such as every other day, then every third day. You move on to less frequent dosing when the hot flashes have subsided on the current dose schedule.

- Adding another prescription medication that is not a hormone, for example, paroxetine, venlafaxine, gabapentin, Neurontin, clonidine, or fezolinetant. This approach relieves hot flashes by a different mechanism. It may supply enough relief when combined with lifestyle modifications after estrogen is stopped completely.

If possible, avoid stopping hormones during the summer (unless you live in a hot climate year-round). If you are going to try tapering off slowly, allow time to get comfortable with a given dose or frequency before taking the next step. Exceptions include an urgent medical problem, such as being diagnosed with breast cancer or a deep vein blood clot, pulmonary embolus, stroke, or heart attack. Women with newly diagnosed breast cancer are advised to stop their estrogen immediately. Some (but not all) breast cancers are sensitive to estrogen and may grow faster if the estrogen is continued. Consider Halal's story.

Halal's Story
QUITTING HORMONES "COLD TURKEY" WAS TOO DIFFICULT

I'm 69 years old and was on Prempro for 20 years when I read the newspaper reports of the WHI study. I stopped taking the pills immediately, but then couldn't sleep due to horrific night sweats. I suffered for weeks before seeing my gynecologist. I had no signs of breast cancer, so my doctor suggested that I taper off the hormones slowly to allow my body a chance to adjust. They understood I was not comfortable stopping the hormones "cold turkey" after all these years. First, over the summer, I took Prempro every Monday, Wednesday, and Friday, instead of daily, and had only a few hot flashes. By September, I was able to reduce the Prempro to every Sunday and Thursday without waking up due to night sweats. By November, I was able to stop the Prempro altogether, and have had only a few night sweats since then, but I associate those with enjoying an occasional beer.

BIOIDENTICAL ("NATURAL") HORMONES

There is a lot of buzz about bioidentical hormones being safer or better for women than synthetic hormones, but this is not the case. The term *bioidentical* is not a medical term with a specific, standardized meaning. The term *bioidentical* was introduced as a marketing term to promote compounded hormones that were close in structure to your own hormones. The term has been used to describe a wide variety of different hormones. In some cases, bioidentical refers to hormones that an individual pharmacist compounds for an individual patient. Or, more generally, it may refer to any hormone derived from plants.

You may request plant-based hormones if you prefer. Not all plant-based hormones have the same safety profile or work better. Your physician may prescribe plant-based hormones that are approved by the FDA. All hormones, even plant-based or bioidentical or compounded, are synthesized.[4,6,7]

> DID YOU KNOW?
> Bioidentical hormones that are not FDA approved may not meet quality and purity standards that are met by an FDA-approved bioidentical preparation. Recently, some online companies offering hormones to subscribers have made efforts to confirm quality and purity standards and have implemented batch testing of their products to ensure that the dosing is consistent and the product meets purity standards.

The appeal of bioidentical hormones is deceptive. Compounded bioidentical hormones are marketed as custom-made to your own body's needs. You are typically asked to have saliva levels, urine levels, or blood tests done to determine the makeup of a compounded hormone preparation that will be prescribed for you.

Why isn't this better? Many of my patients are puzzled that I do not routinely ask them to do saliva, blood, or urine hormone levels. This is because each of you has different levels of hormones at different times during the day, different days of the week, and different times of the month. Your levels will also vary with the stage of perimenopause you are in. Given the fluctuations in hormone levels in one individual over hours, days, weeks, and months as well as between individuals, there is no ideal level of hormones for an individual woman.

So how does a certified menopause clinician or menopause specialist determine the best prescription for you? Typically, joint decision-making works best. The best hormone preparation for you will be easy to use, give you relief from your menopausal symptoms, and cause no side effects. The types of hormones and dosages are adjusted depending on how you feel about the preparation. Consider the following:

- Does it give you relief from hot flashes and night sweats?
- Do you have breast tenderness?
- Do you have headaches?
- Are you sleeping better?
- Has your bleeding pattern changed?
- Has your mood improved? Worsened? Stabilized?

The Menopause Society, the American College of Obstetricians and Gynecologists, and the National Academies of Sciences, Engineering, and Medicine all recommend you use FDA-approved hormones that are plant derived if you choose to avoid hormones synthesized from horse urine. Plant-derived hormones come in many forms, including skin patches, lotions, vaginal rings, and skin sprays, as well as some oral forms such as Menest, Prometrium, and Activella. Hormones that are absorbed through a skin patch, lotion, or spray have fewer risks than those taken by mouth. When hormones are not taken orally, they do not get processed through the liver before they reach the bloodstream, and this decreases the risk of clots.

Low doses of hormones given vaginally are not designed to produce a blood level of estrogen, only a local effect, and do not have the side effects of systemic estrogen. Low-dose estrogen given vaginally for local absorption does not cause breast cancer, heart attacks, strokes, or blood clots.[10]

If you are being treated for breast cancer with an aromatase inhibitor designed to prevent any significant blood levels of estrogen in your body during treatment, your oncologist may advise you to avoid even low-dose vaginal estrogen during active treatment with the aromatase inhibitor. Using vaginal estrogen is important to discuss with your oncologist if you are currently being treated for breast cancer.

The FDA requires that a black box warning with the side effects of estrogen and progesterone hormones be placed on all types of hormones, regardless of the way they are processed or taken. FDA-approved hormones derived from plants carry the black box warning. Compounded bioidentical hormone therapy (cBHT) is not nationally standardized or FDA approved and typically does not receive the black box label. This is not because the black box label does not apply. It is because the pharmacist who compounds a hormone preparation or a hormone preparation sold as a supplement does not have the same labeling requirements and is not required to include a black box warning. Some experts advise doctors to include the FDA black box warning label with their patients' bioidentical hormone prescriptions. This is not yet standard practice. In January 2008, the FDA stated it considers the claims made about bioidentical hormones false and misleading because they are not supported by medical evidence—a violation of federal law.[4] The NAMS Practice Pearl Compounded Bioidentical Hormone Therapy: New Recommendations from the 2020 National Academics of Sciences, Engineering, and Medicine, released December 8, 2020, emphasizes this as well.

What are the other considerations for cBHT versus FDA plant-based hormone prescriptions?

- FDA requires adverse event reporting; cBHT does not.
- FDA requires safety data; bioidentical compounded hormones do not.

- FDA requires high standards of manufacturing with strict guidelines about how much estrogen and progesterone are contained in the preparation; bioidentical compounded hormones currently do not.
- Samples of bioidentical hormones may contain too much of one type of estrogen and not enough of another, not reflected on the prescription label. Variations in amounts of estrogen can cause perimenopause to be more challenging instead of smoothing out symptoms.
- Excess estrogen can cause endometrial hyperplasia, precancer, or cancer of the uterus lining.
- A bioidentical compounded hormone with too little progesterone may cause endometrial hyperplasia, precancer, or cancer of the uterus lining.
- Additives in the bioidentical compounded preparation may not be clearly marked: you may take a preparation that has an ingredient to which are you sensitive or allergic.
- Testosterone pellets have an FDA-approved dosing for men, but implanted compounded bioidentical testosterone pellets often produce 10–200 times normal levels of testosterone in women, causing prolonged high estradiol and testosterone levels. The pellets are also difficult to remove. Prolonged high testosterone levels can result in loss of scalp hair/balding, excess facial hair, lower voice, excess body hair, painful clitoral enlargement, headaches, and weight gain. Some women continue to have unhealthy elevated levels of estrogen, testosterone, or both for a year after pellet insertion.[6,7]

Some of the recommendations for cBHT from the National Academies of Sciences, Engineering, and Medicine include:

1. Consider cBHT if you have a documented allergy to an active ingredient of an FDA-approved drug or need a different dosage than what is FDA manufactured.

2. Check whether your compounding pharmacist/pharmacy is certified by the state and required to comply with FDA inspections. They should provide a standard package insert with product formulation, notification that cBHT is not FDA approved, and a boxed warning identical to an FDA-approved HT prescription. They should also provide production and sales information and submit data regarding potentially serious adverse events.
3. Prescribers and compounders should disclose financial relationships, including ownership or investments in cBHT formulations or companies.
4. More research is needed on the safety, effectiveness, and use of cBHT preparations. This would include clinical research on safety and effectiveness in treating menopause symptoms as well as research on adverse events.

In October 2013, *MORE Magazine* published an article, "The Hormone Hoax Thousands Fall For." As part of the article, a certified menopause practitioner wrote prescriptions for cBHT that were sent to 12 compounding pharmacies nationwide; 2 were brick-and-mortar, and 10 were filled online. The prescription was for Tri-Est: a combination of estranol, estrone, and estriol and progesterone. Each capsule was weighed. The range in weight was 102 milligrams (heaviest) to 80 milligrams (lightest). Numerous health risks were identified when inspecting the prescriptions.[6,7]

Findings included the following:

- There was a lack of uniformity.
- Undisclosed substitutions of ingredients were made.
- Adulteration of ingredients was present, but it was not disclosed on the label.
- Estriol content varied from 67.5% to 89.5% from the labeled amount, indicating estriol was below the labeled potency.
- Two different estrogens were too potent: estrone was 58.4% to 272.5% of the labeled amount.

- Estradiol, the most potent estrogen, was found in excess (95.9%–259% of the labeled amount).
- Progesterone present was 80% of the prescribed amount, and one prescription was less than 60% of the prescribed amount.
- None of these products would pass the FDA requirements.
- FDA mandates no less than 90% and no more than 110% deviation from the prescription the physician sends.

Bioidentical progesterone is made from diosgenin, a plant-derived sterol found in wild yams. The molecular structure is like hormones produced in a woman's body. No head-to-head comparisons of HT and cBHT have been studied. There is only a hypothetical advantage of cBHT that has never been demonstrated.

Both HT and cBHT are synthesized and manufactured. Compounded bioidentical hormones, like HT, involve multiple levels of processing, but cBHT sounds safer and therefore has enjoyed a robust following. After the WHI study was published in 2002, there was a backlash against hormone therapy. Many turned to cBHT instead of FDA-approved HT. cBHT also fits into the antiaging movement. Actress Suzanne Somers kickstarted the cBHT movement with her books and Oprah appearance. In her 2004 book, *The Sexy Years: Discover the Hormone Connection*, Ms. Somers pledged to help women regain their libidos and youthful bodies without the risks of HT. She assured her readers that taking cBHT was not associated with a higher risk of heart attack, stroke, clots, dementia, or breast cancer. This claim is false.[6,7]

DID YOU KNOW?

The illusion of increased safety for cBHT is false. There is no lower risk profile for cBHT and no black box warning to concern you when you open the package. Without the black box warning, many women assume greater safety of their cBHT prescriptions. It is tempting to think that no mention of adverse reactions and no warnings mean that there are none. The misconception that cBHT is safer than FDA-available HT has serious consequences. Unfortunately, the medical risks of hormones are typically not discussed with consumers of cBHT.

Normal estrogen levels post menopause are 0–30 picograms/mL. One woman with a strong family history of breast cancer took cBHT to boost her libido in a new relationship. Her estrogen levels reached 523.8, and she was diagnosed with an estrogen-sensitive breast cancer before undergoing a double mastectomy.

Tri-Est is the most common cBHT prescription. It contains three types of estrogen: estradiol, estrone, and estriol. Estradiol is 12 times as potent as estrone and 80 times as potent as estriol. Estriol, the main estrogen produced by the placenta in pregnancy, is not FDA approved for use in postmenopausal women.

I'll discuss low-dose safe administration of testosterone administered by topical ointment in chapter 7.

CUSTOMIZATION

The promise that cBHT hormones are customized to your body's needs by measuring your saliva, urine, or blood hormone levels is a false promise. Why?

The myth of customization assumes that cBHT can match your individual needs by analyzing costly labs. The reality is that your estrogen and progesterone hormones are secreted in a pulsatile pattern. The hormone levels fluctuate at different times of the day and different times of the month, as well as from year to year. There is no optimal level for each woman: the levels change drastically from one day to the next and even many times of the day until two years into post menopause. With this moving target, customization using lab results is not feasible, practical, or advised.[6,7]

Customization is possible with FDA-approved preparations, including those that are plant-based hormones. The customization process starts with your personal priorities:

- Are you trying to control moderate or severe hot flashes or night sweats?
- Are the sweats or flashes worse during the day or at night or troublesome 24/7?
- Would you prefer to change a patch once or twice a week or take a pill by mouth daily?
- Are you still menstruating?
- Do you or someone in your family have a history of a clotting disorder? (blood clot risk) Once you and your doctor agree on a type of hormone (patch or pill, ring, spray, or lotion) and decide on dose and route of progesterone protection for the uterus lining (if you have a uterus), then the prescription dose can be adjusted up or down to meet your needs.

If you have a uterus, you may choose a patch, CombiPatch, that contains a plant-based estrogen and a plant-based progestin. Or, you may elect to try an estrogen patch along with a low-dose plant-based progestin that you take by mouth (Prometrium, made with peanut oil). If you are allergic to peanuts, do not tolerate progestin, or prefer not to take progesterone by mouth, you may consider a levonorgestrel-releasing IUD (Mirena IUD) that releases small amounts of plant-based progestin into the uterus lining to prevent cancer, precancer, and endometrial hyperplasia.

If you do choose to use a compounding pharmacy, you may check their accreditation by the Pharmacy Compounding Accreditation Board, PCAB.org. They should do skip lot testing on random products monthly as part of their adequate quality control.

Most often, I prescribe bioidentical hormones derived from plants and also FDA-approved. They have been more widely tested than the non-FDA-approved hormones. The medical community would welcome definitive proof that hormones made from plants are safer than synthetic hormones, but the evidence is not there yet.

All hormones are powerful medications, regardless of their source. The Million Women Study showed that many types of estrogen, including estradiol, which is often referred to as a natural or bioidentical estrogen, contribute to an increased risk of breast cancer. If you and your doctor agree you will be taking hormones to control severe hot flashes, you will work together to find the lowest dose that keeps you comfortable.[5]

MAKING THE DECISION

Hormone therapy is still the most effective treatment for certain symptoms of menopause, and today, we are clearer about which menopausal women are most at risk from taking hormones, as well as which women can benefit the most, based on their age and stage of menopause.

If you have symptoms such as hot flashes and night sweats that don't respond to nonhormone interventions and they interfere with your quality of life, you may want to discuss hormones with your doctor, particularly if you are in the low-risk group. Making this decision is a very individual process.

Today, the decision you make about hormone use is less likely to be the same as your friend's, your coworker's, or even your sister's. Your current circumstances and medical requirements are unique and change from year to year. These circumstances are an essential part of your decision process. Consult your gynecologist or clinician to ensure that you get up-to-date advice that is appropriate for you at each annual visit. Information on the internet is not customized and cannot be filtered and adjusted by your age, personal medical history, and family history. Discussion with your doctor is the best way to integrate your personal medical history, family history, and individual circumstances, including how severe your symptoms are and where you are in menopause.

OTHER ESTROGEN-RELATED OPTIONS

When estrogen is combined with a selective estrogen receptor modulator (SERM), the combination with estrogen is labeled a tissue-selective estrogen complex (TSEC). The SERM portion modifies how the estrogen acts in the body to increase safety while retaining the benefit of estrogen, which increases bone strength and stops hot flashes and night sweats. Tamoxifen is an example of a common SERM. Tamoxifen is an estrogen that is modified to block effects on the breast (lowering the risk of breast cancer), but it still acts like estrogen in bone and the uterus lining. SERMs are estrogen agonists/antagonists with a different role in each area of the body and affect different types of tissue in unique ways.

The TSEC I will discuss here is bazedoxifene (Duavee), which contains conjugated estrogens and bazedoxifene, an agonist/antagonist. Bazedoxifene acts two different ways in different parts of the body. It is an estrogen receptor agonist in bone (builds bone health) and an antagonist in the endometrium/uterus lining (protects the uterus lining from estrogen effects). Bazedoxifene is prescribed to relieve vasomotor symptoms. Bazedoxifene (Duavee) is a welcome addition to the toolbox for menopause treatment. It is safe to take for women with a uterus and protects against uterine cancer without requiring a progesterone or progestin with the estrogen due to its mechanism of action that differs in different tissues. [9]

NEW DEVELOPMENTS

Estetrol, a weak estrogen produced by the human fetal liver during pregnancy, has just been released in a new, lower-dose, safe oral contraceptive. It is being considered for development as a new estrogen for hormone replacement. Estetrol is an appealing option for menopausal hormone therapy because it is a weaker estrogen than estradiol (produced by the ovaries during your reproductive years) or estrone (produced by your body during the postmenopausal years). Although it is a weaker estrogen, estetrol promises to help a woman with her hot flashes and bone health without affecting her liver or increasing her risk of breast cancer. If approved for hormone therapy after additional testing, estetrol will have its own new category, "NEST": native estrogen with selective action in tissues. It is longer lasting, with a half-life of 28 hours. Another advantage of estetrol is that it only acts on part of the estrogen alpha receptor and has no active metabolic end product. More research is underway.[8]

IMPORTANT TAKEAWAYS

In summary:

- The decision to take hormones is a very personal one. Only you and your doctor can determine what's best for you.
- Talking with your doctor can help dispel common myths about hormones (and there are many).
- There are many effective strategies to help you stop taking hormones if you choose to do so.
- No data suggests that plant-based hormones are safer or more effective than non-plant-based ones, but many women prefer them, and they are commonly used.
- No data suggests that compounded bioidentical hormones are safer than FDA-approved hormones.
- Hormones that are not FDA approved have not been widely tested and should be used with caution.
- Hormones may be a good option if you don't respond to nonhormone interventions and symptoms of menopause interfere with your quality of life.

QUESTIONS FOR YOUR DOCTOR

1. My sister takes bioidentical hormones for hot flashes and tells me they are safer than FDA prescription hormones. Our mother had breast cancer. What is my safest option for my debilitating night sweats?
2. My friend encouraged me to try estrogen and testosterone pellets. First, I felt great, but now I have headaches, weight gain, and excess growth. What should I do for my hot flashes and low sex drive?

3. I read that hormones help vaginal dryness. I asked my primary care nurse practitioner to prescribe them for me. I took estrogen and progesterone by mouth, but I still have pain with sex. What hormones will help me? I don't want to take a high dose.

4. I have been taking FDA-approved low-dose estrogen and progesterone by mouth for two years and it helped my hot flashes and night sweats. In the last two months, the same dose that worked for two years no longer gives me relief. I don't want to take a higher dose. What are my options?

RESOURCES

Bioidentical Hormonal Therapy: Custom Compounded vs Government Approved. MenoNote from The Menopause Society © 2020

FDA.gov/drugs/compounding/human-drug-compounding-and-FDA-questions-and-answers. Government site with questions and answers about compounded bioidentical hormones

Gallez A, et al. Estetrol combined to progestogen for menopause or contraception indication is neutral on breast cancer. *Cancers (Basel)*. 2021;13(10):2486.

Ramin CJ. The hormone hoax thousands fall for. *MORE Magazine*, October 2013.

www.AICR.org/cancer-prevention/recommendations/limit-alcohol-consumption

The American Institute of Cancer Research has information on risk factors for breast cancer and other cancers, including the influence of alcohol on cancer risk.

www.menopause.org. Bioidentical Hormone Therapy © 2023 contains links to studies and information about different features of bioidentical compounded hormones.

www.nih.gov/PHTindex.htm. Menopausal hormone therapy information (National Institutes of Health [NIH])

www.nhlbi.nih.gov/whi. A government website for the Women's Health Initiative that provides helpful overviews and updates on new studies. Last accessed February 25, 2023.

CHAPTER 4

HEART DISEASE

The Risk of Doing Nothing

Heart disease can sneak up on you. That doesn't mean you can't lower your risk.

MANY OF YOU MAY DISTRUST modern medicine. That's understandable. Recommendations for how to stay healthy change over time as new research emerges. Some people grew up with stoic parents who never went to the doctor, so they think that's normal. Others read about the side effects of taking prescription medications and decide that medications are never to be trusted. And many women believe that since menopause is not a disease, all they must do is let nature take its course—particularly if they feel well.

If you don't visit your doctor on a regular basis, you cannot expect to stay healthy and active in perimenopause and beyond. Choosing to do nothing is risky. Your doctors are qualified to do more than just treat your occasional vaginal itch or bladder infection. They monitor changes in your health from year to year and are skilled at diagnosing all the hidden threats I've mentioned earlier—particularly cardiovascular disease (CVD) that causes heart attacks and strokes.

In this chapter, I'll answer these questions:

- How can women lower their risk of CVD?
- What are the pros and cons of taking aspirin to lower the risk of CVD?

- What are the risk factors for CVD?
- Why does CVD kill women more often than men?
- Why is prevention of CVD so important?

ASSESSING YOUR PERSONAL RISK OF CVD

If you are a woman living in North America, your average life span is 84 years. How can you stay healthy and active for those years?

> DID YOU KNOW?
> Heart disease kills more women than all cancers put together. Fortunately, 80 percent of heart disease is preventable.

Work with your doctor to:

- Determine if you have new risk factors for CVD unique to women
- Establish your personal risk of heart disease and stroke
- Lower your risk of heart disease and stroke

For decades, research on heart disease was limited to men. This was problematic for women as heart attacks and other types of heart disease present differently in a woman. Also, we now know that risk factors for women are specific to the individual. As doctors learn more about estimating the risk of heart disease in individuals, they can design more effective prevention strategies. A prevention strategy that is beneficial for you may be ineffective or even harmful for your friend, relative, or coworker. After reviewing your lifestyle and assessing your personal and family histories of heart disease, your doctors have new tools to estimate your risk of heart disease. The degree of risk influences what prevention strategies will be most beneficial. If you are at low risk, healthy eating and lifestyle modifications may be all that you need to lower your risk of heart disease.

WHY PREVENTION IS SO IMPORTANT

It's a lot easier to prevent heart disease than it is to treat it once it has developed. This is especially true for women because it is challenging to identify heart disease early in women. Also, the rate of disability and death from heart disease is much higher in women than in men, in part due to the unusual way heart disease can show up in women.

> DID YOU KNOW?
> While 1 out of every 25 women will die of breast cancer, 1 out of every 2 women over the age of 50 will die of heart disease/CVD.

Heart disease in women is typically silent. This means if you don't partner with your doctor, you won't even know you have it.

Here are five facts you need to know:

1. CVD is the number one killer of women in the United States.
2. CVD kills more women every year than all types of cancer combined.
3. Half a million women die from heart disease each year.
4. Heart disease is the leading cause of death for women over age 50.
5. More than half of American women will experience a heart attack in their lifetime, most with no warning.

The traditional CVD risk factors, such as hypertension and high cholesterol, do not capture this risk in women and do not adequately predict a woman's risk for heart disease.

Since most women will never be warned before their first heart attack, prevention is key. Neglecting your risk of heart disease can be a fatal mistake.[1,11,14]

WHAT ARE THE RISK FACTORS FOR CVD?

CVD typically progresses by degrees. It begins with early symptoms you can control. Then it moves to the development of hardened arteries to advanced or acute problems. The earlier you intercept this progression, the more successful you will be at restoring your health.

Are you at risk for CVD? Each of the following common risks is a red flag for CVD. If you have one or more risk factors, consult your doctor about detecting and preventing CVD. Note: These guidelines are specific for women.

SMOKING

Smoking increases your risk of CVD dramatically. According to the American Heart Association, smoking:

- Decreases your tolerance for exercise
- Increases the tendency for blood to clot
- Increases your blood pressure
- Lowers your good cholesterol

Women who smoke and use oral contraceptives increase their risk of CVD and stroke. To add perspective, the Women's Health Initiative study initially reported that Prempro increased the risk of breast cancer by 26 percent, increasing the number of breast cancer cases from 33 women out of 10,000 women in a year to 41 women out of 10,000 in a year (or 8 more women per year). Smoking increases the risk of heart disease by 2,400 percent, almost 100 times the risk! An individual that has quit smoking for 12 consecutive months lowers their risk of heart disease.

HIGH-FAT DIET AND PROCESSED FOODS

A high-fat diet that also includes processed foods and only a few fruits and vegetables increases the risk of developing high cholesterol and hardening of the arteries. The typical American diet is high in calories, contains many processed foods, and is low in nutrients.

FAMILY HISTORY OF HEART DISEASE

If you have a family history of heart attacks or strokes, you may be genetically susceptible to heart disease. A first-degree male relative with a heart attack under age 50 or a first-degree female relative with a heart attack under age 60 increases your personal risk of a heart attack or heart disease.

INACTIVE LIFESTYLE

A sedentary lifestyle increases the risk of both stroke and heart attack. Preventive measures to lower the risk of stroke include staying physically active. If you don't get much exercise, increasing your activity level will help alleviate nearly everything that is bothering you! New studies show that exchanging even 10 minutes of sedentary time for 10 minutes of low-intensity activity daily will lower your risk of death by 9 percent.[1]

OBESITY

You are considered at risk for cardiovascular disease if your body mass index (BMI) is over 25. BMI is not helpful if you have a muscular frame. For athletic or muscular individuals, use your waist measurement to estimate heart health. For women, a waist measurement under 35 inches is associated with heart health. Alternatively, you may divide your waist measurement in inches by your hip measurement in inches. If the number is 0.8 or more, you are at high risk for cardiovascular disease and diabetes. It is possible to be underweight or have a low or normal BMI and still have a high risk of heart disease if your waist is over 35 inches or the ratio of waist to hip measurement is over 0.8. The waist circumference reflects the amount of deep fat around your internal organs. Excess fat around the internal organs is a risk factor for diabetes and heart disease. To measure your waist, feel the top of your hip bones, and measure around the smallest part of your abdomen above the hips.

More than 60 percent of American women are overweight. Women who exceed their ideal body weight are at higher risk for heart attack, stroke, and diabetes. Guidelines for determining your ideal body weight and BMI are provided in chapter 12. Although younger women don't always have the medical consequences of being overweight, perimenopausal and postmenopausal women typically cannot avoid them.[11,14]

DIABETES

A family history of diabetes increases the odds that you will develop heart disease. If you have diabetes yourself, it is a risk factor for CVD. Also, if you had gestational diabetes or poor sugar regulation during pregnancy, you are at higher risk of getting diabetes later in life. Even if you are younger, premenopausal, or still perimenopausal, you are at risk for a stroke if you are diabetic. Modifying your lifestyle and eating habits will help you avoid developing complications of diabetes such as poor circulation, leg swelling, open leg ulcers, poor eyesight that cannot be corrected with glasses, or loss of sensation in your feet. When these late complications of diabetes occur, they are not reversible.

HIGH CHOLESTEROL OR ABNORMAL LIPIDS

Your chance of developing cardiovascular disease is increased if you have high total cholesterol (over 200 milligrams per deciliter fasting), your triglycerides are high (over 150 milligrams per deciliter fasting), your high-density lipoprotein protective cholesterol level is low (under 50 milligrams per deciliter), or your low-density lipids are high (LDL). Lowering lipids is a key strategy in preventing cardiovascular disease.

NEWER RISK FACTORS FOR FEMALE HEART DISEASE

If you experience early menopause before age 45 or premature ovarian insufficiency before age 40 (discussed in chapter 1), your risk of CVD will be much higher. Estrogen protects women from a higher risk of CVD before menopause. Losing your natural estrogen early (due to surgical removal of ovaries, radiation, chemotherapy, heredity, or other factors) will increase your risk of CVD even at a younger age.

EARLY MENOPAUSE

Premature loss of estrogen can occur naturally, after surgical removal of both ovaries, during or after chemotherapy, or due to premature ovarian insufficiency (POI).[2] Consider the following facts about early menopause:

- Blood vessel lining impairment (endothelial dysfunction) is more common in young women with no menstruation than in those with regular menstrual periods.[3]
- Doses of hormones in younger menopausal women often need to be higher than standard to ease hot flashes and night sweats.[4]
- Early menopause may occur from ages 40–45 and may be associated with a family history of early menopause or a history of smoking or other lifestyle factors.
- Hormone therapy use lessens CVD risk after surgical premature menopause.
- If there are no contraindications, estrogen-based hormone therapy is advised in women with premature or early menopause until the average of natural menopause. Either oral or transdermal hormone therapy will lower CVD. Estrogen after oophorectomy does not increase the risk of breast cancer in women with a BRCA 1 mutation.
- In monkeys, stress leads to compromised anovulation, high cholesterol, premature bone loss, and premature atherosclerosis.
- In the Nurses' Health Study II, more than 79,000 premenopausal women with no history of CVD cancer or diabetes provided their menstrual history of 24 years. Those who reported irregular menstrual cycles had a higher risk of dying.[5]

- POI or premature menopause (i.e., menopause before age 40) is associated with a 4.5 times higher risk of ischemic heart disease due to premature loss of estrogen. Estrogen replacement with oral contraceptives or higher doses of hormones offsets the risks of premature bone thinning and premature heart disease. The younger the woman, the greater the concern.
- Premature natural menopause is associated with a 36 percent increased risk of CVD.
- Stress disrupts ovarian function. Stress has been increasing for everyone since 2020, and women are more vulnerable to stress than men. Stress affects the functioning of blood vessel lining (endothelial dysfunction), and it also causes inflammation of the blood vessel walls.[6]
- Surgical premature menopause is associated with an 87 percent increased risk of CVD.
- The degree and timing of estrogen loss during a woman's reproductive life span may change her risk for CVD.

HIGH-RISK PREGNANCY

Researchers have found that a woman's reproductive history may help predict her risk of heart disease. More comprehensive research studies looking at larger groups of women over longer periods of time have shown that having a history of preeclampsia or eclampsia puts an individual at three times higher risk for ischemic heart disease in midlife. A history of any of the following features of an individual's pregnancy history puts them at higher risk of CVD in midlife.[7]

- Eclampsia (severe high blood pressure in pregnancy associated with seizures)
- Fetal growth restriction[3]
- Gestational diabetes
- Infertility (associated with future heart failure with preserved ejection fraction)

- Late-life pregnancy
- Preeclampsia
- Pregnancy loss[8]
- Preterm delivery

ONSET OF MENARCHE

Another aspect of an individual's reproductive history, unrelated to pregnancy, is when their menstrual periods first started. Early menarche, or early onset of menstrual periods before age 12, is also associated with a high risk of CVD and a higher risk of hypertension.[9]

POLYCYSTIC OVARIAN SYNDROME

Women with a history of polycystic ovary syndrome are at three times greater risk for type 2 diabetes.[10] They're also at greater risk for the following:

- Carotid plaque associated with atherosclerosis
- Coronary calcium
- CVD
- High blood pressure
- High cholesterol
- Obesity
- Stroke

SHORTENED MENSTRUAL CYCLES IN PERIMENOPAUSE

If your cycle length (i.e., the duration of time between the first day of one bleeding episode to the first day of the next) shortens by more than 7 days or becomes fewer than 23 days in length, you may be at higher risk of CVD in perimenopause and early post menopause.

SEVERE VASOMOTOR SYMPTOMS

Based on new medical research, if you have severe hot flashes or night sweats, this may be a signal that you are more vulnerable to heart disease during perimenopause or post menopause. The

American Heart Association has identified the menopause transition/perimenopause as a period of accelerated CVD risk.

CHANGING LIPID LEVELS IN PERIMENOPAUSE

Independent of changes associated with age, the Study of Women Across the Nation (SWAN study) shows that lipid levels, including total cholesterol and low-density lipoprotein cholesterol (LDL-C), as well as others, increase dramatically from the year before the final menstrual period to the year after it.

CHANGES IN BODY FAT DEPOSITION

Changes in body fat deposition are associated with CVD. Many women get a small fat bulge in their lower abdomen that some have nicknamed the "meno pooch." This lower abdomen fat pocket is associated with increases in risk for metabolic syndrome if it is more pronounced.

CHANGES IN PHYSICAL ACTIVITY

Only 7 percent of perimenopausal women achieve a physical activity level that matches current recommendations.

PREMATURE OVARIAN INSUFFICIENCY (POI)

POI or early menopause (i.e., menopause before age 45) is associated with a 4.5 times higher risk of ischemic heart disease.[2,4,5]

DEPRESSION

Depression is more prevalent in women, and it doubles the risk of ischemic heart disease and POI.

STRESS, THE BRAIN, AND CARDIOVASCULAR HEALTH

Women who are especially vulnerable to stress and stress-related mental conditions experience an increased risk for CVD.

- Brain–heart connections contribute to CVD risk—especially in women.

- Compared to men, women have less plaque in their coronary arteries until menopause.
- Midlife women are especially at risk for CVD due to stress.[6]
- The number of heart attacks is increasing, and more women die of heart attacks than men. Traditional risk factors do not explain the difference. Researchers think stress and other nontraditional risk factors contribute to this risk.[11,12]
- Women experience changes in their microcirculation. Men do not.
- Women with CVD have more symptoms, disability, and worse outcomes.

WHAT IS CVD?

CVD is a general term for diseases that affect the heart or blood vessels, including high blood pressure, coronary artery disease, heart failure, heart attack, and stroke. Some forms of CVD, such as congenital heart problems, are not due to risk factors we can control. Most often, CVD is brought on by a lifetime of habits that are not heart healthy.

HIGH BLOOD PRESSURE

High blood pressure means your blood is pumping through your blood vessels with excessive force. It is considered an early form of heart disease. If high blood pressure is not controlled, it can lead to hardening of the arteries, heart attack, or stroke. According to the newest guidelines from the American Heart Association and the American College of Cardiology's recommendations for Life's Simple 7, a blood pressure goal of 120/80 is desirable. Your blood pressure may be a cause for concern if it is over 120 millimeters of mercury systolic (top number) or over 80 millimeters of mercury diastolic (bottom number). About one in four Americans has high blood pressure. A normal blood pressure reading is 120/80 or under. If you already have diabetes, your doctor may recommend a goal of even lower blood pressure numbers to stay healthy. Your doctor may have a less stringent goal for you depending on your age and individual circumstances.

ARTERIOSCLEROSIS

Hardening of the arteries can occur anywhere in your body. When the arteries carrying blood to your brain are affected, you could have a transient ischemic attack or stroke. When the arteries of the heart are affected, you could have a heart attack. Sometimes arteriosclerosis is associated with an aneurysm, which is a dangerous bulge in the wall of an artery. In women, the hardening doesn't always produce a blockage. The blood vessel function, however, is compromised by small changes in the wall, including calcium in the wall that hardens the vessels, spasm of the vessels, narrowing of the vessels, and reduced blood flow. These more subtle changes are harder to identify and are more common in women than in men.

CORONARY ARTERY DISEASE

The arteries of the heart—the coronary arteries—supply blood to the muscle wall of the heart. If they become narrow due to spasm of the vessel wall, hardened fatty deposits called plaque, or both, the likelihood of having a heart attack is increased. Coronary artery disease may be associated with angina (chest pain). In women, it is common to have atypical pain that may not include chest pain.

STROKE

Strokes are considered a form of CVD. An ischemic stroke occurs when blood flow to the brain is interrupted. This may be caused by a blood clot or by plaque in the blood vessels of the neck or the brain. A hemorrhagic stroke is when a blood vessel in the brain ruptures. Strokes vary in severity, and their consequences depend on the part of the brain that is affected. Loss of function may be temporary or permanent. Some individuals have partial paralysis after a stroke and cannot move an arm or leg. Stroke is also considered a neurological disorder because of the many complications it causes.

HEART ATTACK

When the blood supply to the heart is cut off—for example, when a blood clot blocks the flow of blood through a coronary artery—the muscle of the heart can be injured. The medical term for heart attack is myocardial infarction, sometimes called MI by health care workers. Consider Marsha's story.

Marsha's Story
LOWERING CHOLESTEROL AND HIGH BLOOD PRESSURE WITHOUT PRESCRIPTION MEDICATIONS

I'm a 49-year-old perimenopausal schoolteacher with two teenage children. I have hot flashes that get worse with stress, but I usually sleep well. My menstrual periods are lighter than they used to be and occur once every two to six months. After my children were born, I gained 25 pounds. Most of the weight gathered around my waist. My fasting cholesterol was over 270, and my blood pressure was 140/90—both too high, according to my doctor. I prefer not to take prescription medications or hormones, so when my doctor told me I was at high risk for a heart attack and diabetes, I was very willing to listen to how I might be able to address these problems and avoid prescription medications.

They told me I could lower my blood pressure and cholesterol if I exercised regularly and lost weight. If my blood pressure and cholesterol did not improve, I would need medication. After getting the green light to exercise from my doctor, I began walking every day during my lunch break and started using a weight loss app to track my calorie intake and energy used from exercise. In three months, I lost 10 pounds. My blood pressure returned to normal, and my cholesterol came down 35 points. I have continued to exercise and keep a written food diary, and now my cholesterol is under 200. I'm glad I was able to avoid taking prescription medications, and another great benefit was losing two inches off my waist. I went from 36 to 34 inches. I've now been sticking to my exercise program for over a year.

HEART DISEASE AFFECTS MEN AND WOMEN DIFFERENTLY

CVD is the number one killer of American men and women. But CVD is even more lethal for women; it kills them more often than it kills men. It is more difficult to detect and treat in women.

> DID YOU KNOW?
> Although advances in medical research and treatment have lowered men's risk of dying from a heart attack, women have not yet benefited.

Until recently, medical research was done on white males. Researchers who studied heart disease in men thought their findings applied to both sexes as well as different ethnic groups. Now we know that is not the case. Further research is being done to help us understand the differences between ethnic groups and to learn more about how heart disease differs in women. So far, clinical experience and more sophisticated tests show us that female heart disease looks very different from male heart disease.

HEART ATTACK SYMPTOMS IN MEN VERSUS WOMEN

Many women who have heart attack symptoms experience them differently from men. The typical warning signals of a male heart attack are often completely absent in a female. The tests used to identify a man's heart attack may not identify a woman's heart attack. For example, a woman having a heart attack may not have chest pain, and her EKG may not show changes of a heart attack. The variety of symptoms, as well as the fact that they are atypical and subtle, often causes fatal delays in diagnosis and treatment for women having a heart attack.

> **DID YOU KNOW?**
> If a woman has a heart attack, she is more likely to die from that heart attack than a man. This is true even if she is in perimenopause.

Surviving a heart attack is only part of the battle. Of 100 women who have a heart attack, 38 will die within 12 months. Of those who survive, almost 50 percent will be disabled. That leaves only 31 of the original 100 women alive and unaffected by disability. Consider Hank's story as well as his sister Shondra's story.

Hank's Story
MALE HEART ATTACK VICTIM

"My dad had a heart attack when he was 45. When I was 49, I also had one. Prior to the heart attack, I had cut back on cigarettes but hadn't quit completely. During a particularly stressful day at work, I felt a crushing pain on the left side of my chest. I was sweating and short of breath, and I told my coworkers that the pain was traveling to my jaw. Lucky for me, they recognized these as classic symptoms of a heart attack and called an ambulance. The hospital confirmed I had a heart attack, and I was admitted for treatment and monitoring. After I was stabilized, I went to an outpatient cardiac rehabilitation program, where I learned how to eat a heart-healthy diet and slowly reintroduced exercise until I had more stamina. When my heart muscle healed I was able to exercise safely on my own.

Hank's Sister, Shondra
FEMALE HEART ATTACK VICTIM

One afternoon, when I was 59, I told my daughter I was feeling anxious, and I noticed my heart was racing. My daughter brought me to the emergency room, but they said my heart rate was only mildly elevated. The EKG did not show any changes indicating a heart attack. I was reassured that since my EKG was normal, I was probably having a panic attack. I was given a mild tranquilizer, told to rest, and follow up with my regular doctor. My regular doctor was concerned and ordered an echocardiogram. They also scheduled a Cardiolite exercise stress test, a dye test that studies the heart during exercise. During the Cardiolite stress test, I walked on a treadmill, with monitoring. When my heart was stressed with exercise, the dye study showed areas of weakness in the heart muscle, pointing to a recent heart attack. I had suffered a heart attack, but the medical team did not detect it when I went to the emergency room. Since my symptoms were atypical and I had no chest pain, just irregular heartbeats, I was misdiagnosed with a panic attack. Fortunately, my doctor diagnosed my heart attack and put me on medication for my blood pressure and cholesterol. I am now eating a healthier diet and starting to exercise regularly so I don't go through that again. What a scare!

Amita's story is an example of a young woman aged 45 with early menopause, obesity, and diabetes and no family history of heart disease.

Amita
FEMALE HEART ATTACK VICTIM

By the time I was 45, I was through with my periods. At that age, I was also overweight and had diabetes. My doctor said that although I was young, I was at high risk of having a heart attack, due to the diabetes, obesity, and early post menopause. This was true even though I had no family history of heart disease. One night after dinner, I felt nausea, indigestion, and discomfort under my ribs in my upper middle abdomen. I took antacids, but they didn't help. When I saw my doctor, they did an in-depth cardiac workup. The tests showed I had a recent heart attack. Knowing I had a heart attack led me to focus on getting healthier. I improved my diet, lost weight, and started walking regularly. When I lost 10 percent of my weight, I no longer needed medicine for diabetes and my doctor said I lowered my risk of getting another heart attack and would remain in a lower-risk category if I maintained the new healthy lifestyle.

HEART DISEASE, RISK OF STROKE, AND AGING

Due to the protective effect of estrogen made by the ovaries, young women who still have menstrual periods have a lower risk of heart disease than their male counterparts. Earlier in life, women have fewer heart attacks than their male contemporaries. Perimenopausal women begin to lose that advantage as they begin to lose their estrogen. In post menopause, when the ovaries have stopped making estrogen, the protective advantage is lost. A woman's risk of heart disease rises dramatically when she crosses the threshold into post menopause, increasing the risk by 10 times. After entering post menopause, the risk of CVD rises until, at age 65, CVD occurs as often in women as in men. Strokes commonly affect postmenopausal women.

Women with high blood pressure, a waist measurement thicker than 35 inches, high cholesterol, or diabetes are at even greater risk for heart disease when they lose their estrogen. Addressing these risk factors with lifestyle changes or medication during perimenopause can be lifesaving.

> DID YOU KNOW?
> Once a woman reaches age 50, she has a 50 percent chance of dying from CVD.

Although CVD usually affects women over 50, risk factors such as smoking, diabetes, and obesity can cause the development of CVD in younger women. Once a woman has heart disease, she is much less likely to live a long, healthy life. Once she is diagnosed with heart disease, she has a 50 percent chance it will kill her before age 74. Put another way, half of the women who have heart disease will die before age 74, even though the average American woman lives to 84.

Becoming postmenopausal increases the risk of heart attack 8 to 10 times. Entering post menopause younger than age 40 (premature ovarian insufficiency/POI) increases the risk of heart disease 8 times; entering post menopause between age 50 and 55 increases the risk of heart disease 10 times. Heart disease is the most common cause of death during perimenopause and post menopause, not cancer.[9,11] Consider Vatusia's story.

Vatusia's Story
A WARNING IN THE FORM OF A HEART ATTACK

Last year, when I was 57, I had high blood pressure and was 40 pounds over my ideal body weight. I had a prescription for blood pressure medication but often forgot to take it. That was partly because I was so dedicated to my job and worked such long hours. The job was sedentary and involved lots of meetings. When my doctor advised me to lose weight and exercise more regularly, I rationalized that there was no need to be alarmed because no one in my family had heart disease. I also reassured myself that men were the ones who got heart disease. None of my female friends were worried about heart disease, although several of them had already had breast cancer.

Although I tried different weight-loss diets, as soon as I stopped them, I'd revert to my old eating patterns and regain weight. It was frustrating. I could never find time to exercise because of my busy professional schedule. Eventually, I had a heart attack and required open-heart surgery. I am now in cardiac rehabilitation and out on disability for three months. My perspective on things has changed. I have promised myself, and my doctor, that I will build time for exercise into my schedule when I return to work, and I can now see that's doable. I am now committed to reaching my target weight and following a maintenance program once I do.

WOMEN'S UNIQUE RISK FACTORS FOR HEART DISEASE

As a woman, each of you has unique risk factors related to your reproductive history. These impact your risk for high blood pressure, heart disease, and diabetes later in life. When you see your internist or family doctor, discuss your pregnancy history.[3,8,9] The key elements to mention include the following:

- Gestational diabetes (Note: You have a 10 times higher risk of diabetes later in life.)
- Giving birth to a small-for-gestational-age infant (Note: You have a higher risk of heart disease later in life.)
- Hypertension in pregnancy (Note: This increases the risk of high blood pressure and heart disease later in life.)
- Preeclampsia or eclampsia in pregnancy (Note: This increases a later risk of hypertension and heart disease, especially if these complications developed before 37 weeks in pregnancy.)
- Preterm delivery (Note: This increases your risk of a CVD event by 20–40 percent. The risk is higher if the preterm delivery is prior to 32 weeks.)
- Spontaneous pregnancy loss (Note: You have an increased risk of heart attack by 40 percent for each miscarriage.)
- Stillbirth (Note: You have a 3.5 times increased risk of a heart attack.)

> DID YOU KNOW?
> Pregnancy termination or abortion does not increase the risk of heart disease.

OTHER RISKS FOR HEART DISEASE IN WOMEN

Certain medical conditions are more common in women and contribute to a higher risk of heart disease.

- Autoimmune and inflammatory conditions, such as rheumatoid arthritis and lupus, which are more common in women and result in damage to tissues and blood vessel linings.
- Cancer therapy with anthracyclines or HER2 receptor antagonists (toxic to small blood vessels of heart).
- Depression and anxiety occur twice as often in women versus men and increase the risk of heart disease. Treatment of depression and/or anxiety lowers the risk of heart disease.
- History of radiation therapy to chest or breast (i.e., after breast cancer), higher risk if on left side.
- Rheumatoid arthritis (50 percent higher risk of CVA, two to three times increase in heart attack). Rheumatoid arthritis is more common in women.
- Systemic lupus erythematosus, which typically occurs in women.

WOMEN'S UNIQUE PROTECTION AGAINST HEART DISEASE

So far, in this chapter, I have focused on the unique risks that women have for getting heart disease. Women also have a unique strategy to protect them from heart disease: lactation.

LACTATION

Women have a unique opportunity to lower their risk of heart disease: nursing an infant. Nursing an infant provides the following medical benefits:

- Lower risk of CVD. Reason: there are fewer calcifications in coronary arteries after 3 to 12 months of nursing.
- A lower risk of diabetes is found in mothers who nurse their infants.

- The risk of high blood pressure is lower after 3 to 12 months of nursing.
- Risk of stroke is lower after three or more months of nursing.

OTHER WAYS TO LOWER YOUR RISK OF HEART DISEASE

The American College of Cardiology and the American Heart Association have developed "Life's Simple 7" to lower the risk of heart disease and stroke. Since 80 percent of heart disease is preventable, there are opportunities for risk prevention. Seven areas are targeted to lower the risk of heart disease:

1. Eating a healthy diet
2. Maintaining a normal body weight (i.e., body mass index under 25 or waist under 35 inches)
3. Maintaining normal blood pressure (under 120/80)
4. Maintaining normal fasting blood glucose (under 100)
5. Maintaining normal total cholesterol (updated goal is under 178)
6. Not smoking for 12 months or more
7. Sufficient physical activity (i.e., greater than 150 minutes per week of moderate exercise or more than 75 minutes a week of vigorous intensity exercise)

You can calculate your risk score using the AHA online tool MyLifeCheck: https://www.heart.org/en/healthy-living/healthy-lifestyle/my-life-check%2D%2Dlifes-simple-7.

Want to improve your heart health but not sure where to begin? Consider the following:

- Exercise. Find ways to increase your physical activity on most days. If you are a healthy woman with no medical restrictions from your doctor, you may start with as few as five minutes

daily and gradually increase the amount of time you spend each day. Eventually, work up to 30 minutes of activity four days a week or more. Exercising four days a week for a total of 40 minutes a day will decrease your risk of stroke by 60 percent, and it will also decrease your risk of heart attack.
- Lose weight. To attain a healthier body weight, consider a program with a suitable proportion of healthy fats. Heart-healthy programs include the South Beach Diet, Weight Watchers Core Program with filling foods, a Mediterranean diet, NOOM weight loss app, a low-fat vegetarian option, or a diabetic diet (for more nutrition information, see chapter 12).
- Lower your cholesterol and control your high blood pressure. Although they are beyond the scope of this book, medications can help with both of these risk factors. In some cases, a woman may attain a healthy body weight and exercise regularly but still be frustrated by high blood pressure or high cholesterol. She may have an underlying cause of her high blood pressure, such as kidney disease or a hereditary tendency to have high cholesterol. In those cases, medication may be the best route to tame the high risk of CVD.
- Stop smoking. Smoking causes heart disease, stroke, peripheral vascular disease, and high blood pressure, not to mention cancer. It's never too late to stop smoking, and the benefit to your health begins as soon as you do. Your doctor can help you find a smoking cessation program that's right for you—hypnosis, prescription patch, and chewing gum are just a few of the choices available.

HOW MEDICATIONS MAY HELP

If you don't like taking medications, keep in mind they may be a temporary inconvenience. Some women who develop habits of regular, consistent exercise and maintain a healthy weight can stop some or all of their medications with their doctor's blessing.

With pharmaceutical companies' heavy direct-to-consumer advertising campaigns on television, the internet, and in magazines, it is easy to conclude that we all need prescription medications to be healthy. This is simply not true. Not everyone needs to take a blood pressure medication or a cholesterol-lowering prescription to enjoy good health. Some individuals, however, may not be able to lower their risk of heart disease or stroke without them. Each perimenopausal and postmenopausal woman owes it to herself to learn what medications are available to her. Once you and your doctor review your personal risks and benefits for a specific medication and the medical condition it treats or prevents, you can decide if that medication meets your needs.[14] Consider Jamella's story.

Jamella's Story
REVERSING THE RISK FACTORS FOR CVD

Five years ago, at age 48, I decided to take steps to decrease my risk of heart disease. I work as a customer support representative at a software firm and am on the phone and sitting at my computer all day long. At my last checkup, I had a high blood pressure reading (150/100) and high cholesterol (280). My doctor told me I had a high risk of CVD. They asked me about my general health. I also have indigestion and occasional discomfort in my jaw. Even though I have no chest pain, they recommended I have an exercise stress test to be certain my heart would tolerate an increase in physical activity. Once the test results were back, they gave me the green light to begin moving more. I started a low-fat diet, which means I'm getting less than 20 percent of my total daily calories from fat. I've also switched from saturated fats to healthy oils, like olive oil, as well as adding small portions of avocados and nuts to my routine. I exercise four times a week instead of once or twice. Even if I can't get in a 40-minute workout, I've found I can manage 10-minute mini-exercise routines on those days, which are just as effective in preventing heart disease. There are lots of easy ways to do that.

I walk for 10 minutes at lunchtime whenever I can. I park at the edge of the company lot and walk five extra minutes to and from the corner of the lot to my office, morning and evening. I take the stairs at work and climb them more at home, rather than avoiding them. My cholesterol went down to normal (190) within a year of my lifestyle changes, but my blood pressure did not. Further evaluation showed that I had a kidney problem that caused the high blood pressure. With medication, I'm keeping my blood pressure normal, and that's helping me avoid a heart attack. I feel better now, five years later, than I have in years.

NEW STRATEGIES TO ESTIMATE RISK

Now that research is incorporating unique risks for heart disease in women, tools to calculate these risks are becoming available. These tools are most valuable when you collaborate with your doctor to better understand and leverage the results. That's because the information you collect might affect your health strategy and your doctor's treatment recommendations. For example, if you have a high-risk family history, the tool may not include that in the risk calculation, but it needs to be considered to estimate your true risk of heart disease.

One such tool is the Atherosclerosis Cardiovascular Disease (ASCVD) Pooled Cohort Equations (referred to as the PCE risk estimator here). It was developed by the American College of Cardiology and the American Heart Association in 2013. It has been validated for women and men, whereas other calculators were not accurate in estimating women's unique risks. In addition to heart disease, the PCE includes the risk for stroke and tells you your risk of having heart disease or a stroke in the next 10 years. It is not valid for women who already have had heart disease or a stroke, and it is designed to estimate risk in women without prior cardiac events. The risk tool is available at www.ascvd-risk-estimator-plus.

Your calculator-based risk determines whether you will benefit from taking aspirin to prevent ASCVD and stroke. It also determines whether you will benefit from taking medication to lower your lipids. Consider the following:

- If you are at high risk, you may need medication to lower your lipids.
- If you are intermediate risk for heart disease by the PCE calculator, you may benefit from another test such as a coronary artery calcium (CAC) score to further refine your risk of ASCVD.
- If you have a low risk because of your family history—and the PCE calculator also places you at low risk—you may choose lifestyle strategies.

This is a big advance for women. Your doctor may also recommend another risk calculator, called the Reynolds risk calculator, if your risk is intermediate. The Reynolds risk calculator uses different information, including a family history of heart disease and a high sensitivity C-reactive protein (hsCRP), to estimate your risk of heart disease.

THE RISKS AND BENEFITS OF ASPIRIN TO PREVENT CVD

Taking an aspirin daily has been shown to lower the risk of CVD, but it does not lower the risk of heart attack and stroke in women who are at average or lower risk of CVD. Aspirin therapy has only been shown to lower the risk of heart disease in those at higher-than-normal risk. A doctor can assess your CVD risk and advise you about personal prevention strategies that will be most helpful and beneficial for you. Further, if you are over age 60 and never had CVD, the risk of a bleed and other risks from taking aspirin are typically greater than the benefit. Consider Artemis's and Jordana's stories.[14]

Artemis's Story
ASPIRIN AND HIGH RISK OF CVD

My doctor told me I'm at high risk of heart disease. My mother died of a heart attack at age 52. I'm now 56. I've smoked cigarettes since I was 16. I have high blood pressure and a sedentary lifestyle. My increased personal risk of CVD is based on my family history, blood pressure, lifestyle, and smoking status. Since my risk of heart attack or stroke is high, my doctor strongly advised I take a daily aspirin.

Jordana's Story
ASPIRIN AND LOW RISK OF CVD

My friend Artemis suggested that I lower my risk of heart disease by taking aspirin daily. Her doctor had recently recommended it for her. A month after I started taking a daily aspirin, I developed a painful stomach ulcer that bled. I needed ulcer medication for six months until the symptoms subsided. At my follow-up visit to check how my ulcer symptoms were, my doctor advised I stop taking aspirin immediately. They explained that women like me with a low risk of heart disease do not benefit from taking aspirin and are more likely to experience side effects or problems. I'm a nonsmoker who exercises three times a week. I also have no family history of heart attack, stroke, or diabetes. They told me studies show that preventive therapy with aspirin would not likely lower my risk of heart disease and that the aspirin could actually cause harm. I stopped taking aspirin immediately.

Why are people at high risk of CVD less likely to get ulcers from aspirin? They aren't. Anyone can get an ulcer from taking aspirin. If you are at medium or low risk of getting CVD, the aspirin will not lower your risk of CVD enough to make it worth the potential side effects. In contrast, if you have a high risk of heart attack, you will substantially reduce your risk of CVD by taking aspirin. This substantial reduction in your risk of CVD outweighs the lesser risk of side effects. This is an example of weighing the risks of taking a preventive measure against the benefits. Having a discussion with your doctor that weighs the relative risks and benefits allows you to reach the best strategy to optimize your health.

PROMISING NEW APPROACHES TO FINDING HEART DISEASE IN WOMEN

What are some of the new modalities to learn more about women with an intermediate risk of heart disease? Consider the following new options:

- Coronary computed tomography angiography
- Positron emission tomography
- Stress cardiac magnetic resonance imaging (MRI)

Each of these provides a more discerning approach to diagnose ischemic heart disease, especially the type that affects women most frequently (i.e., disease that does not block arteries and instead affects the smallest blood vessels on a microscopic level).

Another new and promising approach is to look at the calcification in the arteries seen on mammogram, termed breast artery calcification (BAC). A breast artery calcification score done during a mammogram is not yet routinely reported on mammograms but may be a useful approach going forward. Breast artery calcification correlates with coronary artery calcification. If you have a mammogram where BAC is assessed and reported with no BAC found, that correlates with an 81 percent chance of having no coronary artery calcifications.[13]

IMPORTANT TAKEAWAYS

In summary:

- It's easier to prevent heart disease than it is to treat it. Prevention is paramount, especially for women.
- CVD progresses, usually starting with warning signals that may be addressed. There are factors you can control and others you can't.
- CVD may be brought on by a lifetime of habits that are not heart healthy.
- CVD affects men and women differently. Men and women also have different symptoms of a heart attack.
- A woman's risk of CVD and stroke increases with age. Fortunately, there are many ways to reduce that risk.

QUESTIONS FOR YOUR DOCTOR

1. What is my personal risk for heart disease and stroke?
2. What are some ways I can reduce that risk? Should I take medication? If so, what options are available to me, and what are the pros and cons?
3. Should I take a daily aspirin to lower my risk of CVD, or might it cause more harm?

RESOURCES

American Heart Association (www.aha.org)

Hearthub.org (www.hearthub.org) includes tools for risk assessments and a body mass index calculator, as well as other features.

CHAPTER 5

UNDERSTANDING UNEXPECTED BLEEDING

It can be scary. It can catch you off guard. Here's what you need to know.

INTRODUCTION

Unexpected bleeding can be jarring at any age, and it is especially unsettling during perimenopause. The good news is that for many women, unexpected bleeding is normal. But there are times when it is definitely not normal, and it could even indicate a serious underlying health problem.[2] In this chapter, I will answer common questions about unexpected bleeding and dispel myths about this anxiety-provoking aspect of perimenopause, such as:

1. When is it normal to bleed during perimenopause, and when might it be abnormal?
2. Is it ever normal to bleed during post menopause?
3. What are some causes of unexpected bleeding?
4. What tests might I need to undergo to determine the cause of my bleeding?
5. What are some medical procedures that can stop the bleeding? What about other solutions?
6. What can I do to prepare for my doctor's visit? What questions should I ask?

> **DID YOU KNOW?**
> Eighty percent of women have irregular bleeding during perimenopause. It is not always normal, however, and it is wise to talk with your doctor about it.

SORTING OUT THE CONFUSION: WHY IS UNEXPECTED BLEEDING SO COMPLICATED?

Like many problems in medicine, irregular bleeding is a complex puzzle with many pieces that your doctor must take into consideration and evaluate in partnership with you. You have critical information about your bleeding cycles and how they have changed. These pieces include your:

- Bleeding patterns prior to menopause
- Body mass index (BMI)
- Family history
- Personal medical history
- ... and more

BLEEDING PATTERNS

Bleeding patterns and breaks in patterns are particularly significant in determining whether your irregular bleeding during perimenopause is cause for concern. Why? Each woman has a different pattern of bleeding before entering perimenopause. The specifics of how much your menstrual pattern deviates from your former, more predictable cycles determine whether you may need additional evaluation to determine the cause(s) of the bleeding. Here are some questions to consider:

- Is this pattern of menstrual bleeding different from my usual pattern? For example, is it heavier? Lighter? More painful? Am I using a larger tampon or pad? Am I soaking my tampon or pad faster than in the past? Am I filling a

menstrual cup faster? Do I bleed for more days at a time even if it's lighter? Am I spotting between menstrual periods?
- Has the change in my bleeding pattern persisted for three months or more?
- Does the duration or severity of the bleeding keep me from following my usual routine?
- Do I ever soak through a regular pad or tampon in one or two hours (three or four hours for a maxi pad or super tampon)?
- Do I bleed through my clothes without warning or soak through nightclothes or bedding?
- Do I ever rebleed sooner than 21 days from the start of my last bleeding episode?
- Do any of my bleeding episodes last more than eight days, including any spotting immediately before or after?
- Do I bleed or spot between menstrual periods or after sex?
- Have I skipped menstrual cycles for more than three months at a time?
- Have I bled or spotted after 12 consecutive months with no period?
- Have I gained weight, or is my body mass index over 30?

If your answer is yes to any of these questions, consult a gynecologist for a medical evaluation. The gynecologist will use your medical history, specific bleeding pattern, and pelvic examination findings to choose the most appropriate tests.[3,4]

DID YOU KNOW?

Some patterns of irregular bleeding are more worrisome than others. Keeping an accurate menstrual calendar, including how many days you bleed and the cycle length (number of days from the first menstrual period to the next one), is helpful. This can be done on a grid with a box for each day of the month or with a free app on a smartphone. Examples of free apps that include cycle length are Eve, Flow, and Period Tracker.

> **DID YOU KNOW?**
>
> In addition to precancer and polyps, there are other anatomic causes of heavy or irregular bleeding. In 2011, the International Federation of Gynecologic Oncologists (FIGO) updated criteria for evaluating abnormal uterine bleeding with the acronym PALM COEIN.[5]

PALM stands for structural causes: P = polyps (like internal skin tags), A = adenomyosis (back-bleeding into the wall of the uterus), L = leiomyomas (fibroids, mutations that create muscle wall tumors), and M = malignancy/hyperplasia.

COEIN stands for nonstructural causes: C = clotting abnormalities, O = ovulatory disorders, E = endometrial causes such as infection, I = iatrogenic or caused by a medication or device, and N = not otherwise classified.

FIGO also set a new standard that has been upheld. Abnormal uterine bleeding in women over 35 years old or who are overweight should not be evaluated by ultrasound alone. Women with abnormal bleeding age 35 and over should have an evaluation that includes direct visualization. Simply put, an experienced doctor must look directly at the uterine cavity or lining. This usually involves using a hysteroscope, a slender microscope that magnifies the features of the uterine lining tissue.

A detailed menstrual history, medical history, and body mass index (BMI) are important risk factors for your doctor to assess when you have abnormal, heavy, or irregular bleeding. Even after years of heavy or irregular bleeding, or painless bleeding, if you are over 35 or overweight, the bleeding may signal a physical/anatomic problem that may not be identified without a hysteroscopy and biopsy of the uterus lining.

LIFELONG HEAVY MENSTRUAL PERIODS

My patients often say, "I have always had heavy menstrual bleeding. It's normal for me. Why evaluate it now?" While heavy periods in 20- to 30-year-olds do not typically indicate a risk of uterine cancer, heavy menstrual periods during your mid-thirties and beyond may threaten your health. Even painless heavy bleeding may be a sign of cancer, precancer, or an abnormal physical change in the uterus.[2]

> ### HEAVY OR PROLONGED BLEEDING: WHAT ARE THE RISKS?
> Heavy or prolonged bleeding has risks. For example, heavy or prolonged bleeding may cause anemia, poor sleep quality, fatigue, and increased strain on your heart. If you are anemic, your heart works harder to deliver adequate oxygen to your body. Your blood cells cannot load up and distribute enough oxygen to your brain and other tissues. Your doctor will help identify the potentially serious cause(s) of the bleeding and discuss treatment options for you to consider.

SEVERITY OF BLEEDING AND AMOUNT OF BLOOD LOSS

Many women incorrectly assume they'll know whether they're bleeding too heavily. It's not always obvious. For example, even with my advanced training in gynecology, I can personally testify that I couldn't tell when I became anemic in perimenopause. The severity of the bleeding or the amount of blood lost is helpful to know, but it is difficult to estimate. Research shows that women's assessment of the amount of blood they lose during a menstrual period is seldom accurate. The reasons are unclear. One reason may be that blood dissolving into the toilet may give the appearance of a larger loss. Another reason may be that a super tampon, a maxi pad, or an overnight pad can absorb a large amount of blood while giving the appearance of minimal blood loss. Some women are accustomed to losing large amounts of blood with their menstrual periods and do not consider a heavy flow abnormal.[3]

Even if you lose a lot of blood during a menstrual period, you may not see it on a tampon or pad. You may have "back-bleeding," also known as adenomyosis—a form of endometriosis. When adenomyosis is present, the blood pushes backward through the uterus wall instead of out of the uterus through the cervix and into the vagina. This causes the uterus to swell during a menstrual bleeding episode. It may produce a feeling of heaviness or bloating.

ANEMIA AND YOUR HEALTH

If you convince yourself that your bleeding pattern is normal when it is not, you may become anemic. Anemia leads to fatigue, and it places extra strain on your heart. Even if you are accustomed to heavy bleeding, it has a different impact on your health over age 35. Women over 40 already face a higher risk of heart disease over the next two decades of their lives. Becoming anemic over age 40 may add to that risk.

> **DID YOU KNOW?**
>
> You could have anemia without realizing it, especially if you bleed heavily during periods. Conversely, infrequent menstrual cycles may signal a significant problem even if they are not bothersome due to abnormal lining buildup during missed menstrual periods.

IRON SUPPLEMENTS

My patients often ask, "Can I just take iron to solve the problem and fix the anemia?"

It's true that once the cause of the heavy bleeding is identified and treated, taking iron may help fix the problem. But taking iron alone is futile without treating the cause of the heavy bleeding. It is like trying to fill a sink without plugging the drain. If you lose too much blood on a regular basis, taking iron will not correct the anemia or replenish your iron reserves. When it is severe enough, anemia and excess blood loss may put you at risk of needing a blood transfusion or emergency surgery. Consider Tyrona's story.

Tyrona's Story
HEAVY BLOOD: LOSS WITH ANEMIA

I'm 46 and have always had heavy menstrual periods. My gynecologist encouraged me to keep a menstrual calendar, which I've been doing faithfully. It shows that I bleed for 10 days at a time, and I change an overnight pad every three hours for the first 3 days of my cycle. My doctor was concerned by this heavy bleeding and ordered blood tests, which showed that I'm anemic. They recommended further testing to check the causes of the heavy bleeding. I declined to have further testing, since I had been bleeding heavily for more than 25 years. I told them: "This is just me; I can live with it."

My doctor was persistent. At age 46, my risk of cancer and precancer of the uterus is much higher than it was at age 26. I am more likely to have a physical, curable cause for the heavy periods, such as fibroids, polyps, or precancer. I wanted to address the problem by taking daily iron and nothing else. We continued to discuss my options at subsequent visits. When my anemia didn't improve after taking iron for three months, I agreed to have additional blood tests and a pelvic ultrasound. The ultrasound did not reveal any fibroids. My uterus lining was not thick, but my uterus was enlarged, showing there was adenomyosis/back-bleeding. I was also diagnosed with a thyroid disorder. Given the enlarged uterus on the doctor's exam and the ultrasound I agreed to have the uterus lining checked. I had a benign polyp that was removed in the office. I was causing spotting before and after my heavy menstrual periods. After the removal of the polyp and treatment of the thyroid disorder, my periods were shorter and lighter.

DID YOU KNOW?

Women with irregular prolonged spotting are even less likely to be concerned about anemia, especially when the spotting is light. But prolonged spotting—even when it is light—may still cause anemia and signal an underlying problem that needs to be addressed. Consider Ophelia's story.

Ophelia's Story
IRREGULAR PROLONGED SPOTTING WITH ANEMIA

As a 45-year-old woman, I know my body well. In the last six months, I've been spotting five days prior to my menstrual period. Now, two days of the menstrual period flow are heavier than usual. I'm seeing blood clots for the first time. When I spoke to my internal medicine doctor, they said, "Since the spotting is right before your period, it's probably just perimenopause."

I tracked the bleeding another six months, and the spotting got worse. After my menstrual period ended, I only had one week with no bleeding. Then the spotting would start up again. It was exhausting. My internist recommended a gynecologist who specializes in menopause. The specialist did bloodwork and found I was anemic. I not only had a low blood count, but my iron reserves were low. I told the gynecologist I would take iron. The gynecologist said that taking iron alone would not correct the spotting, and they advised further testing. The gynecologist performed a hysteroscopy in his office and removed two polyps. They told me that polyps are soft tissue growths like internal skin tags. He also said that endometrial polyps are usually benign; however, polyps can contain hidden cancer, especially in women over 35. Fortunately, my pathology report said my tissue is benign. After the polyps were removed, I stopped spotting. After taking iron for six months, I have my energy back.

INCORRECT ASSUMPTIONS ABOUT BLEEDING AND OPTIONS TO ADDRESS IT

I've often heard patients say, "I'll just live with my heavy menstrual periods even though they are debilitating. I don't want a hysterectomy." I often advise individuals to consider one of the many nonsurgical, noninvasive options that are available to lessen heavy periods. As a gynecologist, I typically see fewer than six women a year who require a hysterectomy to treat heavy menstrual periods.

Some women also assume it's normal when their periods slow down and get farther apart in perimenopause and eventually stop in post menopause. An irregular bleeding pattern, however, is not reassuring—even when your menstrual periods occur less frequently and are spaced farther apart. If your menstrual periods occur less often, the length of time between menstrual periods matters. Consider Jolene's story.

Jolene's Story
SKIPPING MENSTRUAL PERIODS

I'm 55 years old, and many of my teaching colleagues are in perimenopause and skipping menstrual periods. When my own periods started to become irregular, I didn't worry since so many friends and colleagues had already warned me that this might happen. My menstrual periods were heavier when they occurred, but the spacing changed over time. At first, I bled every two months, then every 4 months, and now I bleed every five to six months. When I saw my gynecologist, they were concerned. I was puzzled and told them that most of my friends and colleagues were experiencing the same pattern of bleeding. They said skipping two months at a time is not usually a problem; however, not bleeding for three consecutive months or more, then rebleeding, was problematic. They told me that three months of no bleeding between menstrual periods allows the uterus lining to build up without shedding. They also said bleeding every three months and less frequent menstrual periods can be associated with endometrial hyperplasia or even uterus lining cancer (endometrial cancer). They advised an evaluation, including a hysteroscopy, during which they took biopsy samples in the office. The pathology report of the biopsies showed I had endometrial hyperplasia. Without treatment, the endometrial hyperplasia could become cancerous. My treatment options included taking progesterone by mouth for six months to rebalance the uterus lining or having a progesterone-containing IUD placed in the uterus. I took the progesterone by mouth and then had repeat biopsies that showed my precancer was fully treated. Then I had a medicated progesterone-containing IUD inserted, and I have not bled again since.

For conditions like these, it is important to collaborate with a doctor to make a diagnosis. Doing internet research and asking friends, coworkers, and relatives about their experiences and opinions is no substitute for a trained clinician's assessment. These individuals mean well, but they are only viewing part of the puzzle. Remember, at times, even clinicians trained in women's health without advanced training in menopause medicine find it difficult to determine which bleeding patterns are normal variants and which are abnormal and warrant further investigation.

For perimenopausal women, irregular bleeding is common but not necessarily normal. For women in post menopause, bleeding is never normal. One in 10 women with postmenopausal bleeding may have endometrial cancer.

> **DID YOU KNOW?**
> A woman is considered postmenopausal when she has no bleeding or spotting for 12 consecutive months.

Causes of postmenopausal bleeding range from noncancerous polyps to life-threatening cancers and other conditions.[4,6,7]

Possible explanations for abnormal bleeding in peri- or postmenopausal women include the following:

- Adenomyosis (back-bleeding)
- Cancer in other genital organs, such as the cervix
- Endometrial hyperplasia (a form of pre-cancer or hormone imbalance in the uterus lining)
- Fibroids
- Polyps
- Sexually transmitted infection of the cervix, such as chlamydia or gonorrhea
- Thyroid disease (more common in perimenopausal women)
- Uterine cancer

BLEEDING AFTER INTERCOURSE

Bleeding during or after intercourse is not normal. If you experience bleeding after intercourse, consult your gynecologist. Possible causes include:

- Precancerous or cancerous change in the cervix
- Sexually transmitted diseases, such as chlamydia or gonorrhea
- Soft growth such as a polyp in the cervix or uterus
- Vaginal dryness and thinning associated with perimenopause or post menopause even if you don't notice the dryness yourself
- Vaginal infection such as yeast or bacterial vaginosis

EVALUATING MENSTRUAL CYCLE LENGTH

Gynecologists evaluate menstrual cycle length from the first day of any bleeding episode to the first day of the next bleeding episode, regardless of how many days the bleeding itself lasts. I recommend you bring your menstrual calendar or a suitable app recording your menstrual cycles to every medical visit during perimenopause. It is an important part of your medical history.

The key to identifying abnormal bleeding is keeping an accurate menstrual chart or calendar. Monitor your bleeding patterns, even when they are still normal. This enables you and your doctor to see immediately if you experience a significant change.

The traditional way to monitor your menstrual cycles is to fill out a grid on paper. The 12 months of the year are stacked on the left, and the days of the month (1–31) are across the top. There's a box for every day. You may put "H" for heavy flow, "S" for spotting, or "SX" to indicate if the bleeding is related to sex.

Another choice is to use an app on your phone. The app should show cycle length. The cycle length is the number of days from the first day of one bleeding episode to the first day of the next.

> **TOOLBOX**
>
> Free apps that show cycle length include:
>
> - Eve
> - Period Tracker
> - Flow

During perimenopause, women who track their bleeding patterns have a baseline for comparison. Begin jotting down your individual bleeding pattern, even if it does not seem unusual right now. When it starts to change, you'll have lots of information to share with your doctor.

Keep a chart or written record including:

- Day your menstrual period begins
- How many days the bleeding lasts
- Whether or not it comes and goes (there are days with no bleeding)
- How heavy it is each day (in pads or tampons per hour)
- Size of the protection being used (for example, super tampon, a maxi thin pad, an overnight pad, or a menstrual cup with size/capacity)
- Date of any spotting or episode of irregular bleeding

- Presence of any blood clots and their approximate size (for example, dime-sized, or the size of a silver dollar)
- Whether the bleeding is related to intercourse

A gynecologist will discuss your personal medical history, family history, and current state of health to determine your risk of having cancer or precancer. If you are overweight, you have a higher risk of endometrial hyperplasia and endometrial cancer even without a family history of this cancer.

Many women who have heavy or irregular bleeding attribute it to perimenopause, but there may be other causes, including polyps, fibroids, or a precancerous condition of the uterus called endometrial hyperplasia. These problems are rare in 20-year-olds but common in 40- and 50-year-old women. Consider Petra's story.

Petra's Story
IRREGULAR MENSTRUAL PERIODS

I'm a 39-year-old artist with menstrual periods that last six days. My menstrual periods themselves are not heavy and have not changed. However, my cycles have become highly irregular. I am a member of an online community that focuses on premenopausal women. It is important to me to be in touch with other women having similar challenges. Most of my colleagues and relatives are much younger than me.

I began my usual menstrual cycle as expected on July 1. The bleeding lasted six days. My mother and older sister went through menopause early, so I wasn't surprised when I started bleeding again July 20 even though I usually have 28 days between the start of one cycle and the next. Many of my online contacts are experiencing these same changes. I had another menstrual period on August 1 as expected, then rebled for 4 days on August 15. Since the menstrual periods were heavier and did not last longer, I attributed the irregular timing to perimenopause. When I spoke to my gynecologist, they said that going from a 28-day cycle to a 19- or 20-day cycle was not just perimenopause, even if the menstrual periods were not heavier. There was too drastic a change from my baseline pattern. After the changes persisted for more than three cycles, they recommended further testing. I ended up having a soft tissue polyp in my uterus. Once that was removed, the early bleeding episodes vanished. My menstrual periods returned to arriving every 28 days, and they lasted 5 days. I did develop a few mild hot flashes and started perimenopause as my mother and sister did at my age, but perimenopause was not the cause of my frequent bleeding.

Now I'd like to discuss a few myths I've heard about menstrual cycle length and clear up the confusion. The myths represent comments I hear from patients and find online. The reality sections represent what evidence-based research shows is often taking place.

Myth: Bleeding every 21 days or less is due to perimenopause and may be safely monitored.
Reality: These types of shortened cycles are often mistakenly chalked up to perimenopause; however, usually, there is another cause.

While an occasional menstrual cycle may start earlier than normal during perimenopause, persistent cycles that begin 21 days or less after the start of the last bleeding episode deserve evaluation.

Myth: Bleeding lightly for more than eight days is not a problem since the bleeding is light.
Reality: Prolonged bleeding is not normal, although it is common in perimenopause.

Prolonged bleeding could signal a change in the uterus lining like a polyp (similar to an internal skin tag in the uterus lining). Polyps can be cancerous or precancerous and need to be evaluated.

Myth: Bleeding every three to six months is not worrisome. It's natural to slow down before you stop bleeding in post menopause.
Reality: Bleeding every three to six months is common but not reassuring.

During this pattern, an individual builds up uterus lining that they are not shedding. This can lead to precancer or cancer.

POSTMENOPAUSAL BLEEDING

Bleeding during post menopause is never normal! Twelve consecutive months with no bleeding signals post menopause. Any bleeding or spotting after that is referred to as postmenopausal bleeding and should be evaluated by a gynecologist. This is the case even if the bleeding is short-lived or a scant amount. Consider Arabella's story.

Arabella's Story
IRREGULAR BLEEDING DURING POST MENOPAUSE

I'm a 54-year-old musician who had a bleeding episode 13 months after my last menstrual period.

I bled every two months or so until I was 53, and then I stopped bleeding for 12 consecutive months. From what I read, I was postmenopausal. The next month (13 months after my final menstrual period), I had a bleeding episode that looked exactly like my previous menstrual periods. I had no pain or cramps. The flow was heavy and lasted five days. My friends said it was just an extra period. My doctor had a different opinion. They advised further testing and ordered an ultrasound of my uterus and ovaries. The ultrasound showed a thick uterus lining in one area. Further testing, including a hysteroscopy and a biopsy of the lining, showed there was a small area of cancer. The uterus cancer was found early and had not spread yet. I had a hysterectomy to remove my uterus with the uterus lining cancer. I did not need chemotherapy or radiation. I was shocked. I had no family history of uterus cancer. I read about the risk factors for uterine cancer, and I do not have any of them. I am not overweight, and I do not have high blood pressure or diabetes. Since I have no risk factors, my doctor suspects a genetic mutation probably caused the cancer.

DIAGNOSING THE PROBLEM: HELPFUL TESTS

Gynecologists start with your medical history. Then they use pelvic examination findings and laboratory results to evaluate whether your current bleeding pattern is a normal variant for you or the sign of a problem. By taking a detailed medical history and performing a careful pelvic exam, a gynecologist can determine which additional tests will help pinpoint the most likely causes of your bleeding.[2,7]

BLOOD TESTS

Your doctor may discuss the following blood tests:

- Hematocrit or hemoglobin (HCT or Hgb). This test indicates your blood count, and it can help your doctor determine whether you have anemia.
- Ferritin. This test indicates your iron reserves over time. Assessing the ferritin level is helpful as the iron reserves may be depleted even when the hematocrit does not show anemia. This scenario of a normal blood count and a low ferritin is most common in women who smoke, but it also occurs in nonsmokers.
- Thyroid test (TSH or thyroid-stimulating hormone). This test checks your thyroid function. Normal thyroid function

is essential for a healthy metabolism. Abnormal thyroid function can cause abnormal menstrual periods of all varieties, and it can mimic perimenopause by causing irregular bleeding, abnormal weight gain (or loss), hot flashes, and fatigue. A sluggish or overactive thyroid may be treated with thyroid medication. An overactive thyroid also causes menstrual irregularities.

IMAGING TESTS

- Sonohysterogram. During this test, the doctor places sterile salt water (saline) in the uterus lining. Then they'll use an ultrasound to visualize the uterus lining. A sonohysterogram is not a definitive test for cancer, precancer, a polyp, or a fibroid; however, it may clarify what additional testing is needed.
- Pelvic and/or vaginal ultrasound. This test uses sound waves to view the ovaries, uterus, and uterus lining. No radiation is involved. An ultrasound may identify ovarian cysts, check the size of the uterus, measure fibroids, and calculate the thickness of the uterus lining from one inner wall to the other. An ultrasound test does not take the place of directly visualizing the uterus cavity. A hysteroscope is a microscope that is introduced into the uterus through the cervix in the office or the operating room and allows the doctor to see the uterine cavity and any abnormalities that might be present such as soft tissue polyps, firm fibroids, or even areas of cancer or precancer. Having an ultrasound does not take the place of a hysteroscopy microscope exam or obtaining an endometrial biopsy.

- *Hysteroscopy*
  During this test, your doctor inserts a hysteroscope into the uterine cavity. Your doctor can see the actual uterine cavity directly to check for polyps, fibroids in the cavity, cancer, or precancer using direct visualization. Hysteroscopy is now

commonly performed in a doctor's office. It may also be done in the operating room.[1]

- *Endometrial biopsy*
  After or during a hysteroscopy, your doctor may take a sample of the uterus lining tissue to ensure they haven't missed any abnormal areas. In the past, endometrial biopsies were done without directly visualizing the uterus lining, and abnormal findings were often missed. New clinical guidelines now advise avoiding a "blind biopsy." You can think of this as a new approach to a "look before you leap" strategy. Typically, a hysteroscopy and endometrial biopsy will identify the cause of the abnormal bleeding; however, endometrial biopsy itself is not a treatment. The definitive diagnosis of endometrial cancer or precancer can only be made by doing an endometrial biopsy and examining the lining tissue under the microscope.

- *Pap smear*
  A Pap smear checks for precancer and cancer of the cervix. Your doctor performs it using a speculum to visualize the cervix and a brush or wand to take cells off the surface of the cervix. The Pap smear is a well-vetted test for diagnosing cervical cancer but is seldom helpful in diagnosing uterine cancer.

- *Swab test*
  A swab test of the cervix can check for chlamydia, gonorrhea, and other infections. During this test, your doctor simply swipes the cervix with a Q-tip swab.

- *Specialized blood tests*
  In some cases, specialized blood tests may help identify the cause of abnormal bleeding or persistent anemia. Blood tests can also identify hereditary forms of anemia, such as thalassemia. Another hereditary condition, Von Willebrand's, impairs the ability of blood to clot in a timely fashion.

Hadina's Story
HYSTEROSCOPY WITH ENDOMETRIAL BIOPSY

I'm 57, and because I still buy sanitary pads for an occasional period, my friends tease me. Even my younger friends have long since stopped buying them. I usually bleed once a month for two or three months, and then I have no period for four months in a row. After that, the monthly bleeding begins again, followed by another stretch of four months with no bleeding, and the cycle repeats itself. This pattern has persisted for five years. I've had a history of uterine lining polyps in the past, which were removed with a dilatation and curettage (D&C) in the operating room. My longtime gynecologist has retired, and I'm seeing a new doctor. They informed me that I am at risk for endometrial hyperplasia and explained how my lining was building up without shedding for four months straight. Even though the bleeding was not heavy at any time, I did become concerned. I had simply assumed the four months of missed periods was a sign that I was getting closer to menopause. Although this is true, my doctor explained how my bleeding history could put me at higher risk for endometrial hyperplasia. My doctor suggested a hysteroscopy with endometrial biopsy, which would allow them to remove polyps if they were present in the upper endometrium. This was performed in their office, and the pathology results showed simple endometrial hyperplasia hiding in the polyp I had developed. The polyp was removed, and I was treated with progesterone by mouth for three months. After I finished the medication, I had another biopsy, which showed the hyperplasia had resolved. I was glad not to have a higher risk of cancer after that.

A few years ago, I met with a 51-year-old nurse who worked in another specialty outside gynecology. She had heavy prolonged menstrual periods. She reviewed her lab results online and saw that she had a normal TSH (thyroid test), ferritin (iron reserves), and hematocrit (blood count) and that her ultrasound showed no worrisome findings. She canceled her follow-up appointment with me since everything was normal in the workup. After our discussion of the potential causes of heavy prolonged bleeding that don't show up on labs or an ultrasound, she agreed to further testing. Hysteroscopy with biopsies in the office showed that her uterus lining was not in sync. Part of her lining was building up while other parts were shedding. This can cause irregular bleeding, heavy bleeding, or both. She and I were both relieved that there was no sign of cancer or precancer. To ease her heavy bleeding and clotting, she elected to have a medicated IUD inserted in her uterus to keep the lining uniform and thinned and slow or stop the heavy prolonged bleeding. It worked well, and her bleeding stopped completely for the next three years.

CAUSES OF ABNORMAL BLEEDING

While it is helpful to be informed, self-diagnosis, self-reassurance, and long-standing myths about abnormal bleeding can be harmful to your health. If you have irregular bleeding, consult your gynecologist sooner rather than later. You will identify the issue earlier, and you may have more options to address it. In some cases, you'll be reassured that you don't have a serious condition.

The following are several myths I've heard from my patients that caused them to delay consulting with a gynecologist.

> **Myth:** My Pap smear has always been normal. I don't have uterine cancer.
>
> **Reality:** The results of your Pap smear are typically not related to the condition of your uterus lining, and your doctor is not able to rely on a Pap smear to detect uterine cancer.

A Pap smear detects abnormal cells from the cervix and is designed to detect only cervical cancer, not uterine cancer. Uterine cancer is much more common in perimenopause and post menopause than cervical cancer.

One exception is when the Pap smear result shows glandular cells. These cells can occur inside the cervix, outside the surface of the cervix, or in the canal of the cervix. When the cells develop abnormal features, they turn into different types of cancer and precancer of the cervix. The presence of glandular cells always warrants further evaluation because those cells could be abnormal and indicate uterine cancer or a glandular cancer of the cervix.

Myth: I don't have any pain or cramps with my bleeding, so I don't have cancer.
Reality: Cancer of the uterus lining is typically painless.

You do not have to have cramps or pain to have early uterine cancer.

Myth: The bleeding I have after menopause looks and feels exactly like the bleeding I had when I was menstruating regularly. Since it is exactly the same, I must not have uterine cancer. Uterine cancer would look or feel different.
Reality: Many types of cancer, such as lung cancer or melanoma, are painless early on.

There is no pain until the cancer metastasizes or spreads widely. Uterine lining cancer is similar in that it is typically painless or silent early on. Bleeding, even normal-appearing bleeding, may be the only early sign the cancer is there. This is true even if the only unusual aspect of the bleeding is its unusual timing.

UTERINE CANCER

Women under 35 seldom get uterine cancer or precancer unless they are significantly overweight. A BMI over 40 (see chapter 12 to calculate your BMI) puts you at higher risk of developing uterine cancer or precancer. Uterine cancer should be identified and treated before it spreads.

ADENOMYOSIS

Adenomyosis is a form of local endometriosis where the tissue lining of the uterus does not stay where it belongs. Instead, it migrates back into the uterine muscle wall instead of passing out the vagina as normal menstrual blood. Adenomyosis may cause pain and swelling of the uterus, bloating, or severe menstrual cramps.

Adenomyosis is difficult to diagnose. Physicians often identify it at the time of hysterectomy when they open the uterus and inspect it for changes deep in the muscle wall. If your physician does not detect other causes of abnormal uterine bleeding, they may determine that adenomyosis is the cause. Keep in mind, however, that adenomyosis may coexist with other causes of abnormal bleeding such as fibroids or polyps.

Women with adenomyosis (back-bleeding) may not be aware of all the blood they are losing. That's because some of it is lost through the abdominal cavity. These women may have bloating as the uterus swells from the extra blood pushed back into the wall. They may also spot between menstrual periods as some of the blood may eventually leak back out into the vagina later and long after the end of their regular menstrual period. They may feel extra pelvic pressure from the swollen, engorged uterus since the extra blood is trapped in the uterine wall and absorbed more slowly than normal. If the pelvic examination shows an enlarged uterus, or there is a discrepancy between the ultrasound and pelvic exam in terms of the uterine size, adenomyosis may be the cause.

Adenomyosis is difficult to identify with the common tests used to check causes of heavy bleeding, a large uterus, and/or anemia. An ultrasound cannot usually identify adenomyosis because it is a dynamic process of back-bleeding and does not leave telltale signs visible on a soundwave test.

In addition, an endometrial biopsy of the uterine lining does not definitively diagnose adenomyosis as the cause of the abnormal bleeding. Also, biopsies of the uterine muscle wall are not practical. Hysterectomy allows the doctor to rule out other causes of abnormal bleeding and deduce if you have adenomyosis. If you wish to retain your uterus, and you're not planning a hysterectomy, magnetic resonance imaging may reveal changes that suggest adenomyosis.

In some cases, all the signs of adenomyosis are present, and nothing else can explain the changes. Consider Antonella's story.

Antonella's Story
ADENOMYOSIS

When I was 46, I started experiencing changes in my menstrual cycles that weren't normal for me. For 30 years, my periods started every 28 days and lasted 6 days. The bleeding was heavy for two of those days. Even when it was heavy, I never needed more than a pad or a tampon in two hours. However, at times, I noticed blood clots. When my periods started changing, I began having periods every 23 days. These periods lasted longer, often 10 days, with heavy bleeding for the first 4 days. When I talked with my gynecologist about this, they updated my medical history, performed a pelvic examination, and ordered blood tests, including hematocrit, ferritin, and thyroid tests. The results showed I had borderline anemia and normal thyroid function. My uterus was slightly enlarged on pelvic examination. My gynecologist scheduled an endometrial biopsy, which, thankfully, showed no cancer or precancerous changes. Since I'm a nonsmoker, she prescribed a low-dose oral contraceptive to control my periods and make them shorter, lighter, and regular, occurring once every four weeks.

After six months using the pills, my doctor and I agreed I would stop them. I was fine for a year, but after that, the periods became heavier again. I was bleeding through a large pad in less than two hours, and the heavy bleeding lasted for more than five days. This time, blood tests showed my hematocrit was low. I was anemic. My doctor had me take iron. During the pelvic examination, they found my uterus was even larger. An ultrasound did not reveal any fibroids. They suspected adenomyosis because the ultrasound did not show any fibroids. I had a hysteroscopy with an endometrial biopsy that confirmed that there were no polyps or fibroids, cancer, or precancer.

My doctor and I discussed the options. They recommended a medicated IUD to decrease the bleeding. That worked for five years by decreasing the amount of bleeding and thinning my lining. At that time I was 51 and wanted to try another solution. My doctor had me consider an endometrial ablation to seal the blood vessels in the uterus lining. Even though ablations are not always effective for adenomyosis, it worked for me. My bleeding stopped after the ablation and lasted until I reached post menopause at age 55.

SIMPLE ENDOMETRIAL HYPERPLASIA

Endometrial hyperplasia is a form of precancer characterized by a microscopic change in the uterine lining, such as glands growing too closely together and forming abnormal clusters. Your physician can detect it through an endometrial biopsy of the uterine lining.

> **DID YOU KNOW?**
> Precancer may remain unchanged, develop into cancer, or resolve on its own. Cancer will not improve without surgical removal, chemotherapy, radiation, or a combination of all three. Precancer is not a type of cancer.

There are different types of endometrial hyperplasia, some more ominous than others. Simple hyperplasia is the most common and least worrisome type. That's because it is the least likely type of hyperplasia to turn into endometrial cancer over time. Women with simple hyperplasia have less than a 5 percent chance of developing endometrial cancer. It is the type of hyperplasia most likely completely cured with oral progesterone medication or a progesterone-releasing IUD (such as levonorgestrel-releasing IUD/ Mirena). Progesterone corrects the hormonal imbalance caused by too much estrogen influencing the uterine lining. If your doctor prescribes oral progesterone, you'll likely take it by mouth for three months. Alternatively, your doctor may suggest a progesterone-secreting intrauterine device that they will place in your uterus lining.

After treatment, it is crucial to resample the uterine lining with another biopsy. This ensures that the hyperplasia has responded to the medication and has resolved. If the hyperplasia persists but has not progressed to a more severe type, your doctor may retry the medication and then resample the lining to see if the condition was cured. After reviewing the results, they may suggest other options for you to consider.

OTHER TYPES OF ENDOMETRIAL HYPERPLASIA

Benign endometrial hyperplasia may occur if a woman is not ovulating regularly or if she has too much estrogen without enough progesterone. The glands in the uterus lining are overactive and multiply too rapidly. The nuclei in the cells do not appear abnormal or atypical.

Endometrial intraepithelial neoplasia shows premalignant changes in the endometrium on an endometrial biopsy. The endometrial glands are even more crowded, and the nuclei of the cells have worrisome changes called atypia. These types of changes are often precancerous or cancerous. They may also be precancerous and coexist or sit next to actual cancer in the uterus lining.

Features of endometrial hyperplasia are not determined by ultrasound measurements or blood tests. It is important to look at the uterus lining directly with a hysteroscope and obtain an endometrial biopsy to get the full story.

RISK FACTORS FOR DEVELOPING ENDOMETRIAL HYPERPLASIA

Hyperplasia of the uterine lining is more common in women over 35. It is also more common in women who are overweight. You may recall from chapter 1 that women make estrogen in their adipose (fatty) tissues called estrone. Women who are overweight make more estrone. This excess estrogen stimulates the uterine lining to thicken and promotes cancer and precancerous changes. Exercising and removing excess weight can decrease the risk of forming endometrial hyperplasia (and endometrial cancer) by decreasing the amount of estrone made in the fatty tissues. Consider Petrova's story.

Petrova's Story
POSTMENOPAUSAL BLEEDING

I'm 55 years old. My periods stopped a year ago when I was 54. I went through the menopause transition smoothly. However, after 14 months with no bleeding, I noticed some pink spotting. The amount was so small that I was tempted to ignore it, but I recalled my gynecologist emphasizing that I should be seen if I bled at all after 12 consecutive months of no bleeding. My neighbor thought I was overreacting since the amount of bleeding was so small. She said, "Why don't you wait and see if the bleeding happens again and then call your doctor? You don't want to be an alarmist." I thought about waiting but then decided to see my doctor. They advised an endometrial biopsy with a hysteroscopy.

The biopsy showed endometrial hyperplasia, a mild precancer. My doctor prescribed an oral progesterone hormone medication to treat the hyperplasia. After taking the medication for three months, I had another endometrial biopsy that showed the hyperplasia had not responded and persisted. Even though it didn't develop into a worse type of hyperplasia, my gynecologist offered me two choices: undergo a hysterectomy or take a stronger medication to try to eradicate the hyperplasia. I tried a stronger oral medication for three months and then had another hysteroscopy and endometrial biopsy. Both showed the endometrial hyperplasia precancerous changes were now gone. The higher-dose progesterone medication had worked. I asked how to lower my risk of the endometrial hyperplasia returning. My doctor said increasing my daily activity and losing weight would lower my chances of getting hyperplasia again. When I asked why, they told me increasing activity and attaining a healthy body weight decreases the amount of estrone my body was making in the excess adipose tissue.

DIAGNOSING ENDOMETRIAL HYPERPLASIA

Diagnosing endometrial hyperplasia isn't always straightforward. On the one hand, endometrial hyperplasia is associated with heavy or prolonged bleeding in women in their mid-thirties and older. On the other hand, it is also found in women who bleed too seldom. A woman who bleeds every three to six months, or even less frequently, does not shed her lining every month. The resulting buildup of tissue can promote hyperplasia. This is common in perimenopause as a woman's cycles become irregular. It can also occur in postmenopausal women who have not bled for 12 consecutive months and then rebleed.

While a transvaginal ultrasound can measure the thickness of the uterine lining, it is not sensitive enough to detect endometrial hyperplasia in its early stages. Therefore, an ultrasound measurement of the uterine lining thickness should not replace an endometrial biopsy or D&C (dilatation and curettage, opening and sampling of the uterus lining) to detect endometrial hyperplasia. That said, an endometrial thickness of over 4 mm measured on ultrasound in postmenopausal women is a warning sign.

Endometrial hyperplasia can also form inside of a soft tissue growth called a polyp. But removal of the polyp does not always ensure that the endometrial hyperplasia is gone for good.

POLYPS

Polyps are mushroom-shaped soft tissue growths that may occur in the cervix or the lining of the uterus. Sometimes they are attached to the uterus or cervical lining without a stalk and are called sessile polyps. They may be benign (innocent), precancerous, or cancerous. Precancerous polyps may turn into cancer over time. If you have polyps, your doctor will remove them to be certain they are not cancerous and to prevent them from turning into cancer.

Polyps may cause bleeding or spotting between menstrual cycles after a few days or weeks with no bleeding. They can also cause bleeding after intercourse. They are common in perimenopause as well as post menopause. They may cause heavy or light bleeding or a combination of both.

The spotting from polyps may occur in the middle of the menstrual cycle when no bleeding is expected. But polyps can also cause spotting before or after a regular menstrual period. The blood loss may not be heavy, but it could still be prolonged, or you could experience irregular spotting. Both are significant and may signal a polyp.

If there is a polyp in the uterus, your doctor may not be able to view it during a routine pelvic exam unless the polyps protrude from your cervical opening. The polyps may also not be visible on an ultrasound study because they're often hidden in the thickness of the lining and look too much like the rest of the lining tissue to stand out. When the uterine lining is measured by ultrasound, polyps can sometimes, but not always, cause the lining to appear thicker.

Your doctor can visualize polyps using a hysteroscope, a microscope introduced into the uterus lining through the cervix, or a sonohysterogram. Regardless of how your doctor visualizes the polyps, they can remove them with an endometrial biopsy in the office or a hospital outpatient setting.

If you have polyps, your doctor should remove them for two reasons:

1. They cause abnormal bleeding.
2. They can turn into cancer. Even though uterine polyps are not commonly cancerous, your doctor will test them for cancer upon removal. Consider Chidinma's story.

Chidinma's Story
IRREGULAR SPOTTING DUE TO A POLYP

At 39, I'd been having heavy menstrual bleeding for five years. I managed the periods well and did not become anemic. My coworkers gave me extra breaks when I needed them. Friends told me my heavy menstrual periods could be a sign of early menopause. Over time, I developed fatigue, and my doctor found I had low iron reserves. My ferritin was only 4. I learned that although the lower end of the normal range is 16–20, most healthy women have a value over 40–50!

I started to have spotting before and after my menstrual period, and then it worsened. I would stop bleeding for a week then have spotting. There were few days of the month when I wasn't bleeding or spotting. During a hysteroscopy and endometrial biopsy, my doctor found polyps in my uterus and removed them. Now, I no longer spot before, after, or between cycles. After taking iron for three months, I am starting to feel more energetic.

FIBROIDS

Fibroids are firm tumors found in the muscle wall of the uterus. They can grow slowly or increase in size very rapidly. Rapidly enlarging fibroids may be cancerous. This type of cancer is called sarcoma. The good news is that sarcoma is rare. Fewer than one in 100,000 fibroids are cancerous (leiomyosarcomas)[8].

Fibroids are common. One out of five women in their thirties has them. Studies show that all women develop fibroids by the time they reach old age.

Fibroids result from mutations. The development of fibroids in the uterine muscle wall over time is analogous to the changes in one's skin over a lifetime. A baby's skin is smooth and clear. As the baby grows, their skin stays smooth and clear into their twenties. At age 40, skin cells no longer duplicate as accurately or as well. Mutations begin to form, and genetic mistakes occur during skin growth. Brown or red dots and areas of discoloration may appear with age. Some women are at higher risk of cancerous fibroids if they have certain hereditary genetic conditions or if they have had radiation to the pelvis.

By the time a woman is in her thirties, her uterine muscle wall cells do not replicate as well. Over the next decade, fibroids may form as firm muscle tumors that look like whorls or gnarls on an old tree. Fibroids begin in the muscle wall of the uterus as tiny nodules, smaller than a raisin. The fibroids may expand or push into the uterine lining, or they may push outward to the surface of the uterus. Fibroids that are not too numerous and not too large may be inconsequential. At times, fibroids may grow as large as a small watermelon. The fibroids are stimulated by estrogen. In chapter 1, you read about the sawtooth patterns of estrogen during perimenopause with erratic peaks of excessive estrogen. High estrogen levels are particularly conducive to fibroid growth.

Large fibroids or too many fibroids may cause pressure and bloating from an enlarged uterus. They may also cause heavy bleeding. A very large uterus may silently press on the ureters (tubes that carry the urine from the kidney to the bladder). In some cases, over time, this pressure can even cause silent kidney failure. More than 20 years ago, women were commonly offered a hysterectomy to remove the uterus with the fibroids to cure the problem of pressure or heavy bleeding. Now there are many other alternatives to treat the problems resulting from a large uterus or heavy bleeding due to fibroids. Examples include medications, focused therapeutic ultrasound, radiofrequency treatment of fibroids through the laparoscope or the cervix, and uterine artery embolization to make a roadblock in the blood supply to the outer uterus.

OUT-OF-SYNC ENDOMETRIUM

The next scenario includes a question I commonly hear from patients:

> I had a hysteroscopy of the uterus lining with a reassuring endometrial biopsy report that confirmed no cancer, no precancer, and no polyps. However, I still have irregular heavy bleeding and anemia. So, what is happening and what are my treatment options?

MY ANSWER?

There are other explanations to consider. One is adenomyosis. The other is an out-of-sync endometrium. When there is an out-of-sync endometrium, the pathology report from the endometrial biopsy may state the lining is dyssynchronous, meaning the lining no longer shows uniform changes throughout the uterine cavity with each phase of the menstrual cycle. The result? Irregular cycles. Estrogen levels are erratic and unpredictable. In response to the mixed signals from the ovaries, part of the uterus lining sheds while another part of the lining is still trying to build up. This differs drastically from the predictable regular uterine lining changes most women experience in their twenties and early thirties. If you have ever listened to a middle school orchestra, you may have experienced something like this. Even if the musicians are playing in tune and in the same rhythm, some of them may have started playing the piece slightly early while others started slightly late so that they are not playing the same part of the piece at the same time.

Treatment options include synchronizing the uterus lining shedding by taking oral contraceptive pills (especially progesterone-only pills) or having a progesterone-releasing IUD inserted inside the uterus (levonorgestrel-releasing IUD).

MEDICAL PROCEDURES TO STOP BLEEDING

Treatment options vary depending on the type of bleeding, its cause, and the phase of menopause. Sometimes observation is a viable option. Other times, it is imperative to treat a woman with medication or a surgical procedure. Surgical intervention may be necessary to avoid the need for a blood transfusion, to avoid taxing the heart from severe anemia, or to prevent the development of uterine cancer.

Many patients tell me they simply want to treat their abnormal irregular heavy bleeding. They often want a hysterectomy, and they're not interested in additional testing to determine the cause of the bleeding.

My response is that treatment options must be tailored to the cause of each patient's bleeding. Even the type of hysterectomy someone undergoes is based on the cause of their bleeding. The surgery that your doctor plans when you have cancer or precancer in the uterus lining is different from the surgical approach planned when no cancer has been found. If cancer is detected in advance, for example, a gynecologist oncologist may perform your hysterectomy.[7]

ENDOMETRIAL ABLATION

Thirty years ago, doctors typically suggested a hysterectomy for women over 35 who experienced heavy or prolonged bleeding. Today, there are other options such as having an endometrial ablation. During this procedure, your doctor seals the endometrium (uterus lining blood vessels) to prevent excess bleeding.

Endometrial ablations have evolved over the past 25 years since they were first introduced. The original ablation techniques to reduce heavy bleeding involved surgically removing the entire uterus lining or cauterizing the uterus lining with cautery or laser. The result was diminished uterine bleeding or even the elimination of uterine bleeding. The downside was that the ablations were performed exclusively in the operating room, where there could be electrolyte and fluid imbalances resulting from the absorption of excess fluid. These earlier techniques also produced scarring of the uterine cavity, making future assessments of the uterus lining challenging. With more research and experience, endometrial ablations have become safe for many women. Yet myths linger about their safety.[7]

I'd like to take a moment to address some common myths I've heard about endometrial ablation.

Myth: An endometrial ablation can hide cancer.
Reality: Be sure to have your uterus lining examined with a
   hysteroscope and biopsied to check for cancer before having

an endometrial ablation. A thorough evaluation of the uterine lining prior to an endometrial ablation includes a hysteroscopy to directly visualize the lining and endometrial biopsies to check for occult cancer.

Myth: An endometrial ablation will distort the uterine lining cavity.
Reality: With some of the newer endometrial ablation techniques, such as hydrothermal ablation (HTA), Minerva, or MARA, there is no distortion of the uterine cavity. If you were to develop cancer or precancer after the ablation, your doctor would be able to diagnose it.

To date, there are only a few isolated cases of endometrial cancer occurring after endometrial ablations. In these cases, women did not have a timely biopsy of the endometrium before the ablation. It is likely that uterine cancer was present but not identified before the ablation was performed.

Myth: Endometrial ablation is not safe.
Reality: Your doctor can safely perform an endometrial ablation in their office.

In some cases, a woman may return to work the same day. Each technique of performing an endometrial ablation has different pros and cons with varied risks and benefits. Your gynecologist can advise you about which technique is better suited to your history, physical examination, and uterine anatomy.

Myth: Anyone can have an endometrial ablation.
Reality: Patients must meet certain criteria before undergoing an endometrial ablation. Consider these questions to evaluate your readiness:
1. Have you had a recent hysteroscopy and endometrial biopsy that show there is no cancer or precancer? This is paramount before sealing the blood vessels that supply the uterus lining.

2. Are you postmenopausal? Endometrial ablation of any type is NOT advised for postmenopausal women.
3. Do you plan to become pregnant in the future? The uterus lining will no longer have a normal blood supply after an endometrial ablation. Pregnancy is not advised after an endometrial ablation because there won't be a sufficient blood supply to nourish a healthy fetus.
4. Are you using a reliable method of birth control? An endometrial ablation will not prevent pregnancy.
5. Are you willing to accept shorter lighter menstrual periods or no menstrual periods? The outcome of a successful endometrial ablation may result in either no menstrual bleeding or short light menstrual periods.
6. Are you aware that the benefits of endometrial ablation may wear off? Endometrial ablations do not always provide permanent relief. It is possible for the endometrial blood vessels to regrow, and the symptoms of heavy or prolonged bleeding may recur after three to five years. Given that an endometrial ablation is not always a permanent solution, it may not be the first choice for a 35-year-old woman if she must consider another treatment option in three to five years. Consult your gynecologist regarding their experience with how long results typically last with the type of endometrial ablation they usually recommend.
7. Younger women may choose a medicated IUD or a hysterectomy to avoid having additional procedures when the endometrial ablation wears off.

TYPES OF ENDOMETRIAL ABLATION

There are many methods of sealing the blood vessels in the uterus lining. Hydrothermal ablation (HTA) using heated water, MARA (water vapor ablation), and Minerva (using radiofrequency and heated water) typically do not distort the endometrial cavity. If your gynecologist advises another type of endometrial ablation, ask them about the advantages, disadvantages, and safety features of the ablation they advise.

Individuals who are pleased with their endometrial ablation procedure report shorter, lighter menstrual bleeding or no bleeding at all. Success rates vary with the type of ablation performed. Consider Venus's story.

Venus's Story
ENDOMETRIAL ABLATION

I'm 49 and have smoked two packs of cigarettes a day since I was 17. I quit smoking once, then took up smoking again after my divorce. About a year ago, I went to my gynecologist because I'd been having unusually heavy periods for over a year. During my annual gyn exam, my doctor told me my uterus was enlarged. Blood work showed my thyroid was normal. Even though my hematocrit was 42, which is well within the normal range, I was exhausted. My ferritin was only 5. The low ferritin showed my iron reserves were depleted and could explain my fatigue. I sought several opinions about how to manage the bleeding and considered a vaginal hysterectomy to remove my uterus. When the pandemic hit, I decided to undergo an office endometrial ablation. The procedure was successful, and within three months, I was having short, light periods lasting only two days. I was able to wear a panty liner for half a day. I took an iron supplement once a day for six months until tests showed my iron reserves were restored to a normal level. My fatigue improved and I got back to my normal energy level after my iron reserves returned to normal.

Many individuals incorrectly assume that an endometrial ablation will put them into post menopause. Even if an endometrial ablation results in no bleeding at all, it will not affect the timing of post menopause, and it will not change your hormone balance or ovary function.

If menstrual bleeding is eliminated by an ablation, the bleeding pattern can no longer be used to determine when an individual enters post menopause. In this case, a hormone blood test may be advised by your doctor based upon your age and other symptoms you may experience.

ANTI-ESTROGEN INJECTIONS

One option for temporary relief of bleeding due to large or numerous fibroids is a medication called leuprolide acetate (Lupron), given as an injection. Within two weeks, Lupron turns off ovarian hormone production, mimicking post menopause. Lupron stops ovarian estrogen production and dramatically reduces estrogen stimulation of fibroid growth. The benefit wears off in one to three months, depending upon the strength of the injection. Side effects include hot flashes. With long-term use beyond six months, osteoporosis becomes a concern. Unfortunately, as soon as the injection wears off, the ovaries become active in releasing estrogen again, and the fibroids regrow. Lupron is not a long-term or permanent solution. Consider Imani's story.

Imani's Story
TREATING ADENOMYOSIS WITH LEUPROLIDE ACETATE INJECTIONS

I've had worsening cramping and heavier bleeding during my menstrual periods for the past three years since I was 41. Now, the bleeding has become so severe I usually need to leave work on the first day of my period. I've kept a menstrual calendar, and it shows my periods are longer and heavier. Between menstrual periods, I spot for more than a week. My gynecologist noted that my uterus is more swollen and enlarged. They ordered an ultrasound that did not show any fibroids or growths in the uterine wall. A biopsy of the uterine lining showed no cancer, polyps, or infection. They said this was typical of adenomyosis. They explained that even though menstrual periods commonly get more irregular during perimenopause, they should not get heavier. My doctor found that my blood count was low, which explained my fatigue. They prescribed an injection of Lupron. I had two injections of Lupron, one month apart. The uterus swelling went down, and my cramps vanished. I continued to take iron once a day, and I felt less tired. However, after two months of Lupron shots, the effects wore off. My doctor suggested an endometrial ablation or a hysterectomy. I chose a vaginal hysterectomy since I didn't want to risk the endometrial ablation wearing off in 3 to 5 years.

HORMONES FOR BLEEDING, INCLUDING PILLS OR A MEDICATED IUD

Perimenopausal women may have the option to try progesterone to rebalance their uterine lining and diminish their bleeding. Nonsmoking perimenopausal women may benefit from the use of a low-dose oral contraceptive to regulate their heavy, prolonged, or frequent menstrual periods. This option is safest after the lining has been biopsied, especially in women over 40.

Another option to control heavy bleeding in both smokers and nonsmokers is the levonorgestrel intrauterine device available by prescription. Your gynecologist places this device in the uterus during an office visit, and the device slowly releases small levels of progesterone into your uterine cavity continuously over five years. It provides reliable contraception and typically decreases heavy bleeding. If you wish to conceive, your doctor can typically remove the IUD in their office. If the bleeding pattern you establish remains stable beyond five years, it is now possible to prolong the use of the levonorgestrel intrauterine device beyond five years, up to eight years with annual reevaluation.

MYOMECTOMY

A myomectomy is a good choice to treat one or two large fibroids that cause pressure or excessive bleeding. During this procedure, your doctor removes fibroids from the uterine muscle wall to preserve the uterus. Years ago, surgeons performed this procedure through an open incision, or cut. Recently, it has become possible to remove some fibroids using a laparoscope. Depending upon the size and location of the fibroids, it may be possible to remove them through an operation using a hysteroscope.

The downside of removing troublesome fibroids is that they often regrow within three to five years of being surgically removed. As a result, myomectomy is not a permanent solution but may be helpful in cases where women want to conceive.

Newer, less invasive methods to remove fibroids include therapeutic ultrasound. Therapeutic ultrasound to treat and shrink fibroids is only available at a few academic centers at this time.

UTERINE ARTERY EMBOLIZATION

Uterine artery embolization (UAE) is a technique that decreases blood flow to the uterus from its outer blood supply. If fibroids are present, reducing the blood supply causes them to shrink. During this procedure, your doctor injects dye into the arteries supplying your uterus to identify them. Then, tiny synthetic particles are passed through a small tube inserted into your groin. These particles block the major arteries that supply the uterine wall and the fibroids. Typically, interventional radiologists are the specialists trained to perform this procedure. Local numbing is used on the skin where the particles are injected. No general anesthesia is needed. It is possible to undergo a UAE as an outpatient. You may also undergo it as an inpatient and remain in the hospital for observation and pain management.

One risk of the procedure is that the blood supply to the ovaries may be affected and compromised, but this is rare. In most cases, the blockage does not affect the blood supply to the ovaries at all. Since the UAE is designed to selectively block the blood supply to the uterus, it does not change a woman's menopause status. Perimenopausal women who undergo a successful UAE procedure usually remain perimenopausal even if they stop bleeding afterward. That's because their ovaries continue to function normally.[7]

A UAE is typically not permanent. Relief from fibroids and heavy bleeding lasts roughly three years. After that, the blood supply may reestablish, and fibroids may regrow.

HYSTERECTOMY

A hysterectomy is a 100% permanent cure for heavy bleeding or fibroids. In a supracervical hysterectomy, however, the body of the uterus is removed, but some or all of the cervix remains. If the cervix remains, Pap smears are still advised to screen for cervical cancer. Bleeding may also recur from the residual tissue at the bottom of the uterus called a cervical stump. Consider Heidi's story.

Heidi's Story
BLOOD LOSS, ANEMIA, AND HYSTERECTOMY

I've always been someone who avoids taking any medication. Shortly after I turned 50, I started having heavier periods. However, the periods remained regular and appeared every 25 days. Eventually, about a year and a half ago when I was 53, the periods got even heavier and then became irregular. I was also passing clots that were larger than a hockey puck. The heavy bleeding was sudden. I would soak through my clothes with no warning, even while wearing overnight pads. These accidents became more frequent and were terribly embarrassing. When I visited my gynecologist, they did a blood count that showed I had severe anemia and had lost the equivalent of at least three units of blood over time! My iron reserves were close to zero.

Taking iron was not going to help me fast enough. They said I was in danger of needing a blood transfusion.

The blood test to check my thyroid hormone was normal. I had a hysteroscopy and endometrial biopsy in my gynecologist's office. A polyp was removed from the upper lining during the procedure and sent to the pathology lab. The pathology report showed complex endometrial hyperplasia, a severe form of precancer. They recommended a vaginal hysterectomy given the cell changes in my uterus lining. I wasn't ready to have surgery, so I took iron for six months, but the bleeding continued, and the anemia persisted.

One day, I passed out due to severe blood loss. I also developed an elevated heart rate from the anemia and required a blood transfusion. That's when I decided to have a vaginal hysterectomy.

After the surgery, the uterus was sent to the lab, and a small endometrial cancer was found next to the complex hyperplasia. My doctor assured me that the hysterectomy had cured me, and I didn't require any chemotherapy or radiation. After I recovered from the surgery, I had no further bleeding. Since the hysterectomy was done through the vagina, I had no incision and healed well. It took a year of taking iron to completely replenish my iron reserves.

TRANEXAMIC ACID

Tranexamic acid promotes blood clotting and temporarily slows down bleeding. It is taken only for a short time—typically three times a day during active menstrual bleeding. It is not safe to take for more than four consecutive days. The risk of taking tranexamic acid in a young woman is low since most young women are at low risk for forming blood clots. This is true even if a woman is on a low-dose oral contraceptive pill. But the risk of a blood clot in the heart or brain in a woman over 40 is substantially higher. For them, tranexamic is a less desirable choice, even in the short term.

BLOOD THINNERS

Women taking aspirin regularly may have prolonged or excessive bleeding and anemia. Aspirin will increase the severity and duration of the bleeding; however, aspirin alone is not likely to cause abnormal bleeding.

Some over-the-counter supplements are known to increase the amount of bleeding or prolong the duration of a bleeding episode. Examples include St. John's wort, ginkgo or ginkgo biloba, ginseng, and dong quai (more details are included in chapter 2).

IMPORTANT TAKEAWAYS

In summary:

- Perimenopausal bleeding is often difficult to interpret. It can look different at different times, and it can present differently in different women. You may experience some or all the bleeding patterns described here during your perimenopausal years. Some of these changes may signal an underlying medical condition.
- Common causes of abnormal bleeding include polyps, fibroids, adenomyosis, dyssynchronous endometrium, endometrial hyperplasia, and cancer.
- It's important to track your menstrual bleeding and discuss it with your doctor.
- Ask your doctor for an evaluation if you have bleeding that is different from your normal pattern or if you bleed again after your final menstrual period.
- Keep a record of your hematocrit, ferritin, and TSH/thyroid hormone values if you have abnormal bleeding. Patients often tell me they don't need more testing if their bloodwork last year was normal. But values are not typically accurate beyond one year if there is active bleeding. Even if you had normal values for these tests 6–12 months ago, they may not reflect your health status in the face of persistent irregular bleeding.

QUESTIONS FOR YOUR DOCTOR

1. What do you think is causing the changes in my bleeding pattern?
2. How can you tell whether it is due to cancer, precancer, or another physical cause?
3. What tests will you do to determine the cause of my bleeding?
4. What treatment options do you offer to treat my bleeding?
5. What risks do I have if I decide not to evaluate or treat my abnormal bleeding?
6. I am skipping menstrual periods and don't bleed for three to five months at a time. Can I monitor this pattern, or do I need further testing?
7. My friend is 37 years old and bleeds every three to five months with her medicated IUD (Mirena IUDTM) containing levonorgestrel. Her doctor does not recommend additional testing. I have a copper IUD that is not medicated, and I am skipping menstrual periods every three to six months and my doctor recommends further testing. Is my doctor mistaken?
8. I always had heavy menstrual periods and soak a super tampon in under one hour for a day or two. Do I need additional testing because I am over 40 years old?
9. I am 35 years old and have gained 40 pounds. My BMI is now over 40. A close friend is a nurse practitioner in gynecology and told me I need further testing for my heaving menstrual periods. Is she right or mistaken?
10. I am 48 years old and went 10 consecutive months with no menstrual bleeding, then rebled. My doctor recommends further testing. I thought I was in menopause. Why should I have testing?

Note: If you do not have an opportunity to review your menstrual history with your current clinician or have these questions addressed, consider another opinion with a gynecologist or menopause specialist.

SPECIAL CONSIDERATIONS

Black women, including women of African or Caribbean descent, are at high risk for getting aggressive uterus cancers that are difficult to identify early. See chapter 13 for more information.

Women who are overweight or obese are at higher risk of getting cancer of the uterus even under age 40. See chapter 13 for more information.

RESOURCES

www.ACOG.org/topics/menopause—American College of Obstetricians and Gynecologists

PATIENT RESOURCES: PAMPHLETS
1. Abnormal Uterine Bleeding
2. Perimenopausal Bleeding and Bleeding in Post menopause

www.asrm.org—American Society of Reproductive Medicine

www.imsociety.org—International Menopause Society information for women and clinicians

www.menopause.org—The Menopause Society

OTHER RESOURCES FOR PATIENTS
1. Menopause and Me
2. The Menopause Guidebook
3. How to Find a Menopause Practitioner
4. Menopause Glossary

www.MenopauseandU.ca—Menopause information for women in Canada

www.Reproductivefacts.org—Patient Fact Sheets and Booklets

www.SOGC.org—Society of Obstetricians and Gynecologists of Canada

CHAPTER 6

COMMON CONCERNS

EVEN IF YOU ENJOY ROBUST health in your younger years, you may experience numerous discomforts as you age. Sometimes it's hard to tell if a problem is vaginal or urinary, gastrointestinal or reproductive. This chapter is designed to clarify some of the common concerns of women over 40 and to give you a framework for approaching your doctor with any further questions you may have. The sooner you visit your doctor, the sooner they will be able to diagnose and treat your problem. In many cases, this can prevent a small incident from becoming a big nuisance.

URINARY PROBLEMS

Postmenopausal women may develop problems with urination. They may urinate too often or lose urine when they cough or sneeze. Sometimes the problem is due to dryness of the vagina associated with the lack of estrogen. Other times, the bladder sits lower in the vagina due to weakening of the supporting tissue. Or there may be malfunctions of the muscles or nerves of the bladder or urethra (the narrow outlet through which urine exits the bladder). It is possible to have one or more of these problems at the same time. Fortunately, there are prevention strategies that lower your chances of having these problems, as well as a range of treatment options available for each.

A gynecologist or urologist (a specialist in the urinary system) can do a specialized evaluation. In some settings a urogynecologist, a gynecologist with additional training in women's urinary problems, will be available.

URINARY TRACT INFECTION OR BLADDER INFECTION

Postmenopausal women are more prone to getting a urinary tract infection (UTI) or a bladder infection (cystitis). Once the vaginal tissues become thinner and less well lubricated with the loss of estrogen, they are more vulnerable to infection.

Symptoms of a bladder infection can include:

- Pain while urinating
- Bladder pain
- Blood in the urine
- Odd-smelling urine
- A sudden, urgent need to go to the bathroom
- Inability to completely empty the bladder
- Needing to void again immediately after voiding

Causes of a bladder infection, in addition to thinning vaginal tissues, comprise:

- Not drinking enough water/dehydration
- Intercourse without adequate lubrication
- Wiping from back to front after a bowel movement (allowing fecal bacteria to get in)
- A polyp or growth in the bladder or urethra
- Kidney stones

Preventive measures include:

- Getting adequate hydration
- Wiping from front to back after urination or a bowel movement
- Urinating immediately before and after sex
- Avoiding the use of soap and washcloths in the vagina and around the urethra
- Using cranberry juice, cranberry supplements, and whole cranberries (to help prevent bacteria from sticking to the bladder walls)

- Taking D-mannose by mouth once or twice a day, as directed, prevents bacteria from binding to the bladder wall lining, lowering the risk of getting a bladder infection. It is available over-the-counter to prevent bladder infections and is safe to take for six months.[11]

While these measures are effective prevention strategies, they are not adequate treatment once a UTI has begun. At that point, antibiotics are needed to eradicate the bacteria. The urinary tract is normally sterile, and bacteria in the bladder or urethra are not normal.

Cheng's Story
URINARY TRACT INFECTIONS

When I was 44, I began experiencing a burning sensation while urinating. I had trouble getting to the bathroom on time and noticed an unfamiliar odor in my urine. Urination was extremely painful, and the color of my urine was darker than usual. When it continued for a week, I made an appointment to see my gynecologist. I couldn't imagine what was going on since I had never had a urinary tract infection. While I waited the three days to see my doctor, I tried drinking cranberry juice, but it didn't help. During the pelvic exam, my bladder was tender. My doctor suspected a urinary tract infection. I left a urine sample, which they said would be used to identify the specific type of bacteria causing the infection. But the doctor said I needed an antibiotic right away to treat my infection quickly and thoroughly. They prescribed an antibiotic to take twice a day for three days. After three doses, which was only half of my prescription, the burning stopped and I felt better. So, I didn't finish the prescription. One week later, the burning sensation during urination returned. When I told my doctor that I had stopped taking the antibiotic after only three doses, they told me that was a mistake. If I had taken the full course of antibiotics, my urinary tract infection would have been gone. They explained that even though the original urine culture showed that I was on the correct medication to kick the infection, I would now need a different antibiotic. What most likely occurred is that the first three doses of the antibiotic wiped out most but not all of the bacteria, which was why I felt so much better. But the remaining bacteria had an opportunity to adapt and become resistant to the antibiotic. My UTI was completely gone after a full course of the second antibiotic. Then, three weeks later, the burning with urination returned.

My doctor was concerned because I subsequently had three urinary tract infections in one month with no history of prior infections. The pelvic examination showed that I had developed a urethral caruncle, a small red piece of tissue that looks like a skin tag, protruding from the opening of the urethra (the urine tube leading out of the bladder). My gynecologist prescribed low-dose estrogen cream to apply to the urethra, and in eight weeks the caruncle resolved. After two additional urinary tract infections, my doctor sent me to a urologist, who performed a cystoscopy to examine the inside of my bladder with a microscope. They found a polyp, a soft tissue growth, protruding from the lining of the bladder. They removed it through the scope. I have not had any further urinary tract infections since then.

INCONTINENCE/UNEXPECTED LEAKAGE

You will undoubtedly be surprised the first time some urine leaks out when you are not near a bathroom. You have lots of company. This is a common occurrence in perimenopause and post menopause.

STRESS URINARY INCONTINENCE (SUI)

This term describes urine loss that occurs when a woman puts extra stress or strain on her bladder. The urine may leak out when you sneeze, cough, laugh, or lift something heavy. In the past, stress incontinence was attributed solely to changes in anatomy resulting from childbirth. More recently, collagen has been implicated. Collagen is a protein-based fibrous support tissue that holds tissues in the body together. It provides strength and flexibility in a variety of tissues, including bones and teeth, as well as soft tissues such as those lining the vagina and supporting the bladder.

COLLAGEN DEGRADES SLOWLY WITH AGE

The quality of collagen varies with each individual. Just as one woman may inherit collagen under the skin of her face that weakens at an early age and forms premature wrinkles, another woman may inherit collagen beneath the surface of her vagina that is less supportive of her vaginal tissues and bladder. In addition, lifestyle choices can influence bladder support. Women who are overweight have more pressure on their bladder and are more prone to incontinence. Fortunately, with weight loss, the incontinence symptoms often improve or even disappear completely.

TREATMENT OPTIONS FOR STRESS URINARY INCONTINENCE

Treatment options for stress incontinence include seeing a certified pelvic physical therapist for pelvic physical therapy, losing weight if you are overweight, and learning Kegel exercises (described later in this chapter). Another option is to have a pessary fit by a gynecologist or urogynecologist. A pessary is a rubber or plastic device that comes in different shapes, such as a ring, cube, or miniature hammock. First, the doctor determines what size and shape will fit you. Then the doctor inserts the pessary in the vagina, under the pubic bone, to support the bladder. It can stay in the vagina for months at a time and then be removed, cleaned, and replaced. Periodic examination of the vaginal tissues in the doctor's office ensures there are no ulcers or sores on the vaginal walls behind the pessary. Finally, a variety of surgical procedures, many of which are performed through the vaginal opening, re-create the original support of the vaginal tissues and reposition the bladder back at the apex of the vagina.[10]

URGE INCONTINENCE

This term describes a bladder that develops "a mind of its own." It may contract and empty at random times whether or not it is full, independent of whether you have chosen to make a trip to the bathroom or not. Bladder irritants can make urge incontinence worse. Avoiding smoking, coffee, alcohol, and soda can help decrease irritation of the bladder. Hydration is also important. Drinking too little water can cause the bladder to spasm. Urge incontinence can also result from problems with the muscles or the nerves that control urination. Treatment approaches include a variety of medications that act on different nerve receptors in the bladder and urethra, either facilitating or inhibiting their function as needed.

Another approach is cognitive behavioral therapy (CBT). After you keep a voiding diary, a trained clinician retrains your bladder with you so that you can urinate at reasonable intervals, when you would normally want to make a trip to the bathroom, as opposed to battling a feeling of urgency every 20 minutes or so. In addition, a newer type of therapy involves using electrical stimulation to control the bladder impulses. Initially, the device to control the electrical stimulation is worn next to the body. Once it is adjusted and proven to be helpful, it can be implanted under the skin to control the bladder contractions long term, much as a pacemaker is implanted under the skin to control an irregular heart rhythm.

Studies show that low-dose vaginal estrogen often alleviates urge urinary incontinence.

Oxybutynin, a prescription medication, alleviates urinary urgency in many women. It is prescribed for overactive bladder and overly frequent or urgent urination. Oxybutynin acts through certain nerves (adrenergic) to relax smooth muscle in the bladder and prevent excess contractions. Side effects include dry mouth and constipation. Some women do not experience these side effects at all; others have them for a week or two, and then the symptoms resolve. For others, the side effects are not acceptable but resolve after stopping the medication. It is typically taken once a day.[3]

BOTOX FOR LESS URINARY URGENCY AND FEWER BLADDER CONTRACTIONS

If medication or vaginal estrogen are not adequate or viable options, Botox injections in the bladder may be helpful. A urologist or urogynecologist may inject the Botox toxin (also used to eliminate wrinkles on the face) into the bladder using a special microscope (cystoscope) to prevent the bladder muscle from over-contracting and causing urgent or too-frequent urination. Relief typically lasts about 12 months, and then the procedure may be repeated.

MIXED INCONTINENCE

This encompasses both types of incontinence, stress and urge. In this case, a combination of treatments may be needed to return to a normal pattern of urination.

Carla's Story
URGE INCONTINENCE

By the time I turned 60, I'd been having difficulty getting to the bathroom "on time" for a while. I have very little warning before I need to go and often leak a little urine before I get to the toilet. The urgency I feel before urinating sometimes involves brief but painful spasms. During my annual exam, I discussed this with my doctor and they said I have a chronic problem of urge incontinence. They ordered a sterile urine test to check for bacteria or a bladder infection, but that and my exam were normal. So, they recommended that I try eliminating coffee, which is a bladder irritant, and that helped. But the problem did not go away completely, so they prescribed a medication to counteract the untimely bladder contractions and spasms. This still was not enough to resolve the symptoms. I also spoke with the nurse practitioner at my urologist's office who helped me with a program of behavior modification and feedback to "retrain" my bladder so I could go to the bathroom at normal intervals without discomfort. I've done well since.

ADDITIONAL TREATMENT OPTIONS FOR URINARY URGENCY

EMSELLA™, KEGEL CHAIR TREATMENTS

The "Kegel chair" or Emsella™ (BTL) is a mechanical device developed in Prague, Czech Republic, by engineers and medical researchers. It is approved by the US Food and Drug Administration for safety. For decades, specialists have recommended pelvic physical therapy to increase the strength of the Kegel muscles and correct instability, weakness, or imbalances in the pelvic floor musculature. Since 2018, the option of the Emsella chair or "Kegel chair" has been available in the United States to strengthen the entire pelvic floor using magnetic energy embedded in the seat of the chair.

WHAT TO EXPECT

After you are positioned on the chair, you sit for a 28-minute treatment that is painless, while the electromagnetic stimulation delivers more than 11,000 supercharged impulses to your pelvic floor, strengthening the Kegel muscles and other pelvic floor muscles. After you complete a series of six treatments, typically over three weeks or so, you find that you have fewer or no symptoms of stress urinary incontinence (losing urine with laughing, coughing, sneezing, motion/exercise) and urge urinary incontinence or mixed incontinence (both). Urine control after an Emsella series of treatments typically continues to improve for six months after the treatment series is completed.

Reschedule your Emsella treatment if you are having vaginal bleeding that day (you may have more cramping). If you have a hip replacement or any metal in your pelvis, you should not have Emsella treatments. If you have interstitial cystitis, defer treatment until you are in remission with no active symptoms.

To get the best results, do not wear any kind of pad, pessary, tampon, or vaginal ring during treatment. A plastic IUD (i.e., Mirena IUD) is safe for this treatment but not a copper-containing IUD or other metal IUD. You may be clothed during the treatment, but avoid wearing leggings and any clothing containing Lycra, spandex, or metal as they alter the magnetic path of the treatment. Treatments are typically twice a week, at least two days apart, for three weeks. A booster every 6 to 12 months may be used to maintain the benefits of the treatment and keep pelvic muscles strong. There is also a setting to enhance sexual response that is available after the first initial series is completed. Additional larger studies are underway.[4]

OVER-THE-COUNTER KEGEL TREATMENTS

A number of do-it-yourself Kegel treatments are available on the internet. Some have controls embedded in bike shorts to wear and stimulate the Kegel muscles. These devices are not well studied and have not been compared to each other regarding effectiveness. Some do not have full-text scientific studies evaluating them, and others have small numbers of participants in their studies. More research is needed.[8,9]

MEDICATIONS THAT CAN CAUSE URINARY SYMPTOMS

If you have bladder symptoms, the doctor will review the list of medications you are taking, looking for those that can cause urinary problems. For example, some medications for glaucoma (an eye condition) influence bladder function and urination because they work through the same part of the nervous system. Some allergy pills or over-the-counter decongestants also work through the nervous system and affect the nerves in the bladder that influence urination patterns and even cause vaginal dryness.

WHEN INTERNAL SUPPORT WEAKENS

Earlier, you read that weakened collagen may cause the support of the bladder to weaken. Weak collagen, surgery, childbirth, and other factors may result in the supports of the uterus, bladder, rectum, or even the vaginal walls themselves weakening and bulging into the vaginal canal. At times, the weak tissue may extend outside the vagina, where it may be seen and felt.

CYSTOCELE

A bladder that is no longer well supported high in the vagina, or that has "dropped," may be another cause of problems with urination. The bladder can be repositioned; this can be achieved with a pessary (a ring or other device placed in the vagina to hold up the tissue). Alternatively, surgery may be used to restore bladder support and return the bladder to its normal position in the vagina. This is a common problem that probably has a hereditary component. Some women have weaker connective tissue than others. The connective tissue helps keep the bladder and pelvic organs suspended in place at the top of the vagina. Over time, if the connective tissue weakens, the uterus, vagina, or bladder can drop lower into the vagina.

Kegel exercises help strengthen the tissue and muscles supporting the bladder. To see results, Kegels must be done at least three times a day on a regular basis. It may take three to six months to notice an improvement. The technique for doing Kegel exercises is to identify the muscles by stopping the flow of urine while you are on the toilet. Then, when you are not urinating, squeeze the muscles 10 times, three times a day. Hold the squeeze for three seconds. You can do the Kegel exercises standing, sitting, or lying down, and no one can tell you're doing them. I suggest you pick triggers to remind you to do them: for example, waiting in line at the bank, while on hold on the telephone, while downloading email, at red lights, and so forth. Avoiding weight gain also helps prevent pressure on the pelvic organs and bladder.

Isabel's Story
HELPING URINE LOSS WITH KEGELS

I considered myself to be a youthful 47, so when I started noticing that I accidentally leaked a little urine when I laughed, coughed, or exercised, I was distressed. When I had my annual exam, I told my doctor about the problem and that it had worsened over the past 10 months, to the point where I experienced chronic urine loss. I did not have any burning sensation or trouble getting to the bathroom on time. During the pelvic exam, my doctor noted that my bladder was positioned lower in the vagina. They said it was sinking slightly into the top of my vagina and was sitting lower in the vaginal canal than it had three years ago. The vaginal roof, instead of being flat, was shaped more like a hammock. If the bladder drop worsened, or if I experienced uncomfortable pressure, my doctor said I could try a pessary or surgical repair of the problem. My doctor taught me how to do Kegel exercises, and after doing them three times a day for three months, urine loss is extremely rare for me. I was glad not to have to consider additional treatment.

RECTOCELE

The roof of the rectum lies under the floor of the vagina. When the support tissue weakens, the rectum bulges into the weakened vaginal floor, forming a rectocele. Some women develop this over time and need to press down on the floor of the vagina with their fingers to help a bowel movement to pass. Problems passing stool due to a bulging rectocele may be eased with over-the-counter stool softeners, adequate hydration with water, increased fiber consumption, and increased daily physical activity as well as achieving a healthy body weight. Constipation and inactivity aggravate rectocele symptoms. Also, excess body weight puts pressure on the supporting tissue that can aggravate a cystocele or rectocele. If the conservative measures just mentioned do not provide adequate relief, or the rectocele worsens or interferes with intercourse, it can be corrected with a surgical procedure in the operating room called a posterior repair or rectocele repair. Another option is to have a noninvasive radiofrequency treatment of the vaginal walls. ThermiVA technology is noninvasive and restores collage support, making a cystocele or rectocele milder by increasing the blood supply to the underlying collagen. It is a painless procedure with no downtime. ThermiVA radiofrequency treatments have no reported side effects and are FDA approved for safety. They are discussed in more detail later in this chapter, as ThermiVA treatments are also used to treat vaginal dryness and laxity of the vaginal walls.

UTERINE AND VAGINAL PROLAPSE

The attachments or ligaments that hold the uterus in place can loosen over time and weaken. They may be affected by inherited weaker collagen, collagen weakened by age, smoking or poor nutrition, childbirth, surgery, excess weight gain, chronic cough, or long-term heavy lifting. This can be alleviated with a pessary or corrected surgically. Protrusion of vaginal tissues may also occur for similar reasons. The loosened vaginal walls may be associated with the loss of other support for the uterus, bladder, or rectum. A gynecologic exam can help determine which organs have lost their natural support. While a pessary may help in some cases, others require a surgical repair to restore the normal anatomy.

PROBLEMS THAT CAUSE VULVAR AND VAGINAL DISCOMFORT

If you have itching or discomfort in the genital area, you owe it to yourself to have a gynecologic exam to determine the cause. Self-diagnosing an itch as "just a yeast infection" may mean missing a bacterial infection, a sexually transmitted disease, vaginal dryness and thinning, a skin condition, or even a precancerous change. Even prolonged scratching can cause problems with the skin outside the vagina. And choosing to live with discomfort may make the problem harder to diagnose or treat over time.

At times it can be difficult to pinpoint where the problem of itch or discomfort originates. Some infections affect the skin outside the vagina inside the pubic hair or the smoother tissue closer to the vaginal opening. Or, the itching may be only in the vagina itself. At times, the infection may affect both the outer skin and inside the vagina.

Vaginal dryness occurs when estrogen levels drop. The vagina is usually very elastic, able to easily stretch for sex and childbirth. It is also a self-cleaning organ, providing its own lubrication for sex as well as for cleansing purposes. But as estrogen levels go down, the vaginal walls get thinner and lose some of their elasticity. The vagina also becomes drier and takes longer to become lubricated (for more on vaginal dryness, see chapter 7).

Atrophic vaginitis can be caused by lower estrogen levels after menopause. Symptoms include dryness and irritation. There may even be a dark yellow or mustard-colored discharge.

Options for vaginal dryness, including hyaluronic acid and low-dose vaginal estrogen, are discussed in detail in chapter 7. If you have vaginal dryness, or the inside of your vagina feels like sandpaper, or you have discomfort from dry vaginal walls while walking or exercising, this is troublesome even if you are not having intercourse. Newer options are available, and their role, effectiveness, and side effects are still being explored. They include the following options.

Radiofrequency treatment of the vaginal walls with ThermiVA restores moisture, elasticity, and comfort without using vaginal estrogen. This option may be elected by women who are breast cancer survivors and want or need to avoid all estrogen prescriptions or those on aromatase inhibitors (i.e., letrozole and anastrozole) designed to eliminate all estrogen from the body to lower the risk of breast cancer. More information is included in chapter 7, including study references. ThermiVA typically improves vaginal dryness and helps symptoms of stress incontinence and urge incontinence. Stress incontinence improves when the blood supply to the collagen tissue behind the vagina wall and the blood supply to the Kegel muscles is enhanced. The urge incontinence often improves when moisture and elasticity to the vaginal wall lining are restored.

CO_2 lasers are being used to restore vaginal health without hormones. They are not yet approved by specialty societies such as the American College of Obstetricians and Gynecologists for this purpose, nor are they endorsed by The Menopause Society. Studies thus far are limited by small size. Some studies show lasers are effective in treating vaginal dryness, but the degree of improvement they demonstrate is very small. The CO_2 laser works by drilling tiny holes in the vaginal mucosa layer and then generating a healing response. At times there can be scarring and worse symptoms.[5,6,7]

VAGINAL SYMPTOMS THAT INDICATE A VISIT TO THE DOCTOR IS IN ORDER

The symptoms of very different problems may be similar. Only a doctor can correctly identify the underlying problem and prescribe appropriate medications. Schedule a visit to your doctor if you have any of these symptoms:

- Odor
- Irritation
- Itching
- Discharge

A fishy or ammonia-like odor may be a sign of a bacterial infection. Irritation or burning also may indicate bacterial infection, atrophic vaginitis (thin dry vaginal walls) now referred to as genitourinary syndrome of menopause (GSM), or both.

Vaginal infections may produce initial pain or irritation with sex. Although yeast is the most well-known vaginal infection, it is not the most common type. The most common type of vaginal infection is Bacterial vaginosis. Different types of vaginal infections include:

- Yeast infections
- Bacterial infections
- Sexually transmitted diseases

It is also possible to have a combined type of vaginal infection such as yeast and bacterial vaginosis. Each of these infections is discussed separately in the pages that follow.

YEAST INFECTIONS

A yeast infection inside the vagina is called Candida vaginitis. If it occurs on the skin outside the vagina, on the vulva, it is called Candida vulvitis. Often, both the vagina and the vulva are involved, and that is called Candida vulvovaginitis.

Yeast infections in either or both locations are common after taking antibiotics. The antibiotics alter the normal complement of bacteria that are supposed to live in the vagina. When healthy, the vagina is acidic. That is one reason that using soap to clean the vagina goes against your body's natural way of keeping the vagina clean and healthy. Soap is basic—it has a higher pH than the vagina's low acidic pH. The soap disturbs the natural pH balance of the vagina. Basically, soap cleans out the bacteria that are supposed to stay. As a result, the vagina's natural barriers are compromised, allowing bacteria that do not belong there to enter.

Many women are brought up to believe that their vulvas and vaginas are "dirty" and therefore must be thoroughly scrubbed and cleaned. This is unfortunate since the vagina is a self-cleaning organ, just like the eyeballs. Your eyeballs do not require scrubbing or the application of soap, and neither does your vagina. Similarly, the mouth has bacteria that normally live there, and the saliva keeps the sides of the mouth lubricated and clean (although not the teeth and gums).

Different kinds of yeast can cause vulvovaginitis. The most common types of yeast respond well to over-the-counter anti-yeast preparations. Other types of yeast may grow, requiring a different treatment approach. And a yeast infection may occur with other types of infection that require different treatment.

It is reasonable to use an over-the-counter preparation to treat yeast if you have taken an antibiotic in the past six weeks or so, but if you do not get completely better, see your doctor. Also, be aware that if you have itching on the vulvar skin outside the vagina, using a vaginal yeast cream or suppository inside the vagina will not cure the vulvar yeast infection. You will need to apply the yeast cream directly to the skin outside the vulva to get relief.

BACTERIAL INFECTIONS

Bacterial vaginosis is the most common vaginal infection in women. It can occur at any age, from the teen years to the nineties. It is usually not contracted from a sexual partner.

Bacteria from the rectum may settle in the vagina and cause a fishy or ammonia-like odor. There also may be irritation or burning at times and dryness or discomfort with sex. Examination and evaluation of the discharge will reveal the type of infection to be bacterial vaginosis, not yeast. Over-the-counter yeast medications or douching will not clear this infection and should be avoided. Bacterial vaginosis requires an antibiotic to correct the problem.

One common way to acquire bacterial vaginosis is to wipe the wrong way and bring bacteria from the rectum into the vagina. Wipe from front to back to avoid this risk. Also avoid introducing soap or a washcloth into the vagina, which can sweep in the wrong kind of bacteria (see Vaginal Health, below).

While yeast will respond to over-the-counter treatment, a bacterial infection requires prescription antibiotics to resolve. Bacterial vaginosis is only relieved by taking antibiotics by mouth or placing them directly in the vagina. Both oral and topical antibiotics are obtained by prescription. If the bacterial infection persists or recurs after treatment with antibiotics, the woman's sexual partner should also be treated with antibiotics to prevent passing the infection back and forth.

Every year, I see many women like Valerie.

Valerie's Story
SAME SYMPTOM, DIFFERENT CAUSE

I'm 54 and have been married for 30 years. I made an appointment to see my gynecologist between annual exams because I was experiencing pain with intercourse and had vaginal burning at other times. I had tried an over-the-counter yeast medication, but the symptoms did not improve. At my annual exam four months earlier, I was fine. I thought it must be part of post menopause. I told my doctor I was concerned about vaginal dryness. As it turned out, that wasn't my problem. The pelvic exam revealed vaginal discharge with an atypical color and odor. The discharge was analyzed under a microscope and revealed bacterial vaginosis. My doctor explained the importance of wiping from front to back, which may have been the source of my problem. They prescribed an antibiotic, Metronidazole (Flagyl), and gave me some information about vaginal care to prevent further episodes.

Six months later, I was back because of burning inside the vagina, which I'd been experiencing for three weeks. I was concerned that the bacterial infection had returned. During the exam, I told my doctor that I had taken antibiotics for bronchitis a month before. The pelvic examination and laboratory tests showed that I had a yeast infection, and my doctor advised me to buy an over-the-counter antifungal treatment that included a suppository or cream for the vagina. They said the yeast infection was unrelated to my bacterial vaginal infection, but rather was related to the antibiotic I had taken for bronchitis. Instead of buying the preparation she suggested, I used an over-the-counter medication I already had in my medicine cabinet: Vagisil. I learned it is not a medicine that specifically treats yeast infections. The itch and burn lessened but never completely disappeared. Because my symptoms felt somewhat better, I didn't call my doctor. But the infection persisted and then worsened.

I developed burning and itching of the skin outside the vagina. At that point, although I didn't know it, I had an even more extensive yeast infection, affecting not only the vaginal canal but also the vulva. Now I would need to use an antifungal treatment with an insert for the vagina and cream for the skin. My doctor explained that treating a vaginal yeast infection does not treat a vulvar yeast infection on the skin outside the vagina. Even though these infections felt similar to me, they required different treatment. Neglecting the first yeast infection led to a more extensive problem.

DESQUAMATIVE INFLAMMATORY VAGINITIS

Desquamative inflammatory vaginitis (DIV) is the least common type of vaginal discharge and the least well understood or studied. It may be caused by a change in immunity. Signs of DIV include a purulent or pus-like discharge that is not caused by any other type of infection, including bacterial vaginosis, trichomonas, gonorrhea, or chlamydia. There may be redness and tiny pinpoint red dots on exam, as well as swelling of the vaginal walls of the vulva. Treatment is not well studied but usually involves intravaginal clindamycin gel or cream (prescription antibiotic vaginal cream) or vaginal steroids.[1,2]

SEXUALLY TRANSMITTED DISEASES

Postmenopausal women can still acquire sexually transmitted diseases even though they are no longer fertile or having periods. Many of these sexually transmitted diseases will also cause pain or discomfort. The sexually transmitted diseases that can plague any woman earlier in her life may still descend on the menopausal woman.

Herpes

Women who have intercourse are at risk for herpes, a virus that produces painful genital ulcers. Herpes pain may be alleviated with antiviral medication to shorten the duration of symptoms.

Genital Warts

The human papillomavirus (HPV) causes genital warts, or condyloma. One out of three young women (in their late teens and early twenties) now carries this virus. There are more than 300 DNA types of HPV. Once infected with this virus, you can harbor it for the rest of your life. It is not known how many postmenopausal women have been exposed to HPV. You can acquire the virus earlier in life, or from a partner, and not know. For example, you may have had a wart on your hand or foot as a child. This means you were exposed to HPV then. The virus may remain dormant for decades.

The virus may produce raised white cauliflower-like lesions, which may occur on the hands, on the feet, or inside or outside the genital area in men or women. If you contract the wart virus, it may result in an abnormal Pap smear of your cervix. If you had a wart on your hand and then wiped or cleaned your genital area, you could acquire genital warts without having them sexually transmitted. Wart virus is acquired and spread by skin-to-skin contact.

Women of any age may show signs of wart virus on their Pap smear, even if they have not been sexually active for years. They should be examined by a gynecologist and treated for the virus if it produces abnormal precancerous changes on their Pap smear. At this point, if wart lesions are found, they are treated. Or, if the HPV causes a change in the cervix, such as dysplasia or precancer, that may be treated to prevent progression to cancer (see chapter 13).

If you have ever had warts, inform your doctor and be certain to have regular Pap smears. The wart virus may produce precancer or dysplasia of the cervix, which is typically found on a Pap smear. Treating the precancer of the cervix will prevent it from progressing to cervical cancer in the future. Once precancers are found on a Pap smear, a microscope exam of the cervix (colposcopy) and a cervical biopsy in the office may identify abnormalities of the cervix that require treatment. It is possible to test for HPV with a swab test or during a Pap test (for more information, see chapter 13).

At present, researchers are looking for a vaccine to treat wart virus. Your doctor will keep you posted. Currently we have a vaccine to prevent cervical cancer due to HPV wart virus that is given to young men and women up to age 27 in the United States.

HIV/AIDS

Menopausal women may also contract human immunodeficiency virus (HIV/AIDS). Using condoms will help prevent this possibility.

Chlamydia

This is an infection of the cervix that can spread to other pelvic organs and cause pain with intercourse, abnormal bleeding, or vaginal discharge. It is diagnosed using pelvic examinations and cultures or microscope analysis and is treated with antibiotics.

Sonya's Story
CHLAMYDIA

As a 54-year-old woman in post menopause, I was not concerned about getting pregnant and did not use a condom with my new sexual partner. Unfortunately, I began to experience bleeding and deep pain during intercourse. My gynecologist performed a history and physical examination. The chlamydia test came back positive. I took antibiotics, and my partner was tested for chlamydia by their doctor. Although their test came back negative, they also took antibiotics. I was retested after treatment, and the bleeding and pain stopped.

Gonorrhea

Gonorrhea can infect the cervix and must be treated with antibiotics. It is diagnosed using pelvic examinations and cultures or by microscope analysis. While postmenopausal women with new partners need not be concerned with contraception, they may consider using condoms to help protect against gonorrhea, chlamydia, and HIV.

Trichomonas

Trichomonas infections produce a characteristic foul odor with an irritating discharge and red swollen surfaces inside the vagina. It is usually sexually transmitted. It may cause burning or odor and a green watery vaginal discharge. Analyzing the discharge under the microscope and identifying the organism that causes the infection (a protozoan or type of microorganism related to algae) clinches the diagnosis. Treatment consists of a prescription antibiotic. The sexual partner should also receive treatment. If untreated, trichomonas may cause an increased chance of abnormal Pap smears.[1]

VULVAR CHANGES

Postmenopausal women are more vulnerable to vulvar problems. Itching and burning may be chalked up to a yeast infection but not be caused by yeast at all, nor are they always associated with an infection. A wide variety of problems may be causing the itch and warrant a different approach to treatment.

Skin problems elsewhere on the body, such as psoriasis or eczema, can also occur on the vulva. Sometimes psoriasis or eczema shows up on the vulva before it appears anywhere else. Treatment includes prescription-strength creams prescribed by a dermatologist, gynecologist, internist, or family doctor familiar with this condition.

Other skin disorders unique to the vulva can cause swelling, pain, itching, burning, and pain with intercourse. If neglected, the swelling can be severe enough to make sitting or walking difficult. Distinct features of the three common vulvar skin conditions can be diagnosed by medical history and physical exam.

CONTACT DERMATITIS

Contact dermatitis is an irritation of the skin that results from exposure to a particular substance such as a scented product. Soap, fabric softener, detergent, dryer sheets, douches, wipes, pads, lotions, creams containing alcohol, and panty liners are all possible offenders. Vagisil, an over-the-counter product sold to help vulvovaginal symptoms, is itself a common cause of dermatitis. It contains Benzocaine, an allergen. Other products contain preservatives or perfume that may not agree with you.

Treatment includes stopping contact with the offending product or additive. It also involves stopping the vicious cycle of itching that produces more scratching. Infections need to be treated, but the inflammation resulting from the irritation and scratching often points to the need for a mild steroid cream such as triamcinolone. Why not treat this yourself, using over-the-counter steroid cream? If you use steroid cream and have a yeast infection, the infection will get worse. It is important to get a doctor's evaluation, including a careful history and physical examination, to prescribe the most helpful treatment and not worsen the condition. If contact dermatitis occurs in the setting of incontinence, topical estrogen may help as well.

LICHEN SIMPLEX CHRONICUS

This condition occurs when chronic itching leads to more scratching and more itching over a period of time. It worsens with hot, humid conditions, as well as stress and irritants. It is common in women with conditions such as psoriasis or contact dermatitis. The itching that results is difficult to tolerate. On physical examination, the skin is thickened from repeated scratching. One or both sides of the vulva may show differences in color as the pigment in the skin evaporates. There may be scratch marks or hair loss. The doctor will check to be certain that the only cause is prolonged scratching and to ensure there are no precancerous areas present. They can look similar. At times, a biopsy is needed to identify the cause of the changes.

LICHEN SCLEROSIS

Lichen sclerosis (LS) is a chronic condition that occurs only on the vulva; it does not involve the vagina. It is caused by an immune response that produces changes in the vulvar skin that include white areas, tissue thinning, and scarring. It can also cause red areas near the white patches or white areas as well as fissures. The white areas, red changes, and fissures characteristic of LS may be mistaken for changes associated with vulvar yeast or Candida vulvitis. Lichen sclerosis can cause burning or itching, pain with urination, and pain with sex.

Sometimes, lichen sclerosis is asymptomatic and silent, causing the vulva to shrink, thin, scar, or even fade away without a warning pain, burn, or itch. I have seen vulvar scarring in women who did not know that they had the changes of lichen sclerosis. Those not familiar with this condition may attribute the vulvar thinning and scarring to old age. While there is some loss of the fat pad under the vulvar skin with age, the tissues of the vulva, including the covering of the clitoris, are not designed to vanish or scar over with age. Even in the absence of itching or burning, vulvar scarring may result if you have lichen sclerosis that is neglected.

Pelvic exams that identify asymptomatic LS early allow for treatment before the vulva shrinks, thins, scars, or fades away, especially if there are no warning symptoms. For those who do get them, it is important to get a pelvic exam to avoid falsely attributing these symptoms to a yeast infection. Once the type of vulvar dystrophy is identified, special ointments may be applied to the area to reverse the changes and treat the symptoms. Many months of treatment are usually needed to treat these types of skin changes. Hygiene changes are also advised.

While there isn't proof that lichen sclerosis causes vulvar cancer, squamous cell cancer is more likely to develop in women with a diagnosis of lichen sclerosis. There is a genetic predisposition, such as thyroid disease or lupus; almost half of the women with lichen sclerosis have auto-antibodies, and many have an actual autoimmune disease, such as thyroid and lupus.

VAGINAL HEALTH

Proper care of the genital area can prevent many common problems. In my experience, women have many misconceptions about vaginal care. Sometimes their efforts to stay clean and fresh actually do more harm than good. Here are up-to-date guidelines that will help minimize any episodes of vaginal discomfort.

- Wipe from front to back—all the time, whether you have urinated or moved your bowels. Wiping from front to back will prevent the bacteria in the rectal area from getting into the vagina. This will also help prevent urinary tract infections. Healthy urine is sterile and contains no bacteria.
- Use unscented, plain white toilet paper.
- If you use pads or tampons, avoid the type with deodorant.
- Avoid dryer sheets and fabric softeners. They have strong chemicals in them that are harsh for menopausal skin.

Many women get rashes and itching from using these products.
- Wear all-cotton panties (not nylon with a cotton crotch). Avoid thong underwear; they track bacteria from the rectum forward into the vagina.
- Avoid wearing tight jeans or slacks.
- Avoid wearing pantyhose under slacks. Even though they are called "pantyhose," wear all-cotton panties underneath.
- Put your underwear through an extra rinse cycle in your wash to avoid detergent residues that may irritate your skin, or use half the amount of liquid detergent recommended so there is less soap residue. Use liquid rather than powder; it will dissolve more thoroughly. When you do the laundry, dissolve the detergent in the machine water before adding your clothes.
- Do not clean the vagina with a washcloth. It will disturb the protective function of the vulvar and vaginal surfaces. No matter how carefully you use the washcloth, it will also spread bacteria from the rectum into the vagina since they are often less than an inch apart.
- Avoid deodorant or antiperspirant soaps in this area. They have harsh, irritating chemicals. Try using mild glycerin soap for the hip, lower stomach, and groin area.
- If you have a handheld shower head, do not point the nozzle into your vagina when showering. Use a sitz bath to clean the genital area (see below).
- If you are traveling and cannot use a sitz bath, consider carrying the over-the-counter product Balneol, a perineal lubricant and cleanser. Put a dime-sized dab of the lotion on clean toilet paper, wipe front to back, and then continue to wipe with clean pieces of toilet paper until they are no longer soiled. This also helps clean around hemorrhoids.

> **DID YOU KNOW?**
>
> **VAGINAL DOUCHING IS NOT ADVISABLE**
>
> Despite the many products available online and at your local drugstore, do not douche. The vagina has a delicate balance of acidity (pH). The normal vaginal pH encourages healthy bacteria to live in the vagina and discourages foreign bacteria from inhabiting it. Commercial products or douches cannot mimic or improve nature's own balance. Douching is now suspected of causing serious infections of the fallopian tubes and ovaries, as well as abnormal Pap smears. The lining tissue of the vagina is similar to the lining tissue of the mouth. You wouldn't use soap to clean out the inside of your mouth. It isn't necessary to douche or use soap inside your vagina, either.

HOW TO USE A SITZ BATH

Sitz baths are plastic basins that look like bedpans. They may be purchased at your pharmacy without a prescription. Raise the toilet seat the way men do. Put very warm water in the sitz bath and place it on the base of the toilet bowl. It will not touch the toilet water. Sit in the sitz bath for a few minutes. (You do not need to use the plastic tubing that comes with the sitz.) Spread the folds of the vulva apart and cleanse the area.

A sitz bath cleanses the skin outside the vagina without moving bacteria in the wrong direction. It rinses away sweat and secretions without harming the body's natural balance. A sitz bath with warm water will not irritate any dry areas or aggravate other skin conditions. It is also effective for soothing and preventing hemorrhoids.

IMPORTANT TAKEAWAYS

Chronic vaginal discharge is not always from an infection like yeast or bacterial vaginosis. Have your clinician check for infection, and if there is no infection or the infection is treated, see a gynecologist or menopause specialist to evaluate you for genitourinary syndrome of menopause/GSM, formerly called vaginal atrophy. There are safe hormonal and nonhormonal treatments available. A more detailed discussion of treatment options is included in chapter 7.

White changes on the skin outside the vagina (vulva) or itching do not always represent yeast. If yeast medication on the vulva does not relieve the discomfort, consult a dermatologist, gynecologist, or menopause specialist to evaluate you for other vulvar skin changes.

Leaking urine and/or urinary urgency and frequency do not always indicate a urinary infection in perimenopause and post menopause. If you do not have a urinary infection and you have urinary issues, consider consulting a gynecologist, menopause specialist, or urologist for diagnosis and treatment options.

Feeling a heaviness or low tissue in the vagina may or may not require surgery. Nonsurgical options are available for addressing a low uterus with weak ligaments, or a "bladder drop" or loosening of the wall of the rectum. Consult a gynecologist, urologist, or menopause specialist to discuss the type of low tissue you are experiencing and options to treat it or increase your comfort with other strategies.

QUESTIONS FOR YOUR DOCTOR

1. I have chronic yeast with vaginal discharge that does not respond to over-the-counter Monistat or an oral Diflucan prescription from my primary care doctor. What else could it be, and what are my treatment options?
2. I have white changes and itching on the skin outside my vagina that does not respond to yeast medication. What could this be? What are my treatment options?
3. I leak urine when I laugh, cough, run, jump, or lift. It is interfering with my work as well as my ability to exercise. What nonsurgical options should I consider?
4. I urinate too often, frequently get the urge to urinate, and don't always get to the bathroom in time. What are my treatment options?

5. I feel a ball of tissue low in my vagina. It is uncomfortable. What is it from and what can I do about it?
6. I have frequent urinary tract infections. What options do I have to address this?

RESOURCES

The American College of Obstetricians and Gynecologists (www.ACOG.org) has a patient information pamphlet on urinary incontinence available at www.acog.org/publications/patient. It may also be available at your gynecologist's office.

The American Urogynecology Society (www.AUGS.org) has information on what a urogynecologist can do to help with bladder and pelvic support issues, how to find a urogynecologist, and patient information sheets.

www.AUGs.org has patient fact sheets.

CHAPTER 7

SMOOTHER SEX

You want—and deserve—enjoyable sexual experiences. Here is what you can do to get them.

FROM A MEDICAL PERSPECTIVE, thinking about sex is daunting. Sex is such a personal private matter with individual preferences and needs. Sex is not a part of your life that you or your doctor wants to "medicalize." In other words, most people want to have a normal sex life without medication or a doctor's input. That said, if or when you notice a change in the way you feel or function sexually, and this change bothers you, you deserve medical help. Unfortunately, 9 of 10 clinicians are not accustomed to asking you about your satisfaction with your sexual function. According to surveys, most women are reluctant to bring up this topic during a medical visit.

In this chapter, I will answer the following questions:

- What are some potential causes of sexual problems in peri- and post menopause?
- What are the strategies and treatments to address these sexual problems?
- What type of medical help is available to help you enjoy smoother sex?

Note that the medical treatments discussed in this chapter are studied in heterosexual women and those in same-sex relationships. There are a few small studies designed to understand the challenges transgender individuals face in peri- and post menopause. While some of the information discussed here will be helpful to transgender individuals, they will likely benefit from additional specialized expertise that is beyond the scope of this chapter.

EVOLVING VIEWS OF FEMALE SEXUALITY

When I wrote the first edition of this book more than a decade ago, I asked a respected colleague in oncology to comment on the cancer prevention chapter. I also asked another respected female colleague in psychiatry to comment on the mental health chapter. They each laughed and said they only read the sex chapter. This was interesting to me, and it proved my theory that sex is an incredibly important topic to women of all ages. It's also a challenging topic to discuss.

To frame the discussion, I would like to briefly review different medical views of female sexuality as they developed historically. Initially, doctors and researchers used the Masters and Johnson model developed in the 1960s. This model was designed explain a four-stage sexual response in men and women. It was a linear model:

1. Interest, arousal, and excitement build.
2. Feelings plateau.
3. Orgasm occurs.
4. Feelings resolve, and arousal decreases.

Helen Singer Kaplan then modified the model and incorporated the component of sexual response to create a three-phase model with desire, excitement, and orgasm. In 2000, Dr. Rosemary Basson developed a circular model that experts agree better represents the female sexual response. Basson's circular model incorporates biological and psychological aspects of sexuality. Her model recognizes spontaneous sexual drive separate from sexual arousal, sexual stimuli, and emotional intimacy. The model also includes emotional and physical satisfaction. Basson's model allows that desire may not be the only prompt for sexual activity. Feelings of emotional intimacy with one's partner may lead to being more open to sexual stimulation. Basson's construct is also more complex, and offers more flexibility—it allows for the concept that sexual arousal and desire occur together and may come after sexual stimuli. Basson's insight is that arousal and desire do not need to occur to initiate sex and that sexual stimuli can get things going. For Basson, desire does not need to precede arousal. Research supports her framework.[1,2]

Why are these insights helpful? Researchers need a framework to study women's sexuality. They must start somewhere. Sexual behavior and sexual encounters vary between individuals and even in the same individual. Yet researchers and clinicians need to identify parameters to make comparisons and recommendations when interpreting results. The questions researchers ask women influence the answers and results they obtain.

In addition, aspects of different models may apply to different women at various times in their lives. For example, one study showed postmenopausal women are more likely to agree with the Basson model.[4] Additional research is needed for specific ethnic groups, different age groups, and individuals in the LGBTQ community. A few previous studies report that over time, women in same-sex relationships have better sexual function and satisfaction compared to heterosexual women.[5] Risk factors for sexual dysfunction in lesbian women and heterosexual women are similar: aging, relationship dissatisfaction, mood symptoms, and one partner wanting more sex than the other partner.

If a female's sexual function bothers them, then it is termed *female sexual dysfunction* (FSD). There is no dysfunction if an individual has a low sex drive or does not wish to have sex as often and it does not bother them. If an individual and their partner both agree not to have sex, there is no FSD or issue with that decision from a medical standpoint.

DID YOU KNOW?

Only issues about sexual function that bother you or cause you significant personal distress are considered medically concerning.

One study showed 43 percent of American women report a sexual problem, but only 12 percent of these women have sexual problems that cause them significant distress.[3] As women age, they are more likely to report sexual problems; however, these reports of sexual problems peak at midlife, then taper off.

Many individuals assume that sex will become painful and less pleasurable with age. In fact, for many women, sex becomes more pleasurable. The worries about an unplanned pregnancy are left behind. Typically, there are fewer responsibilities for young children and potentially less pressure on the job. All of this translates into less anxiety and more opportunities for fun. Part of this increased enjoyment of sex may stem from the fact that some women simply become more comfortable with themselves over time.

This chapter should reassure you that menopausal women do not have to suffer with "drying up" and having pain with intercourse. Many women enjoy intercourse in their postmenopausal years without pain or dryness. Although some women experience temporary decreases in their libido, research in this area is encouraging. In fact, researchers are finding women reporting more satisfaction with their sex lives after menopause than before.

The good news is that for most postmenopausal women, the sexual response is healthy and intact. Postmenopausal women are responsive. They can still enjoy orgasms if they were orgasmic before. They can learn to be more responsive if they so desire. Individuals' actual enjoyment of intercourse or being intimate need not diminish with post menopause. Women in their fifties, sixties, seventies, and beyond can (and do) enjoy a healthy sex life. This chapter is not intended to encourage self-diagnosis or treatment. It is an introduction to a complex topic and provides an overview of issues and questions that you may wish to discuss with your physician.

AGE-RELATED PHYSICAL CHANGES THAT CAN AFFECT SEX

Intermittently low levels of estrogen can cause changes that may affect sex, as can a long-term lack of estrogen. With lower levels of estrogen, there is less blood flow to the vagina. With less estrogen, the vagina becomes less acidic. Less acidity makes the vaginal tissues more susceptible to infection. Vaginal wall thickness and elasticity are also lost. Less lubrication is generated, and achieving lubrication during sexual activity takes longer. The vaginal tissues typically atrophy (thin). While the walls become thinner and dryer, the length of the vagina may become shallower, and the width may become narrower. More stimulation may be required to achieve arousal. Over time, response to vibration may be greater than to light touch. Less estrogen also affects the pelvic floor muscles and may lead to an increase in muscle tone that is responsible for deep pelvic pain.

THE IMPACT OF SOCIAL CONTEXT

If you are distressed by a change in sexual function, it is helpful to factor in changes in your social circumstances and, if you are comfortable, share them with your doctor. Consider these questions:

1. Do your children or grandchildren live with you?
2. Has there been a change in the quality of the relationship with your partner?
3. Has your partner experienced health changes?
4. Have there been changes in your health?
5. Have you experienced the loss or absence of your sexual partner?
6. Have you recently experienced financial strain? What about insomnia, depression, stress, or anxiety?

All these changes (and more) can affect your libido. Consider Tabitha's story.

Tabitha's Story
CONCERNED ABOUT HER LOSS OF LIBIDO

I am in my late 50s and work three jobs. I drink about 12 cups of coffee daily. My relationship with my partner of five years is good. In the last year, I noticed my sex drive is low, and this concerns me. It is an important part of my relationship with my partner, who is five years younger. My doctor assured me that low sexual desire is the most common sexual concern women report. I sleep less than six hours a night and never feel rested when I wake up. I have no downtime. I expected my gynecologist to prescribe a medication to restore my sex drive. Instead, they recommended lifestyle modifications. At first, I was not receptive. I wanted a pill to take, and I might even inject a medication like my friend did. When I thought about it more, I decided to try lifestyle modifications. I tapered my caffeine intake. I now sleep seven hours a night and wake up rested. I have built in some downtime, 30 minutes a day just for me—it is not much but it is more than I had. And finally, I decided to work two jobs, not three. After one month of the new routine, my sex drive started to re-emerge, and I told my doctor I would not need to bother with a pill or a shot to increase my sex drive.

Long-term lack of estrogen may also affect the central and peripheral nervous systems, changing your experience of sensation, touch, and vibration. This compromise in nerve function is more commonly seen in diabetics whose nerves are affected by their condition.

Other physical changes in post menopause include thinner skin over the clitoris. This offers less protection and can result in increased sensitivity of the clitoris. Loss of fat in the thickness of the vulva, or folds of skin outside of the vagina, occurs over decades. Pubic hair loss also occurs. The remaining pubic hair usually turns gray. The degree of these changes varies among individuals.

> **DID YOU KNOW?**
> A woman's physical health and well-being impacts her sexuality.

Fatigue, chronic pain, depression, limited mobility, and incontinence of urine or stool may also impact sexual health. Diabetes may affect autonomic nerve conduction and compromise genital sex response. Body image can be affected after a mastectomy or a hysterectomy. In addition, a woman's sex responses are negatively affected by a male partner's sexual dysfunction, such as premature ejaculation or inability to have an erection.

AGE-RELATED PHYSICAL CHANGES IN MEN (AND THE IMPACT OF THOSE CHANGES ON FEMALE PARTNERS)

As men age, they experience an increase in erectile dysfunction. Fortunately, there is no corresponding sexual dysfunction in women as they age, although there is a subtle decrease in desire with age and menopause. Despite the changes in women's genitalia with age (i.e., there is less volume of clitoral tissue and less vascularity in the vulva and vaginal areas), these changes do not usually correlate with sexual symptoms. The increase in congestion around the vagina in response to erotic stimulation is similar in women with and without estrogen.

There are now prescription medications to address erectile dysfunction, including Viagra and Cialis. But women do not automatically get an increase in sexual enjoyment and satisfaction when a male partner uses Viagra or Cialis. Using these therapies may result in less foreplay. Surveys questioning women in healthy marriages report foreplay as the most satisfying component of partner sex. If a woman has some genital atrophy and her partner uses Viagra, she may need more time for foreplay and stimulation prior to intercourse. Men who use Viagra to attain an erection can adjust the timing of taking the Viagra to match the needs of their partner. Viagra produces a rapid erection without allowing a female partner to have the time she needs to lubricate. One strategy for such couples is to encourage foreplay prior to the male partner taking Viagra. Couples may try to be intimate together first and allow time for the woman to enjoy foreplay prior to the man taking Viagra. This puts less pressure on the woman to have intercourse before she is well lubricated and ready. Otherwise, the woman is not likely to be satisfied with the sexual outcome.

The same strategy is advised for couples where the man has a penile implant to treat erectile dysfunction. Some men have erectile problems due to the medication they take to control high blood pressure. They may benefit from a new blood pressure medication that does not affect sexual function. A medical evaluation will define which options have the best chance of working.

Spending more time on foreplay is helpful. Different positions may be more comfortable or pleasurable. These include the woman positioning herself on top, next to, or in front of her partner so she can control the depth of penetration. Women's genital anatomy is not structured for maximum sexual stimulation with penile-vaginal intercourse, especially in the missionary position with the woman on the bottom and the man on the top. For most women, orgasm is most easily reached through direct vulvar stimulation, not by intercourse (in contrast, the neuroanatomy of men's genitals results in intercourse providing a very efficient way to stimulate the nerves around the tip of the penis).

FIVE CATEGORIES OF CHANGE IN SEXUAL HEALTH

There are five categories of female sexual health disturbances for which therapeutic strategies are available. These sexual health disturbances are recognized by medical professionals and have corresponding diagnostic codes that insurers recognize. Note the following five categories and proactive strategies to address them:

1. Low libido/low sexual desire
   - Consider off-label testosterone in low doses.

- Consider bupropion to treat depression instead of an selective serotonin reuptake inhibitor if the SSRI is causing low libido.
- Consider sex therapy and counseling.
- Identify medications that curb sex drive (e.g., certain antidepressants and certain blood pressure medications) and discuss alternative medications with your doctor.
- Identify turnoffs and how you can eliminate or address them.
- Take stock of your relationship.
- Try yoga to increase sexual desire.

2. Vaginal dryness and thinning
   - Ask your doctor to check your pelvic examination for signs of infection or sores or other physical findings that may explain your symptoms.
   - Participate in regular sexual activity or stimulation, including masturbation, to promote blood flow and vaginal health.
   - Ospemifene (Osphena) is an option to consider; it is taken by mouth daily.
   - Prasterone, vaginal DHEA (Intrarosa), is a vaginal insert used at bedtime every night to restore vaginal wall health.
   - Using low-dose vaginal estrogen as a cream, ring, or vaginal tablet typically restores vaginal health and eliminates thinning and dryness.
   - Use vaginal moisturizers regularly (but not during sex) to increase moisture.
   - Using a vaginal lubricant before or during intercourse offers some temporary relief and typically lowers the risk of vaginal tears.

3. Arousal difficulties

    If an individual has a lack of sexual interest or arousal or a significant reduction in sexual interest or arousal, their

doctor may ask if they have a decrease or absence of three of or more of the following:
- Erotic fantasies or thoughts
- Initiation of sexual activity or responding to a partner's attempts to initiate sex
- Pleasure and excitement
- Response to sexual cues
- Sensations during sex
- Sexual interest

Arousal difficulties may be addressed with:
- Off-label bupropion
- Off-label Viagra-like drugs to increase blood flow to the clitoris (not yet approved by the US Food and Drug Administration [FDA] for women for arousal difficulties in the United States)
- Sex therapy and counseling
- Topical treatments for vaginal dryness and atrophy discussed above
- Using a vibrator or other device
- Yoga

4. Pain during penetrative sex

Do you notice that your pelvic floor muscles tighten when your partner attempts vaginal penetration? Or do you have pain, burning, or tension when your partner attempts vaginal penetration? If you answered yes to one or both questions, do the symptoms persist or recur?

The approach to treating pain on penetration varies by the location and timing of the pain. Consider the following:
- Antibiotic pills or creams for vaginal infection
- Kegel exercises (Note: Ask your doctor or physical therapist to check and make sure you are performing Kegels correctly.)
- Low-dose vaginal estrogen or other prescription medication

- Pelvic floor physical therapy for deep pelvic pain or muscle spasms
- Prescription topical lidocaine gel applied at the vaginal opening 10 minutes before sex, which may decrease pain with penetration at the vaginal opening
- Sex therapy and counseling
- Vaginal dilators to gently stretch the opening over time
- Vaginal moisturizers and lubricants
- Yoga

5. Orgasm difficulties
    Consider the following questions:
    - Do you have orgasms that are less intense, occur less often, or take longer to achieve?
    - Do you notice a change in your orgasms 75 to 100 percent of the time?
    - Have you stopped having orgasms with intercourse? Will masturbating no longer produce an orgasm?

If you answer yes to any of these questions, talk to your doctor about how sex therapy, counseling, or yoga can help.[10,11,12,13]

Other aspects of your health history are important and may influence your sexual function, including your surgical history, the amount and quality of your sleep, depression and anxiety, your alcohol consumption, and any other substances you use besides prescription medications. If you feel unsafe in your current relationship, that should also be addressed. In addition to reviewing your medical and social histories, having a thorough pelvic exam is important for a doctor to identify physical changes that you may not feel or see yourself.

MEDICATIONS THAT CAN AFFECT SEX

ANTIBIOTICS

One common side effect of taking antibiotics is that you develop a yeast infection inside the vagina, outside the vagina, or both. Yeast infections can produce itching, burning, or irritation. The discomfort may occur days or even weeks after taking the medication. Yeast infections that are not detected or treated may cause vaginal dryness or discomfort with sex.

> DID YOU KNOW?
>
> If you have taken antibiotics in the past two months, you may be more susceptible to developing a yeast infection.

ANTIHISTAMINES

Prescription or over-the-counter antihistamines may cause dryness of the vaginal tissues and a dry mouth. Lubrication is reduced, causing pain with intercourse. Drying effects from antihistamines may also cause constipation, resulting in deep pain with intercourse.

BLOOD PRESSURE MEDICATIONS

Diuretics push fluid out of the blood vessels. Beta-blockers (such as atenolol) work by slowing the blood flow and reducing the pressure in the blood vessels. Both types of blood pressure medication may reduce blood flow to the pelvic organs enough to reduce sensation during sex or to suppress orgasms. Changing to a different type of blood pressure medication may result in a return to normal sexual arousal and orgasms.

ANTIDEPRESSANTS

In most studies, depression is tied to impaired sexual desire. Unfortunately, some antidepressants are also associated with sexual dysfunction and lack of sex drive. This paradox is frustrating. Fortunately, certain antidepressant medications will not disturb a healthy sex drive. You may find your sex drive dampened by one antidepressant but not by a sister medication in the same class. If changing to another antidepressant is not an option, some doctors recommend a "drug holiday" where you stop taking the antidepressant medication for the weekend to improve your sex drive and then resume taking it. This strategy must be used with a knowledgeable doctor since stopping certain antidepressants without medical supervision can produce severe side effects.

> **DID YOU KNOW?**
> Women with impaired desire are twice as likely to have a history of major depression. Chronic anxiety is also linked to impaired sexual function and low desire.

There are a variety of options to counteract a low sex drive related to taking an antidepressant. The sexual side effect of an antidepressant may occur with arousal, desire, or orgasm. One option is to use bupropion or mirtazapine as a first-choice medication for depression for those at risk for FSD. Sexual side effects are more common with certain selective serotonin reuptake inhibitors (e.g., paroxetine), serotonin-norepinephrine reuptake inhibitors (e.g., citalopram), and tricyclic antidepressants (such as amitriptyline [Elavil], desipramine [Norpranin], and nortriptyline [Pamelor]). Sexual side effects such as low libido are common on these medications and may improve after the first one to two weeks using the medication.

If the sexual side effects do not improve, additional medication (e.g., bupropion) may be added. Lifestyle modification can be used by introducing or increasing the amount of exercise or adding a new type of exercise. You can also schedule sexual activity, therapy, and/or vibration stimulation. If your arousal changes while you are on the medication, you may be a candidate to try sildenafil, testosterone, or acupuncture before changing to an antidepressant with a lower chance of sexual side effects.[9,10,11]

MEDICAL CONDITIONS THAT CAN AFFECT SEX

Sexual changes may be due to other changes in your health or personal situation. For example, sometimes a problem, such as a vaginal infection, can affect sex. Your doctor can easily diagnose and treat this during an office visit. Survivors of child abuse, rape, posttraumatic stress disorder, or chronic pelvic pain require longer-term treatment.

> DID YOU KNOW?
> Medical conditions affect the amount of energy you have for sex, your physical response during sex, and your physical comfort during sex.

RECTOCELE, CYSTOCELE, UTERINE, AND VAGINAL PROLAPSE

Loosening of the vaginal wall tissues, the uterus, or the bladder support is common in postmenopausal women and may influence their experience during sex. A gynecologic exam helps determine which organs have lost their natural support. Options to correct the problem include using a pessary to support the loose tissue or a surgical repair to restore the anatomy.

A newer option that is FDA approved for safety is radiofrequency treatment. Radiofrequency is gentle heat applied to the tissue behind the vaginal wall to increase the blood supply to the vaginal wall and increase collagen to support the wall. ThermiVA is an FDA-approved radiofrequency device to restore collagen and support of the vaginal tissues under the bladder (cystocele) and over the rectum (rectocele). ThermiVA may also increase support of the side walls of the vagina.[18]

ThermiVA was FDA approved for safety in 2015. ThermiVA uses ultrasound gel to protect the surface of the vagina while heating the tissue behind the surface. ThermiVA typically reduces a cystocele or rectocele and increases support of the entire vaginal wall by using heat to increase underlying collagen. If there is uterine prolapse, however, it is unlikely to have much impact: uterine prolapse is related to weak ligaments. Small studies have shown safety and effectiveness; larger, more long-term studies are needed. The initial series of radiofrequency treatments is typically three treatments spaced three to six weeks apart. The effects of radiofrequency treatment typically last 9 to 12 months. Then a single booster treatment maintains or restores the improvements. ThermiVA treatments are not associated with burns or adverse events. (Vaginal burns have been reported for laser treatments.)

OVARIAN CYSTS

Another cause of deep pain with sex is ovarian cysts. Ovarian cysts form regularly during the reproductive years when women are still menstruating. A small cyst forms during the middle of the menstrual cycle at the time of ovulation or egg formation. Another cyst forms just prior to the menstrual period itself. These types of cysts are referred to as physiologic, or cycle, cysts. These small cysts usually do not enlarge and are considered a variation of normal. They dissolve shortly after they form while the cyst is still small.

When a cyst gets too large or persists too long, it may cause pain. Some cysts develop abnormal features and no longer look clear and simple inside as a physiologic cyst would. These cysts may persist as tumors or even become cancerous. These must be watched carefully by a gynecologist or, in some cases, surgically removed. Consider Bathsheba's story.

Bathsheba's Story
PAINFUL OVARIAN CYST

I am 43 years old and have premature ovarian insufficiency. I stopped menstruating at age 35. My mother and sister also went into menopause early. I use low-dose vaginal estrogen to avoid painful sex, and it works well for me. My doctor encouraged me to also use systemic plant-derived estrogen and progesterone in a patch form to lower my risk of heart disease, stroke, and osteoporosis in addition to controlling my hot flashes and night sweats. So, I was surprised when I had pain while using a sex toy with my wife that was worse on my right side. I had my appendix removed in my twenties, so I did not understand why I would have pain there. The pain worsened over the next two hours, and my wife took me to the emergency room. When they did an ultrasound, they found a leaking ovarian cyst on the right. They told me the ovary looked healthy, and the clear fluid would reabsorb. They suggested ibuprofen for pain and a heating pad. The pain subsided, and I have felt well since.

DID YOU KNOW?

While postmenopausal women are not expected to bleed or cycle, they may still form ovarian cysts.

BARTHOLIN GLAND CYST

Another cause of initial pain or discomfort with sex is a Bartholin gland cyst. This is a swelling of the lower vulva, the skin just outside the vaginal opening. The gland deep in this skin may get blocked off. When a cyst forms, it may fill with fluid, become painful, and cause a partial blockage. The cyst may cause pain when sex is initiated and at other times. If it enlarges enough, it can even make walking or sitting uncomfortable. A Bartholin gland cyst can become infected, requiring antibiotics and, at times, drainage in a doctor's office or emergency room. A gynecologist can tell if it needs to be drained to release the fluid or to control the infection. A doctor can prevent the cyst from recurring by using a simple surgical technique called marsupialization.

SKIN CHANGES OF THE VULVA

Another common cause of pain or discomfort with sex in women over age 40 is skin changes of the vulva. Thinning of the skin, raised or thick areas, or white or red color changes may be found on exam. Types of discomfort that may be attributed to these changes include dryness, itching, or burning. Many of these types of skin changes will be diagnosed as vulvar dystrophies such as lichen sclerosis, discussed in chapter 6. Other changes of the vulva skin (e.g., eczema or psoriasis) may echo changes elsewhere on the body. For many women, yeast infections will also produce red itchy changes of the vulva in addition to vaginal discharge.

DIABETES

Whether you are slender, average weight, or over your ideal weight, you may develop diabetes. Diabetics are predisposed to yeast infections inside and outside the vagina. Dryness, burning, itching, and actual pain during sex may result. Women with long-term diabetes may have less blood flow to the pelvic organs. Your doctor can diagnose diabetes by checking your blood sugar level or testing your urine for sugar. Diabetes runs in families but also occurs in those who do not have a family history of diabetes.

THYROID PROBLEMS

As you read in chapter 2, thyroid problems are more common in women than in men, and thyroid disease is more common with increasing age. When thyroid function becomes overactive or underactive, it affects metabolism and sex drive as well as lubrication. Once the thyroid gland abnormality is diagnosed and treated, the related problems usually resolve. Body weight can normalize over time, sex drive may return to normal, and the rest of the body rebalances.

URINARY PROBLEMS

A urinary tract infection can cause pain with sex. Once treated, the problem resolves. Women who leak urine when they laugh or cough may also leak urine during sex. The approaches to this problem are discussed in chapter 6.

VAGINAL INFECTION

As you read in Chapter 6, distinct kinds of infections can cause vaginal discomfort and pain with sex. It is important to have a doctor check for a vaginal infection and treat it before assuming that you have pain with sex due to vaginal dryness.

CONSTIPATION

The most common cause of deep pain with sex is constipation. The intestines surround the pelvic organs. A large stool can back up and cause pressure and pain in the pelvic organs. Even if you move your bowels every one to three days, you may still suffer from a large amount of backed-up stool pressing in your pelvis, especially if your colon or intestinal tract is large.

Sufficient water intake daily is more important than ever. You may avoid drinking water to stop running to the bathroom too frequently or at an inconvenient time. There are ways to work around this. If you have trouble with urination, either urinating too frequently or not being able to make it to the bathroom on time, you can train your bladder to work more efficiently (see chapter 6). Try drinking 48 to 64 ounces (about 1.89 L) of water a day. Additional water might be needed if you exercise, live in a warm climate, or are taller or more muscular.

Coffee and sodas are bladder irritants and may force the bladder to empty prematurely or more often. Try to get most of your fluids as water. If you like carbonated drinks, look for seltzer with no sugar, salt, or artificial sweetener.

Exercise can provide dramatic relief from constipation or backed-up stool. Be certain to drink adequate fluids daily to get the full benefit in eliminating the bulk of the stool.

A high-fiber diet is helpful. Many Western diets have less than 10 grams of fiber a day, while an ideal amount is 20 to 30 grams. Most processed foods have little fiber. Fruits and vegetables eaten raw or cooked have good fiber content. Fruit juice does not have fiber because the fruit's natural fiber is removed during processing. Brown rice, whole-grain products, and beans have a healthy amount of fiber. You may also use a product like Konsyl, Per Diem, Metamucil, or Citrucel. Use these as directed, and make sure to drink extra water. Otherwise, these products will not be effective. Try them for six weeks or more and then continue if you have relief.

Avoid regular laxative use. Laxatives are not a healthy long-term alternative and can cause problems when they are stopped.

The bulk agents in dietary fiber and the over-the-counter products listed above draw water into the colon to move the stool in a healthy way. Do not be concerned that these agents may cause diarrhea. They seldom do. Even those with irritable bowel syndrome or those who alternate between diarrhea and constipation can usually use these bulk agents without problems. Consult your doctor if you are unsure.

VAGINAL DRYNESS

Many causes of dryness are not related to age or menopause. The good news is that these causes are treatable. Estrogen may provide relief to those women who do not have other causes for their discomfort, but not every woman must take estrogen to continue to have enjoyable sex in menopause.

The first step is to have a gynecologic history and exam to identify the reasons for the dryness. This is not an area for self-diagnosis. There are many causes of vaginal dryness and many effective treatments once the specific cause is identified. An expert examination will go a long way to helping you address the problem that you have, not the problem you think you have.

> **DID YOU KNOW?**
> The first thing that comes to a woman's mind when she experiences vaginal dryness is, "I am drying up; it must be age." Fortunately, that is not always the case. And if it is, it can be addressed. Vaginal dryness due to age, menopause, or both can be treated.

If the cause of your dryness is a vaginal infection or a reaction to a scented hygiene product, you can expect to return to your normal level of lubrication after the infection is treated or the hygiene routine is modified. You can become sensitive to certain products even if you used them without problems when you were younger. Eliminating the use of scented soaps, dryer sheets, and fabric softener may reduce irritation and dryness outside the vagina and at the vaginal opening. On the other hand, if the dryness is due to perimenopause or postmenopausal estrogen deficiency, there are many safe options for you to consider.

Vaginal dryness or discomfort with intercourse is a problem that may begin during perimenopause, but it more commonly surfaces during post menopause, especially when months or years go by without intercourse. Intercourse or masturbation twice a week may maintain vaginal lubrication and vaginal health without the need for supplemental estrogen. If you have intercourse on a regular basis, you may not notice dramatic changes that produce dryness or discomfort, even if you do not take estrogen. Extended periods of abstinence may make the changes more pronounced, but they are still reversible. Consider Lorinda's story.

Lorinda's Story
NEW-ONSET VAGINAL DRYNESS

I am a 54-year-old widow and had not has sex for three years. My last menstrual period occurred when I was 51. Recently, I started seeing someone. When my new male partner and I tried to have sex, I had pain and dryness. Even with lubricant I could not get comfortable. When I saw my doctor, they said I have two problems. First, my vaginal opening had narrowed so there was a mismatch at the start of intercourse. Second, my vagina became very dry with no estrogen and no intercourse for three years. They recommended low-dose vaginal estrogen twice a week at bedtime in addition to a lubricant for the dryness. I had a choice of a cream or vaginal tablet. I was concerned about breast cancer, but my doctor said the vaginal estrogen levels are so low they do not appear in the blood and do not cause breast cancer. For the narrow opening, my doctor prescribed vaginal dilators that have a flat bottom. They are made of silicone and look like dildoes with a flat bottom. I was advised to sit on them daily for at least 30 minutes and more if possible. When the dilator gets loose, I use the next size if I am comfortable. It took four months for my vagina to feel normal again and to have intercourse with no discomfort. My doctor said it may take even longer for some women.

If no other cause of vaginal discomfort is identified, over-the-counter preparations to decrease friction during intercourse are helpful. A water-soluble lubricant is one excellent option. Other options include silicone-based products to reduce friction during intercourse. Some women elect to use coconut oil. Examples of vaginal lubricants sold over the counter are Astroglide, Lubrin, Slippery Stuff, Uberlube, and K-Y Jelly. When used at the time of intercourse, these lubricants often decrease pain or discomfort. Avoid Vaseline. Do not use hand cream or other products containing perfume or alcohol because they may damage the vaginal wall tissues. Vaginal lubricants may be used even if you are using other products to moisturize (e.g., estrogen cream), but do not apply the lubricant and other product at the same time. Estrogen cream for vaginal use is not a vaginal lubricant and should not be used during intercourse, but only at bedtime.

Vaginal Moisturizers

Vaginal moisturizers are used regularly to restore the thickness, elasticity, and moisture of the vaginal wall tissues. Moisturizers are not designed for use during sex. They work at other times to promote healthy vaginal wall tissues. Examples of over-the-counter moisturizers include Replens, RepHresh, and K-Y Long-Lasting Vaginal Moisturizer. In addition, there are now hyaluronic acid-based moisturizers that help the vaginal walls hold more moisture without using vaginal hormones. Options in the hyaluronic acid group include HyaloGyn and Revaree. All vaginal moisturizers just listed, including the hyaluronic acid-based preparations, are safe for individuals who are not sensitive to any of the ingredients. They are also safe for cancer survivors. You may find adequate relief with the use of a vaginal moisturizer or require prescription estrogen, Prasterone, or Ospemifene to get adequate relief and comfort.

Hormones for Vaginal Dryness

Women who take estrogen in pill form, as a skin patch, or as a lotion may or may not also require vaginal estrogen, lubricants, or moisturizers. Regardless of whether you use systemic estrogen, you may benefit from low-dose vaginal estrogen at some point in your life. If you feel dry or are uncomfortable urinating, are prone to frequent urinary tract infections, or have itching in the vagina not associated with a local infection, you may get relief with low-dose vaginal estrogen. On exam, your gynecologist can detect the degree of vaginal dryness or elasticity of the vagina by doing a simple speculum exam in the office and correlating this with your medical history and your report of comfort during sex and at other times. While the degree of discomfort you experience may match the physical findings of a medical pelvic examination, the discomfort may not match the physical exam findings. At times, I see women who are uncomfortable and feel quite dry, but their vaginal walls do not yet show severe changes of menopause. On other occasions, I see women who are not troubled by more than mild occasional discomfort or dryness, but the changes on their physical examination suggest they will have worse symptoms sooner than later. Consider Trina's story.

Trina's Story
MISMATCH BETWEEN SYMPTOMS AND THE PHYSICAL EXAM

I am 64 years old and newly remarried. I rarely have any discomfort with sex. Usually using a lubricant during sex does the trick. I did not see a need for any unnecessary medication. I was divorced, then single for 10 years before marrying my second husband. My gynecologist told me they saw menopausal changes and is concerned I will start having pain with sex if I do not use low-dose vaginal estrogen. I was not convinced since I feel well. We talked about alternatives. I agreed to use a nonhormonal vaginal moisturizer containing hyaluronic acid twice a week regularly and consistently using a lubricant for intercourse. After six months, I feel well and have no discomfort with sex or any other time. I agreed to reconsider low-dose vaginal estrogen if I become prone to frequent urinary tract infections or develop more severe discomfort.

If vaginal thinning has taken place, local estrogen restores the elasticity, strength, and moisture of the vaginal walls. Estrogen for this purpose is now available in a vaginal tablet, a vaginal insert, a cream, and a ring. Once the vaginal walls are healthier, some women can maintain their own vaginal health over time, even without continuing to use estrogen. Others continue to benefit from vaginal estrogen use. Vaginal estrogen has fewer side effects than estrogen taken by mouth or other routes and does not produce a significant blood level of estrogen. Vaginal estrogen prescribed for vaginal dryness or pain does not cause dementia, breast cancer, heart attacks, strokes or blood clots. Unfortunately, the package insert does mention these risks even though they apply only to women taking systemic estrogen designed to give them a blood level of estrogen.

Vaginal Tablets

After an initial nightly dose for two weeks, low-dose vaginal tablets are typically inserted into the vagina with an applicator twice a week (Monday and Thursday) at bedtime. These vaginal tablets improve the quality and function of vaginal wall tissue. Vaginal tablets are available by prescription (Vagifem, Yuvafem, and estradiol 10 mcg). They come with an individual applicator to use for each insertion.

There are also low-dose vaginal estrogen inserts available in two low doses, 4 mcg and 10 mcg. These inserts have a similar dosing regimen to vaginal tablets. You insert them at bedtime. No applicator is needed, and the insert may be placed in the lower third of the vagina at bedtime (Imvexxy 4 mcg and 10 mcg).

The newest option for a vaginal insert is vaginal prasterone (Intrarosa). Prasterone contains the hormone DHEA, dehydroepiandrosterone, that is processed by the vaginal walls (not the liver) and broken down into low-dose estrogen and testosterone locally in the vagina. Levels of these hormones are low in the vagina and do not produce significant levels of estrogen or testosterone in the blood. Prasterone (Intrarosa) is inserted every night at bedtime. It is not a lubricant and is not designed to be used before intercourse. Rapid improvement may be seen in women who use prasterone in the vagina every night. It is not necessary to balance a low dose of vaginal estrogen with progesterone as it has not been associated with a thick uterine lining or uterine cancer. Prasterone does not have a black box warning in the FDA information packet, but it is metabolized locally to estrogen and testosterone. If you are a breast cancer survivor or have another estrogen-dependent cancer in your history, consult with your oncologist.[14]

Low-Dose Vaginal Estrogen Cream

Vaginal estrogen cream is available by prescription. It is placed in the vagina with an applicator at bedtime. It typically restores elasticity to the vaginal lining tissue and eliminates vaginal dryness over time. If you had pelvic radiation or have spent many years without estrogen from your ovaries or hormone therapy, it will take longer to restore vaginal lubrication.

Several types of prescription-strength estrogen creams are available. Your doctor will advise you regarding how much to use based on your history and examination. They will also tell you how often to use the cream. At times, you may bleed or get irritated from the tip of the plastic applicator. If this happens, see whether your doctor recommends applying the cream with clean fingers until the vaginal walls get stronger and until you can use the applicator without discomfort. Be sure to tell your gynecologist about any vaginal bleeding, especially if you take estrogen. Consider Hagit's story.

Hagit's Story
UNCOMFORTABLE WITH REASSURING EXAM

I am 31 years old with premature ovarian insufficiency. Early menopause runs in my family. My menstrual periods stopped two years ago. My doctor put me on a birth control pill to lower my risk of premature heart disease, but I still feel dry. My vaginal dryness affects my ability to exercise. It is just so uncomfortable. Sex is unpleasant even with lubricant. My doctor said the vaginal tissues look normal, and the physical changes of menopause are minimal so far. Since my symptoms are severe, they prescribed a low-dose vaginal estrogen cream. My wife read the package insert and did not want me to use the cream even though it would help me feel better and improve our sex life. I called my doctor. They explained that the package insert for low-dose vaginal estrogen is not accurate. It is the same black box warning included for systemic estrogen, but it does not apply to low-dose vaginal estrogen. Low-dose vaginal estrogen does not get absorbed into the body enough to raise the level of estrogen in the bloodstream. If they measured my blood estrogen level after using low-dose vaginal estrogen, it would not be elevated and would not increase my risk of breast cancer. After I shared this information with my wife, we both decided using low-dose vaginal estrogen made sense. After two months of using it, I felt like myself again, could exercise comfortably, and sex was no longer painful.

Vaginal Ring

Your doctor may prescribe vaginal estrogen in the form of Estring, a silastic ring that releases small doses of estrogen slowly to the vaginal tissues over 24 hours, seven days a week, for three months while the ring is left in place. This soft plastic ring sits inside the vagina, away from the opening. It slowly releases a small amount of estrogen into the vaginal wall tissues. The amount of estrogen is so small that it does not get into your bloodstream. For most women, the Estring vaginal ring is a safe alternative even if they have had breast cancer or have other reasons not to take estrogen in other forms. The estrogen ring is available through your gynecologist by prescription. After you have a medical exam, your doctor will insert the ring. They will also recheck it within the first two weeks to ensure there are no ulcers or sores under or behind it. Once this initial check has taken place, you can insert a new ring yourself every three months. Alternatively, your doctor or other clinician can change it for you. The Estring ring stays in place during intercourse. You can use it as your only form of estrogen or in conjunction with estrogen by mouth or in patch form. Many women prefer the estrogen vaginal ring to vaginal creams because there is no leakage of cream.

The estrogen ring is a breakthrough for many women who have survived breast cancer or other estrogen-sensitive cancers. The estrogen ring offers local delivery of estrogen while protecting the rest of the body from receiving any significant amounts of estrogen. Postmenopausal women who do not take estrogen often have a blood level of 20 picograms per milliliter of estrogen. Studies of women using Estring show blood levels are also 20 picograms per milliliter and not elevated due to Estring usage. In view of this, some gynecologists, surgeons, and oncologists are comfortable prescribing Estring for breast cancer survivors who have vaginal dryness and pain with intercourse because their blood levels of estrogen remain low with this dose and form of estrogen. The common exception is if you take an aromatase inhibitor, such as letrozole or anastrozole, designed to eliminate even tiny amounts of estrogen from your system. In this case, your oncologist may not approve a prescription for Estring or another low-dose vaginal estrogen until you have finished taking the aromatase inhibitor medication. The goal of taking the aromatase inhibitor is to eliminate all estrogen in the body, so introducing estrogen in the vagina, even in low doses, is frowned upon by oncologists.

Oral Medication for Vaginal Dryness

One oral medication is FDA approved to treat vaginal dryness: ospemifene (Osphena). It is a selective estrogen receptor modulator, or designer estrogen. In this case, estrogen is modified so it does not increase the risk of breast or uterine cancer. While it acts only in the vagina, it may cause a slight increased risk of developing deep vein blood clots in the legs or lungs. But the actual increased risk is small (i.e., the increase is less than 1 case of blood clots in 1,000 women per year, less risk than the risk of blood clots during a normal pregnancy). Ospemifene may not be taken with oral or transdermal estrogens.

LIFESTYLE FACTORS THAT AFFECT SEX

Ask a friend or partner: What is the most important female sex organ? Even medical professionals often answer this question incorrectly. Contrary to popular belief, it's not the clitoris or G spot. The most important female sex organ is the brain. What you think and how you feel about yourself and your partner (if you have one) influences your sexual experience.

> DID YOU KNOW?
> The most important female sex organ is the brain—not the clitoris or G spot.

Many aspects of your life will affect your attitude toward sex, your motivation to have sex, and your physical experience when you do have sex. Analyzing these factors is a complex process. Our understanding of what contributes to sexual experience is still developing. This is an exceedingly difficult subject to research, as women vary widely in their experiences and expectations. Currently, there is a great emphasis placed on hormone levels, including estrogen and testosterone, but the key to sex in post menopause goes beyond achieving an optimal balance of hormone levels. These are other key areas that influence female sexuality, including the following:

- Alcohol. Alcohol loosens inhibitions, relaxes us, and makes it easier to enjoy sex. Ironically, alcohol also chemically dampens sex drive and decreases sexual responsiveness. Finally, alcohol disturbs deep sleep. Less quality rest leads to a lower libido and compromised sex drive.
- Personal time. Do you have any? A hectic schedule with no private time or couple time is not conducive to a healthy and

pleasurable sexual experience, particularly in perimenopause and post menopause. Changes in your routine can affect your sex drive or motivation to have sex.
- Physical exercise. Exercise enhances blood flow throughout the body, including the pelvic area. Exercise also decreases stress by releasing endorphins, the "feel-good" hormones. If exercise came in pill form, doctors would prescribe it for every patient in post menopause, including those with decreased libido. Exercising regularly will enhance your sex drive as well as your sexual experience. The exercise program does not have to be a formal one. Gardening, walking, and even housework can be part of your exercise routine. (For more information, see chapter 12.)
- High stress levels. Individuals with high stress levels and busy schedules with no downtime may find it challenging to maintain or restore their libido. Some unscheduled time or time for self-care for reflection may help. Keeping a diary or tracking how you spend your time each day for a day or two may be a revelation, and the insights you gain may prove helpful. It may be possible to reclaim some time you currently commit to projects or other people and use it for yourself and your relationship instead.

SEEKING MEDICAL CARE WITH CONCERNS ABOUT SEX

When seeking medical care with concerns about sex, it is helpful to organize your thoughts beforehand. List any medications you take, including the dosages, and note how long you have been on each medication. Also, think about these questions:

- Are you experiencing muscle spasms due to fear, anxiety, or anticipation of pain?
- Can you pinpoint the specific change that has happened?
- Do you enjoy sex when you have it but no longer want to initiate sex with your partner?

- Do you have physical discomfort or pain in your abdomen, pelvis, or joints?
- Do you not want to have sex?
- Do you notice a difference in your sex drive?
- How long have you been noticing a change in your sex life?
- If so, is it during foreplay, initial penetration, or deep penetration?
- Is the pain triggered by certain positions and not others?
- Is there pain or discomfort during sex?
- Is your desire or motivation to have sex waning?

These questions may be embarrassing or difficult to consider. But your doctor needs to have this information to help pinpoint what is causing your problem so they can address your concerns. Consider writing down your questions or concerns before your doctor's visit so you do not forget them. That way, you can hand the doctor the written questions at the start of your visit or refer to them during your visit.

If your doctor feels they are not the best person to evaluate these problems, you may be referred to another specialist. Depending on your doctor's specialty and training, they may use a formal questionnaire, their clinical judgment, or both to assess your concerns while trying to pinpoint which areas of sexual function are relevant to designing a helpful approach.

Different areas of concern suggest different medical approaches. Is desire or motivation for sex affected, or has arousal or the physical response to stimulation changed? Ability to achieve orgasm and satisfaction is another key area in addition to physical comfort during sex. Issues of pain or lubrication are fully evaluated using findings on pelvic examination and your personal history.[10,12]

DID YOU KNOW?

Even though pain during sex is a separate issue from sex drive, they are intertwined.

If your sex drive is initially intact, but you experience pain rather than pleasure with sex, your sex drive will suffer. Expect a time delay even after the cause of the pain is treated. It takes time for the brain to process that there is no longer going to be pain with sex. After the brain has reprogrammed, and there is consistently no more pain with sex, pleasurable sex can return.

Whether your concern is how to maintain your sex drive and sexual function or how to enhance or improve your sexual function, it is important to schedule regular gynecologic exams. This will enable you and your gynecologist to be certain that you are physically healthy. If changes do occur in your body, your doctor can help you to address them early before the changes become more severe. As current information is available, you and your physician can talk about what is best for you to maintain a healthy body that functions well for you.

HOW INTERESTED ARE YOU IN SEX?

Libido, or sex drive, does not necessarily diminish with age. As the North American Menopause Study (now The Menopause Society) showed, most women in their fifties, sixties, and seventies are delighted or at least satisfied with their sex drive and sexual function.

A British researcher recently found that for women, libido decreases after the first two years of a relationship regardless of a woman's age. A 60-year-old woman in a new relationship will have an intact sex drive for the first two years of that relationship, just as she would if she were 30. Despite this research, there are women with long-term partners who remain delighted or satisfied with their sex drive and sexual function in their fifties and well beyond.

Be ready to adjust your expectations of your spontaneous sex drive during the perimenopausal years. Researchers tell us that women should adjust their expectations of what a normal female sex drive looks and feels like before, during, and after menopause. One author suggests that women should not expect to "get horny" as frequently as they might have in their twenties or early thirties.

Women often retain the ability to enjoy sex once it is initiated. Those women who were orgasmic prior to post menopause continue to be orgasmic. For this group of women, the enjoyment of sex remains the same once they get going. The difference is that their motivation lags, and they are less likely to initiate sex. Experts suggest that you plan to have sex. Waiting to feel motivated in your mature years may leave you without sexual experiences. Here is an analogy I use with my patients:

Are you always hungry when you make reservations to go out for dinner? Not necessarily. During perimenopause and post menopause, you may want to "schedule" sex with your partner just as you would make dinner reservations in advance. If sex has been a welcome part of your relationship, do not wait for spontaneous opportunities to arise or until you are in the mood. While it is still terrific to have spontaneous sex if you are in the mood, don't count on that alone. Scheduling sex with your partner, even if the biologic urge is dormant, may help you weather perimenopause and early post menopause.

If you experience pain or discomfort, see your gynecologist to identify physical changes that may be diagnosed and treated. If you have a partner with a medical or physical condition that imposes limitations on your sexual activity, be open to other forms of sexual experience that do not include intercourse itself for a brief time or as a long-term approach.

LOWER LIBIDO

For women, two factors predict whether sex will be a satisfying experience: feelings for their partner at the time of the sexual interaction and emotional well-being. Typically, men do not operate the same way and may have a wider disconnect between their feelings, emotional well-being, and sexual function at times. For example, when women experience chronic stress or lack of sleep, they may lose their sex drive. In fact, lack of sexual responsiveness may be a normal, adaptive response. This means women may be able to improve sexual function by addressing their emotions and the negative aspects of their environment. In the past, clinicians and researchers tried to pinpoint a biological or psychological cause of sexual dysfunction. It is important to look at environmental stresses and how they impact a woman's physiology to see whether the environment is conducive to a positive sexual encounter.

Especially during perimenopause and post menopause, women may not engage in sex for reasons of desire. It is not clear whether changing hormone levels are the cause of this temporary dampening. Lack of desire may be a consequence of stress, lack of private time with a partner, lack of exercise, or lack of personal time. Family pressures or illness of a parent, relative, or friend may influence sex drive or experiences. Financial pressures, empty nest syndrome, or caring for grandchildren may dampen sexual desire or enjoyment. Still, other menopausal women are inhibited by the presence of teenagers or adult children in the house. The good news is that the stimuli and context of the occasion can change a woman's neutral sexual stance to a responsive one. An individual's view of themselves is also a factor. Some may feel old or undesirable over time. Others may have unrealistic expectations of what is sexually appealing to their partner, judge themselves, and feel that they are falling short. Some individuals are more critical of their appearance than their partner is. Physical changes that bother an individual may not be important to their partner. Based on conversations with my patients, I find these questions helpful to ask yourself:

- Are you bored?
- Do you have a critical or unsupportive partner?
- Do you lack stimulation or variety in your routine?
- Is your partner verbally or physically abusive?

If you are comfortable discussing these issues with your doctor, they may suggest other experts or resources to help you address them.

Remain open to the other aspects of your health that impact your sex drive and sexual function, such as regular exercise, adequate hydration with water, and enough rest and relaxation with a reprieve from stress. Allow more time for vaginal lubrication to take place. Monitor your overall health. Sleep deprivation, common with hot flashes or night sweats, will make you more irritable and may affect your sex drive.

What concerns you more—changes in your sex drive or discomfort during sex? The more specifically you can pinpoint your concerns, the more readily your doctor can determine the questions to ask. Your doctor can also provide a more targeted physical exam and decide what tests, if any, to order. If your doctor cannot address all your questions, they will refer you to colleagues who can address them.

> DID YOU KNOW?
>
> Enhancing the quality of sex in a relationship cannot be separated from enhancing the quality of the relationship itself. This becomes even more important in the menopausal years.

The physical and psychological changes that individuals experience in their forties, fifties, and sixties are different from those they had in their twenties and thirties. Some partners no longer sleep in the same room. They evolve away from intimacy, and their ties with each other are no longer close physically or emotionally. In the past, women in this circumstance would be labeled as having a problem with sex. Now, with a broader understanding, it is viewed as a problem with the relationship and intimacy, not just a problem with sex.

In the menopausal years, several aspects of the relationship become more important. The quality of emotional intimacy is more critical. There may be fewer work and family distractions than there are for younger couples. Each partner may find it helpful to maintain some independence while still staying connected as a couple, and each needs the ability to manage stress.

For example, I have worked with traditional female homemakers married to a husband who works outside the home. In that role, the homemaker may enjoy the support of her friends and volunteer activities. When the husband retires and is home full-time, away from his network of work associates, he may demand more of her time. As a result, the wife may not be able to access her friends. This can tax the relationship and cause imbalance as each person in the couple no longer has the same routine with colleagues or friends. This same scenario could play out similarly with a stay-at-home father and a spouse who works outside the home or a same-sex couple.

Some couples, whether same-sex or heterosexual couples, enjoy being empty nesters and find that adult children and/or grandchildren returning to live at home "cramps their style." Each of these factors contributes to the quality of the sexual relationship. A woman's expectations of herself and her partner may not be realistic. Studies have shown that having a youthful body is not required to have enjoyable sex. Pressuring oneself to attain a "normal" frequency of sexual intercourse is also damaging. Such norms do not exist. Furthermore, they should be irrelevant to you.

> **DID YOU KNOW?**
>
> Although sex continues to be a part of many mature couples' relationships, it is not a part of every healthy relationship. If a woman and her partner are content without having sex, that is fine. Having sex once a month, once a year, or less often is fine if that works for both partners.

Some individuals are motivated to have sex but do not have a partner. They may choose to masturbate. Still, other women are in a relationship with someone who has medical problems or a disability that precludes them from having penetrative sex. They may be open to different forms of intimacy and adjust by expanding their sexual repertoire. Options to consider include massages, caressing, mutual masturbation, oral sex, and taking baths or showers together. This reduces the pressure on both individuals to have penetrative vaginal sex and maintains closeness and intimacy.

For women, feelings about their partner and pleasure are paramount. Concern about the physical sexual response has less influence on a woman's views on sex than her perception of the relationship and the pleasure she derives from it in a multitude of areas. Brain studies that image women during sexual arousal show that areas in the brain responsible for emotional response and cognitive appraisal are activated separately from areas that perceive genital responses. Women's physical response does not necessarily correlate with their subjective arousal. This differs from similar studies in men.

For most women, sexual desire itself is not a frequent reason to engage in partnered sexual activity. Instead, reasons women cite include increasing emotional closeness to their partner and enhancing their sense of well-being. Women can enter a sexual experience feeling neutral but willing to become aroused. Well into the experience, they may then feel sexual desire. If the experience is enjoyable and the outcome is rewarding, women will find it satisfying.

Motivation to have sex and the mental processing of sexual stimuli are influenced by the larger context of a woman's life and the immediate potential sexual experience. Longer-term menopausal studies emphasize the importance of a woman's feelings for her partner in influencing her sexual appetite and responsiveness. Relationships with others and the demands of those relationships, as well as her feelings about them, also influence her sexual experience and frequency, as do society's standards.

If your emotional well-being is compromised, it is a strong predictor that you will have sexual stress. Worry, anxiety, low self-esteem, and guilt are all emotions and experiences that dampen sexual response and desire. Addressing these areas may enhance your sex life.

Your sexual pleasure is also influenced by the expectations you have of your relationship. A sexually exclusive relationship has been found to be important to both men and women in a long-term relationship. It is tied to their emotional satisfaction and their physical pleasure from sex. A woman who expects her relationship to last indefinitely has more emotional satisfaction with sex.

MEDICATIONS TO IMPROVE LOW SEX DRIVE

Many women seek a "magic pill" that will restore their sex drive. Wouldn't it be wonderful if there truly were such a pill? In fact, most women do not need to resort to this. Researchers find that some women who have intercourse regularly maintain vaginal health after perimenopause. They do not necessarily need hormones or other medications to enjoy sex. There are circumstances, however, where hormones may be helpful.

TESTOSTERONE

This male hormone is made in every ovary, even during post menopause, when the ovary stops making estrogen. Another source of testosterone in healthy women is the adrenal glands, positioned on top of each kidney. The production of testosterone by the adrenal glands is not affected by the ovary's production of testosterone. Enzymes in the skin also convert other hormones into testosterone.

Testosterone influences sex drive and motivation, but it is not the only influence. Circumstances, relationship issues, comfort during sex, stress levels, outlook, and many other forces influence sex drive.

Testosterone can be measured in the saliva or blood. Methods for measuring testosterone vary greatly and cannot be reliably compared to each other. Testosterone is difficult to measure accurately regardless of the testing method. As a result, normal levels of testosterone in healthy perimenopausal and postmenopausal women are not well established.

Adding testosterone improves sex drive in some women, but side effects of excess testosterone may include the following:

- Increase in hair growth on the face, chest, or belly
- Male-pattern balding
- Painful enlargement of the clitoris
- Weight gain

In addition, a woman's voice may become permanently lower from using testosterone, making it an unacceptable choice for some.

Although testosterone is touted for its ability to revive one's sex drive, the FDA has not approved it for this purpose in women. In the past, testosterone was only approved for treating severe hot flashes that did not respond to estrogen replacement. Therefore, if your doctor prescribes testosterone in a pill, patch, or cream form to enhance your sex drive, they are prescribing it off-label, meaning not for its original intended use. If your doctor is comfortable prescribing testosterone, it should be used as 1/10th the male dose. Less than one fingertip of testosterone ointment can be applied to the vulva, and some doctors prescribe it to enhance sex drive. Newer guidelines from The Menopause Society recommend doctors check blood levels of testosterone to avoid toxicity.[6,7,8]

> **DID YOU KNOW?**
> It is important that a woman have enough estrogen in her system when she is taking testosterone. Testosterone is not effective if a woman is lacking estrogen.

Women with elevated cholesterol or abnormal liver function should avoid taking testosterone by mouth. It can cause liver damage and worsen lipid levels. Doctors can check liver function and cholesterol blood tests before prescribing oral testosterone.

Women with normal cholesterol levels and liver tests who elect to try testosterone should continue to monitor their cholesterol and liver function to ensure they are not adversely affected. Those who develop abnormal blood levels of cholesterol will be advised to stop testosterone. At present, there is not much research on the long-term use of oral testosterone beyond three years. More information about safety is needed.

Dr. Jan Shifren, a clinical researcher and menopause specialist, published her findings about testosterone patches in the *New England Journal of Medicine*. First, she studied women who had complete hysterectomies and removal of both ovaries with the uterus. These women reported improved sex drive, improved sexual response, and a better sense of well-being after using testosterone patches. Subsequently, she published her study of the testosterone patch improving sex drive for women who still have their own uteruses and at least one ovary. The women ranged from age 40 to 70 and were distressed about their lack of desire. They reported improved sexual function, frequency, and drive after using a testosterone patch.[6]

The testosterone patch has been reviewed by the FDA but still has not been approved for use in treating low libido in women. Although women benefit from much lower doses of testosterone than their male counterparts, testosterone patches at low strengths suitable for women are not yet available.

Topical testosterone creams can be applied to the outer genital area to increase sex drive. Specialized pharmacists can compound these creams with a doctor's prescription. Well-controlled medical studies have not been done, and there is no proof that this cream is effective. In tiny amounts, the cream is unlikely to affect your voice, your cholesterol levels, or your blood liver tests. One known side effect of testosterone cream is painful clitoral enlargement.

Testosterone can be compounded with petrolatum (like petroleum jelly) to produce an ointment that can be rubbed into the clitoris and vulva to enhance sexual response. We do not have studies on large numbers of women to assess how well this works and what doses are most helpful.

In Europe and Canada, a more specialized form of testosterone, Andriol, is prescribed and has fewer side effects for many women. It is not yet available in the United States.

EstraTest is the only FDA-approved oral testosterone preparation available in the United States. It was taken off the market for many years and is now available as a prescription. Each EstraTest pill contains both estrogen and testosterone. Individuals with a uterus must take progesterone to safely benefit from EstraTest and avoid a higher risk of uterine cancer.

For years, women have been asking for testosterone to reverse their lagging sex drives. It is unwise to use testosterone supplementation without a thorough gyn exam and pre-treatment blood levels as a starting point. A thorough history and physical examination with targeted testing will provide context.

Remember, testosterone will not help you if your relationship with your partner is not working for you. The other components of a healthy relationship need to be in place for testosterone to be successful. The relationship does not have to be perfect, but there must be more potential than two people who are not even glad to spend time together in nonsexual settings. Consider Alexandra's story.

Alexandra's Story
DISTANCING AND HOSTILITY IN A LONG-TERM RELATIONSHIP

At 59, after 30 years of marriage, I went to my doctor to request testosterone to help improve my sex drive. Before writing the prescription, my doctor asked about my relationship. I admitted that my husband and I did not sleep in the same bedroom, and we no longer enjoyed each other's company. My husband has a prescription for Viagra. My doctor advised me that a prescription for testosterone would not likely help my sex drive if I did not want to be in the same room as my husband. They made a referral to a marriage counselor instead. My husband and I agreed to see the marriage counselor and found it helpful. We reestablished a bond. After we worked with the marriage counselor, I approached my doctor about testosterone, and they gave me a prescription that helped us reestablish our sex life. Now we get along better inside and outside our bedroom.

DEHYDROEPIANDROSTERONE

Dehydroepiandrosterone (DHEA) is a hormone made by the adrenal glands. DHEA does not drop suddenly during post menopause. Instead, it diminishes gradually over decades in both men and women. Its role in sexual function is not yet well defined.

Despite the lack of thorough research studies, DHEA has been touted as a cure for low sex drive. No large, well-controlled studies show DHEA is safe or effective in improving sex drive. As a result, most physicians believe oral DHEA supplements are unlikely to make a difference.

ESTROGEN

As you read in chapter 1, estrogen is still produced by the ovaries in perimenopause as estradiol. During this time, its production becomes very erratic before shutting down in post menopause. Estrone, the principal form of estrogen produced in post menopause, is synthesized in fatty tissue. Estrone is a weaker estrogen than estradiol. Even though estrone is a weaker estrogen, it may influence bleeding patterns in perimenopause and affect the uterine lining after menopause. The role of estrone in maintaining libido or vaginal health or in controlling hot flashes has not been well studied.

VIAGRA FOR WOMEN

Researchers are studying Viagra to determine whether it helps women during intercourse. Viagra and other similar medications, such as Cialis, help some men who have otherwise lost the ability to attain an erection. The preliminary data for women suggests that very few women have more satisfying sex using Viagra. At present, studies show that the women who benefit from Viagra are those who have had spinal cord injuries and therefore have compromised blood supply to the pelvis. Additional studies are underway.

PROGESTERONE

Progesterone may help revive a suppressed sex drive. Progesterone comes in pill form, a skin cream, and a vaginal cream. There are several types of progesterone hormone available. In your body, some progesterone made by the ovaries is naturally converted into testosterone. If your doctor feels that progesterone is safe for you, and you are not enthusiastic about trying testosterone, progesterone may be a viable option.

Some concerns have been raised about Provera (medroxyprogesterone) because of its potentially undesirable effects on the heart or the breast tissue, but these are not common concerns at low doses. Prometrium, a plant-based progesterone, is well tolerated by many women. Prometrium is made from peanut oil. Avoid Prometrium if you are allergic to peanuts.

ORAL ESTROGEN

Indirectly, estrogen replacement may help with sex drive. If your sex drive is low due to poor sleep from hot flashes or night sweats, estrogen may improve the quantity and quality of your sleep, increase your sense of well-being, and allow your sex drive to return. Estrogen replacement may also help you when the cause of your low sex drive is related to vaginal dryness and poor lubrication. Discomfort is not conducive to pleasurable sex, and it will affect your sex drive.

Oral estrogen is processed in the liver. There, oral estrogen increases sex hormone binding globulin (SHBG), a protein that binds sex hormones in the blood. When estrogen and testosterone hormones are bound to the SHBG protein, there is less free hormone in the blood that is active, and the sex hormones are less available to the body.

Over time, women who take estrogen by mouth increase the amount of SHBG in their bodies, making estrogen less available to the body and less effective. In these cases, individuals may feel more improvements from their estrogen prescriptions by changing to a form of estrogen that is not taken by mouth, such as a patch, cream, lotion, or vaginal ring.

EXAMPLES OF OTHER TREATMENTS FOR HEALTHY SEXUAL FUNCTION

If your desire for sex is waning, and this decrease disturbs or distresses you, you may consider asking for testosterone ointment off-label as discussed above. You can also ask for flibanserin. Flibanserin (Addyi), also known as the little pink pill, can be taken daily to help restore low sex drive in perimenopausal women who have a healthy relationship and had a previously intact sex drive. When initially introduced on the market, it was not to be taken with alcohol due to a risk of low blood pressure and fainting. Now, with further study, this restriction has been modified. You may take flibanserin if you wait two hours after having two servings or less of an alcoholic beverage. Flibanserin is only FDA approved for use in perimenopausal women. Doctors who prescribe flibanserin to a postmenopausal woman are prescribing it off-label. Women taking flibanserin may experience one to two additional satisfying sexual encounters per month.[9]

Another medication available to boost sex drive is bremelanotide (Vyleesi). To use it, inject yourself under the skin in your belly or thigh area. It is self-administered as a subcutaneous injection 45 minutes before intercourse. Use is restricted to once in a 24-hour period. Consider bremelanotide if you have low sexual desire that is troubling to you and is not related to relationship issues or medications. The most common side effects are nausea (40 of 100 women), flushing (20 of 200 women), and headache (11 of 100 women) or vomiting. Avoid bremelanotide if you have slow stomach emptying, liver or kidney disease, uncontrolled high blood pressure, or cardiovascular disease.[15]

If you have difficulty becoming aroused, sexual aids such as a vibrator may be helpful to increase sensation. If you have difficulty reaching orgasm, a therapist may use directed masturbation or sensate focus therapy that focuses on responses to touch and may reestablish a positive mind–body connection during intimacy. Sexual aids may also be recommended.

Sexual aids or medical sexual devices, previously referred to as sex toys, may be used to address common complaints such as low libido, lack of arousal, absent orgasms, or painful sex. They may include devices such as dildos, vibrators, or graduated dilators. More than 50 percent of women in the United States have used a vibrator, and more than 75 percent of women who have sex with women have used a vibrator. In a 2009 study, 52 percent of women incorporated a vibrator during sexual activity and up to 41 percent included a vibrator with partner sex. By 2022, 80 percent were reporting vibrator use. One prospective study of women showed using a genital stimulation with a vibrator improved arousal, orgasm, sexual function, and satisfaction and decreased sexually related distress. Vibrators and dilators may also be used by pelvic floor therapists to improve pelvic floor issues as well as pelvic and vulvar pain. Individuals may consider incorporating sexual toys if they are curious or interested in trying a device solo or with a partner or to address sexual distress or dissatisfaction with arousal, orgasm, pain with sex, lack of or diminished desire, or a need for additional stimulation.[16]

If you have pain or discomfort, it is important to treat any thinning of the vaginal tissues with moisturizers or low-dose vaginal estrogen, vaginal DHEA (prasterone), or oral Ospemifene. If these are contraindicated, consider using a hyaluronic acid–based vaginal moisturizer.

In addition to treating genitourinary syndrome of menopause as detailed above, a prescription for topical lidocaine applied before intercourse at the lower vaginal opening has helped some women. A tricyclic antidepressant or gabapentin has helped others with nerve pain.

For deep pain with sex, consider working with a trained pelvic physical therapist to loosen tight muscles in the pelvic floor.

For breast cancer survivors, other cancer survivors, and individuals who cannot or choose not to take estrogen, research on lasers to restore vaginal health is in its early phases. The CO_2 laser burns holes in the vaginal tissue. As the tissue regenerates to heal, more collagen is created. Side effects include discharge for two weeks or more and narrowing of the vagina or scarring. The procedure can be painful. In trained hands, women get relief. The frequency of the treatments and the long-term consequences of using vaginal lasers to restore vaginal health are not well studied. Small studies are underway.[17] ThermiVA, a noninvasive radiofrequency treatment using heat, has also been used to restore vaginal health, including moisture and elasticity. No adverse events have been reported to the

FDA from ThermiVA treatments at this time. ThermiVA is discussed in more detail earlier in this chapter.[19]

For relationship challenges, cognitive behavioral therapy, mindfulness-based therapy, and interpersonal therapy are helpful in addition to working with a certified sex therapist.

Reading erotic books or stories and watching erotic videos geared to a women's viewpoint may also be helpful.

IMPORTANT TAKEAWAYS

In summary:

- For many women, sex becomes more pleasurable as they age. But even if it becomes less pleasurable, women can take proactive steps to improve it.
- Various age-related physical changes, medications, and medical conditions can affect sex.
- Vaginal dryness due to old age and menopause is common but not inevitable, and certain causes of dryness are treatable with lubricants, moisturizers, hormones, estrogen cream, and more.
- Lifestyle factors such as stress, lack of personal time, alcohol, and lack of physical exercise can all affect sex.
- Libido doesn't necessarily diminish with age, but if it does, there are ways to address it—particularly by improving the quality of your relationship. Certain medications can also improve sex drive.
- The more information you can provide to your doctor about your sex-related concerns, the more effectively they will be able to help you or refer you to someone who can.

QUESTIONS FOR YOUR DOCTOR

1. I am less interested in sex. What suggestions do you have?
2. Sex is painful, and I even feel vaginal dryness when exercising. What treatment options do I have?

3. I have pain before we even get started, and the opening feels small. What can I do?
4. I have deep pain with sex that lingers. What are my treatment options?
5. I have sex with men and women. What testing do I need to stay safe?

RESOURCES

www.aasect.org—American Association of Sexuality Educators, Counselors and Therapists, a nonprofit organization, has a list of sex therapists in your area

www.acog.org—The American Society of Obstetricians and Gynecologists has information for women on sex in menopause

http://isswsh.org—International Society for the Study of Women's Sexual Health includes resources for lay readers and professionals as well as sex therapists by location

www.kinseyinstitute.org—The Kinsey Institute podcasts from the sexuality research center at Indiana University, including some that cover sex and menopause

www.MedAmour.com—Contains resources and medical tools that are reviewed and recommended by medical professionals

www.menopause.org—The Menopause Society has resources about sex for women in peri- and post menopause

www.nia.nih.gov—National Institute on Aging has sections for consumers on sexuality in later years

www.OMGYes.com—A website featuring research and approaches to enhance female pleasure and sexuality developed by Indiana University and the Kinsey Institute. It is designed to be used by women alone, women and men, or men who are interested in female sexuality. There is a one-time fee to access the site. It also gets updated as new research findings become available.

www.sexualityandu.ca—Sexuality and U is maintained by the Society of Obstetricians and Gynaecologists of Canada and has a consumer section on sex over 50.

BOOKS

Casperson Kelly J. *You Are Not Broken*. Yanb Media; 2022. A female urologist discusses female sexuality and anatomy.

Hague M, Hague N, Smith JA, Smith J. *Start Talking Intimacy: A Couples' Guide to Discussing Sex*. Xulan Press; 2015. A female obstetrician-gynecologist, her husband and a licensed sex and family therapist and his wife educate readers with language and approaches to discussing sex in a relationship.

Goldstein A, Brandon M, Marianne B. *Reclaiming Desire: 4 Keys to Finding Your Lost Libido*. Rodale Books; 2009. A gynecologist and a psychologist discuss restoring libido.

Komisurak B, Beyer-Flores C, Whipple B. *The Science of Orgasm*. Johns Hopkins University Press; 2006. This award-winning book is written by a PhD neuroscientist, a PhD endocrinologist, and a PhD RN sex researcher.

Streicher L. *Sex Rx Hormones, Health, and Your Best Sex Ever*. Harper Collins; 2015. A board-certified gynecologist and certified menopause practitioner discusses natural hormone changes and medical issues that can affect your sex life.

Westheimer R, with Lehu PA. *Dr. Ruth's Sex After 50: Revving up the Romance, Passion, and Excitement!* Quill Driver Books/Word Dancer Press; 2005. "Dr. Ruth" is the first expert who comes to mind, both within medical circles and outside them, when discussing women's sexuality.

CHAPTER 8

COMPATIBLE CONTRACEPTION

The good news? You have options. The bad news? You have options, and it can be overwhelming to choose. Here's some guidance.

INTRODUCTION

The sheer number of options available for contraception can be overwhelming for women. This is especially true for women in perimenopause, many of whom may assume they don't even need to use it. In this chapter, I'll explain why contraception is important during perimenopause and what methods are currently available. Throughout the chapter, I will answer common questions such as:

- Why are unplanned pregnancies in perimenopause so risky?
- If I become pregnant during perimenopause, is there anything I can do to increase my chances of having a healthy pregnancy and a healthy baby?
- If I don't want to become pregnant, what are my options for contraception? What if I prefer not to use a hormonal method of birth control?
- Are there any methods of contraception that can help with heavy, prolonged, or irregular menstrual periods? What about hot flashes and night sweats?

Each week, I meet with women in perimenopause. Some of these women would like to become pregnant, and others would not. If a woman is in a heterosexual relationship and has intercourse once a year or more, I'll ask her if she wants to become pregnant in the next year. If she says no, I'll ask what contraception she prefers. What are the responses I hear most often? "I don't want to take anything." Or "I don't think I'll get pregnant."

Unfortunately, the reality is different. Women in their 40s are more likely to have unplanned pregnancies than women in any other age group except for teenagers. The pregnancy termination rate for women over the age of 40 is 35 percent. It's even higher for women over the age of 45. The only group with a higher rate of pregnancy termination is preteens. Nearly half of all pregnancies in the United States are unplanned, and the rate of unintended pregnancies in perimenopausal women is particularly high.[1]

Why does the high rate of unplanned pregnancy in perimenopause worry doctors and midwives? There are two reasons:

1. Unplanned pregnancies are riskier than planned pregnancies for both mother and baby.
2. With increasing age, a woman's chance of having a healthy pregnancy and healthy baby diminishes.

One myth I hear often is this: "I am in menopause; I will not become pregnant because I am already skipping menstrual periods." In fact, many women in perimenopause have unplanned pregnancies even as they are experiencing hot flashes, irregular menstrual periods, or missed periods. You can ovulate, not see a menstrual period, and still get pregnant. Younger perimenopausal women may find that their menstrual periods start up again after a gap of 10 or 12 months. Your doctor can advise you when you can safely stop using contraception.

> DID YOU KNOW?
>
> If you are age 40 or older, an unplanned pregnancy puts your health at greater risk than using some form of contraception. An unplanned pregnancy is also risky for your unborn child.

BECOMING PREGNANT DURING PERIMENOPAUSE

Pregnancy after age 40 is riskier for the mother and her baby than pregnancy in women under age 35. With that said, I know patients, friends, and relatives who conceived their children at age 40 or older. Thankfully, they each had healthy pregnancies and healthy babies. Your odds of having an uneventful, healthy pregnancy and delivering a healthy baby, however, decrease as your age increases.

Is there anything you can do to increase your chances of having a healthy pregnancy and healthy baby after age 40? Yes. Consider these strategies:

1. Take folate 400 mcg by mouth once daily or take a prenatal vitamin. Folate lowers the risk of birth defects in the spinal cord and is available over the counter.
2. Update your immunizations, including rubella, tetanus, and COVID-19 vaccination.
3. Avoid alcohol. The baby's organs begin to develop very early in the pregnancy—even before a positive pregnancy test. Alcohol increases the risk of birth defects.
4. Avoid undercooked meat, poultry, and seafood as well as unpasteurized milk. Undercooked meat or seafood can lead to an infection with *Toxoplasmosis gondii*. Toxoplasmosis is a protozoan parasite that a mother can transmit to her fetus. It affects the fetal nervous system, causing birth defects and other medical problems.
5. Avoid changing cat litter. This, too, can cause *Toxoplasmosis gondii* infection.
6. Wear gloves while gardening. Women can get infected with *Toxoplasmosis gondii* from contaminated soil or water.
7. Avoid over-the-counter medications such as Aleve, Advil, Motrin, and ibuprofen because they compromise normal development of the baby's heart and lungs.

8. Check if your prescription medications and supplements are safe during pregnancy.
9. Attain a healthy weight and blood pressure.

PREVENTING PREGNANCY DURING PERIMENOPAUSE: WHAT WORKED IN YOUR YOUTH WON'T WORK NOW

Unfortunately, strategies to avoid becoming pregnant in earlier decades of life may not be as effective now. Consider the following.

"RHYTHM METHOD"

The rhythm method attempts to avoid conception by restricting the timing of sexual intercourse to the times of the menstrual cycle when ovulation is least likely to occur. Even individuals who successfully used the rhythm method of birth control during their twenties or early thirties and were meticulous about tracking changes in their cervical mucus to determine their fertile time will discover that this method is ineffective in the mid- to late thirties or forties. In perimenopause, the menstrual cycle can change with no warning. While the expected mucus changes may not appear, you may still ovulate anyway and be able to conceive. This is one reason the rhythm method of birth control is not considered reliable in the perimenopausal years. Irregular cycles and absent or disguised signs of ovulation make the failure rate of the rhythm method of birth control high. This is true even for women who are experienced in using this method. But if you are open to becoming pregnant and delivering your baby at any time (not at a certain time of the year), the rhythm method is still a viable option. The same is true for using the withdrawal method as described below.

"WITHDRAWAL METHOD"

Withdrawal (i.e., removing the penis from the vagina before ejaculation) is not a reliable method for preventing pregnancy at any age. That's because small amounts of sperm can be released before ejaculation. That's why withdrawal has a 50 percent failure rate. If you are open to conceiving, the withdrawal method may be used to shift the timing of when you might conceive.

PREVENTING PREGNANCY DURING PERIMENOPAUSE

WHAT WORKS

Now I'll discuss viable options to consider if you don't want to become pregnant in perimenopause.

OVER-THE-COUNTER SPERMICIDES

The use of over-the-counter spermicides alone has a high failure rate, although spermicides used with a condom or a diaphragm are effective methods for preventing pregnancy. Condoms also help to prevent sexually transmitted infections.

ON-DEMAND BIRTH CONTROL

Do you prefer a method that you only use before intercourse and not every day? *On-demand birth control* is a term I'll use to discuss pregnancy prevention options that fit this preference. The following options are all nonhormonal and only used when you need them.

The newest option for "on-demand" birth control is a combination of lactic acid, citric acid, and potassium bitartrate (i.e., Phexxi), a nonhormonal vaginal gel. You may use Phexxi before intercourse by inserting the contraceptive gel in the vagina. Use it before intercourse any time during your menstrual cycle. Phexxi works by changing the pH of the vagina, making it more acidic. When the vagina becomes more acidic than normal, it is temporarily less hospitable for sperm, and sperm are unlikely to thrive or fertilize eggs in this unfavorable environment. Phexxi does not prevent sexually transmitted infections. It differs from over-the-counter spermicides because it is designed to be used alone, not with a condom or diaphragm. Your doctor can prescribe Phexxi for you. It is not available over the counter.[2] Consider Zia's story.

Zia's Story
HAS USED THE RHYTHM METHOD OF CONTRACEPTION FOR 25 YEARS AND PREFERS NO HORMONES

I am a 48-year-old woman with two children who has used the rhythm method successfully for 25 years and would like to continue using it. I do not want to take a birth control pill, and neither I nor my husband wants to get a sterilization procedure. I also do not want an intrauterine device (IUD). Condoms do not appeal to us either. I used a diaphragm in my early twenties and then became pregnant with my second child. My body changed after giving birth to my first child, and my diaphragm was not refit. When my doctor presented me with the high failure rate of both the withdrawal and rhythm methods, I agreed to try Phexxi during my perimenopausal years and have been happy with my choice.

BARRIER METHODS

Barrier methods are effective regardless of where you are in your menstrual cycle, and they do not affect your bleeding pattern. You only use a barrier method when you actually having sex, and there are no hormones involved. The two most common barrier methods are condoms (for men) and the diaphragm (for women). Both also offer varying degrees of protection against sexually transmitted diseases such as HIV/AIDS and others. When using a condom or diaphragm, it is important to use spermicide as directed.

FEMALE CONDOMS

A female condom is also available, and women wishing to prevent pregnancy should wear it before sex at all times—not just before sex when they're ovulating. The female condom has a pouch that rests inside the vagina and a wide rim that presses against the outside of the vagina and covers much of the vulva. It is visible to your partner because part of it is outside the vagina. Extensive testing in Africa and Mexico shows that the female condom prevents sexually transmitted infections, including human papillomavirus, HIV, and other infections such as gonorrhea, chlamydia, and syphilis.

MALE CONDOMS

Condoms for men are 98 percent effective in preventing pregnancy if they are used correctly and reliably. This means using them correctly all the time before intercourse with no exceptions as well as not reusing them. In real life, the failure rate is higher due to inconsistent or incorrect use.

> **DID YOU KNOW?**
> Asking your male partner to use a condom only during certain times of your menstrual cycle is unreliable as a means of birth control. This is especially true during perimenopause when menstrual cycles may not follow any type of regularity.

During perimenopause, your menstrual cycle can become irregular with no warning. If male or female condoms are your birth control method of choice, here is some advice:

1. Ask your male partner to use a condom at all times.
2. Use a lubricant that is compatible with the type of condom you are using. Some spermicides or lubricants are not compatible with latex condoms. Also, select a lubricant or spermicide with as few additives as possible.
3. If you are sensitive to latex products, be certain to select a nonlatex condom.

4. Avoid scented products. Some women are sensitive to benzocaine or other additives included in some spermicides. Try a small amount of the product to be sure you are not sensitive to any of the ingredients. Do allow extra space at the tip of the condom by pinching the end while applying it. It will be less likely to break.
5. Do not reuse condoms.

In addition to preventing pregnancy, condoms also help prevent the spread of sexually transmitted infections, including human papillomavirus that can cause genital warts, abnormal Pap smears, and, in some cases, even cervical cancer.

DIAPHRAGM

A diaphragm may appeal to you if you or your partner dislikes condoms or wants an on-demand method you can control. You may choose to insert a diaphragm many hours before having sex, but you'll need to add more spermicide without removing the diaphragm if more than one hour has passed since you inserted it. Before intercourse, the diaphragm (coated with spermicidal cream or gel) is inserted into the vagina by the woman or her partner. The diaphragm should remain in place six to eight hours after intercourse. When properly fitted by a clinician, it will cover the cervix and the upper vagina, preventing sperm from entering the cervix. It should always be used with spermicide, which forms a seal around the inside rim of the diaphragm. You can have a diaphragm fit in your doctor's office, then get a prescription for the size and type of diaphragm that fits your body best. A new diaphragm, Caya, does not need to be fit by a clinician and can be purchased over the counter in some pharmacies, or by prescription.in others. More information about Caya can be found at www.Caya.usa.com.

DID YOU KNOW?
You may be due for a refit of your diaphragm. The size and fit of your diaphragm may change after giving birth, nursing, and weight gain or loss of seven pounds or more. The diaphragm protects the cervix from sexually transmitted diseases, but it doesn't protect the vaginal cavity or the vulva outside the vagina. The diaphragm should be cleaned after each use and checked for holes by holding it up to the light for a visual check and by filling it with water to see if the water leaks through.

CERVICAL CAP

The cervical cap covers only your cervix and uses suction to remain in place. It is smaller than a diaphragm, and it does not rest on the bladder as some diaphragms do. Some physicians are trained to fit a cervical cap for you. You may prefer the cervical cap since it fits differently and is smaller. It is removed within six to eight hours after intercourse and should be used with spermicide.

"MORNING AFTER PILL"

The "morning after pill," also known as "Plan B," is available as a backup method only. It is not suitable for regular, frequent, or routine use. It is not designed to be used for contraception to reliably prevent pregnancy over time. Plan B is a last-ditch method to prevent pregnancy after having sex. It does not cause an abortion or pregnancy termination.

DID YOU KNOW?
The "morning after pill" does not cause an abortion or terminate a pregnancy. It simply reduces the chance of pregnancy after unprotected sex by delaying ovulation, the release of the egg from the ovary.

When might Plan B be helpful? One scenario is after a condom breaks or tears. Another is in the devastating instance of a rape. I recommend that patients keep the "morning after pill" in mind as a back-up method if they are using a barrier method.

You can purchase Plan B over the counter at a pharmacy; you don't need a prescription. The Plan B kit includes two progesterone pills that you'll take by mouth 12 hours apart. Side effects do not always occur, but you may experience include nausea or vomiting, stomach pain, breast pain, headache, dizziness, diarrhea, fatigue, or menstrual changes. Do not use Plan B if you are already pregnant.

> **DID YOU KNOW?**
>
> Taking Plan B within 72 hours (three days) after unprotected intercourse will prevent pregnancy more than 90 percent of the time. Plan B works best if taken within the first 24 hours after unprotected sex.

If you are unable to purchase Plan B, your doctor may recommend that you take a certain number of pills from a regular birth control pill pack also within 72 hours after unprotected sex to achieve the same result of delaying ovulation. The earlier you take Plan B, the better it works. That's why it's important to contact your doctor as soon as possible. The dosage will differ depending upon the type of pill being used. Keep in mind that what worked for a friend may not work for you. It's very important to talk with your doctor about a specific pill regimen based on your unique circumstances. In some instances, insertion of a copper-bearing IUD within five days of intercourse provides emergency contraception that is 95% effective in preventing pregnancy..

"SET-AND-FORGET" OPTIONS

This category of contraception options includes methods such as an IUD, vaginal ring, a contraceptive patch, or an intramuscular Depo

Provera injection. I will review the vaginal ring and contraceptive patch in the next section, which includes hormonal contraception options. With all of these options, you don't need to do any preparation immediately before intercourse. The protection is already in place.

IUD

The IUD is a desirable choice for some women who want a reversible method that requires no preparation before intercourse. The IUD acquired a bad reputation among some baby boomers due to the Dalkon Shield, an outdated IUD that was designed poorly, caused pelvic infection, and is no longer in use. The Dalkon Shield was taken off the market more than 40 years ago due to a high risk of pelvic inflammatory disease. Since the 1970s, the IUD has been redesigned and is now safe for women. Different types of IUDs are designed to protect against pregnancy for different lengths of time, ranging from 3 to 10 years. If you have an IUD in place but decide to conceive, you can ask your doctor to remove it so you can become pregnant.

There are distinct kinds of IUDs—ones that secrete hormones and ones that do not. An IUD that has no hormones will not decrease prolonged or heavy bleeding. A hormone-secreting IUD (e.g., Mirena, Kyleena, Lyetta, or Skyla), however, releases progesterone directly into the uterine lining/cavity. This helps reduce heavy or prolonged bleeding while simultaneously providing contraception. A hormone-releasing IUD is also used to protect the uterus lining from uterine cancer in menopausal women who are taking estrogen who cannot tolerate oral progestin. The low dose of progesterone released by the hormone-secreting IUD is not designed to produce hormone levels in the blood. It is typically safe for women with a history of breast cancer who wish to avoid hormones. Other IUDs may have no progesterone or contain copper. These nonprogesterone types of IUDs may be associated with heavier, prolonged, or irregular bleeding; however, they still provide "set-and-forget" contraception.[3]

> **IS AN IUD RIGHT FOR YOU?**
> You should not consider an IUD if:
> - You have a history of an ectopic or tubal pregnancy.
> - You have had a severe pelvic infection such as pelvic inflammatory disease.
> - You or your partner have untreated gonorrhea or chlamydia.
> - You have multiple partners and will not be using condoms consistently.

The IUD is inserted into the uterus in a doctor's office. Removing an IUD can typically be done in a doctor's office, especially if the string is still visible in the vagina.

DEPO PROVERA

Medroxyprogesterone acetate for injection (Depo Provera) is a long-acting birth control method that is reversible. It is administered as an injection of progesterone into the arm muscle or buttock every three months. There is no estrogen in the preparation. Depo Provera injections may produce light or irregular periods or result in no menstrual periods at all. Depo Provera is not a suitable long-term choice for a perimenopausal woman because it is associated with bone thinning when used for more than a year in this age group.

ORAL CONTRACEPTIVES

Birth control pills can help you weather perimenopause while also providing contraception. They may ease hot flashes and night sweats, and in some cases, they may even help regulate irregular menstrual cycles. Most nonsmoking perimenopausal women over age 35 can safely take the newer, low-dose birth control pills. These newer pills have lower levels of estrogen, and as a result, the risk of heart attack, stroke, and blood clots is much lower. Most of the low-dose birth control pills contain small amounts of estrogen and progesterone. A few oral contraceptives contain progesterone only, and these progesterone-only pills are safe for individuals over 35 who smoke. All of the low-dose birth control pills have higher amounts of estrogen to prevent pregnancy than the amounts of estrogen provided by hormone replacement options.

> **DID YOU KNOW?**
> Oral contraceptives are not appropriate for women in post menopause or women who smoke. The risk of heart attack, stroke, and blood clots is too high for women over 35 years old who smoke. Even low-dose contraceptives contain estrogen that will add to that risk. In addition, the oral contraceptives deliver hormones in a cyclic fashion that does not match the biology of the postmenopausal woman.

Even if you're in perimenopause, you may need to avoid taking contraceptives containing estrogen. More specifically, do not take contraceptive pills with estrogen if you:

- Are over the age of 35 and smoke. You are at higher risk of stroke, heart attack, and deep vein blood clots.
- Have migraine headaches with aura. You are at higher risk of a stroke.
- Have untreated high blood pressure. Note: Your physician may be comfortable prescribing a low-dose estrogen-containing oral contraceptive if your blood pressure is well controlled on medication, or they may be comfortable prescribing a progesterone-only oral contraceptive pill..
- Have high lipids such as cholesterol or triglycerides. These lipids will worsen on oral contraceptives containing estrogen. Checking baseline lipids and rechecking them on oral contraceptive pills is helpful.
- Have a personal history of heart attack, stroke, deep vein clots, or pulmonary embolus

- Have a personal or family history of clotting disorders or factor V Leiden
- Have a personal history of liver disease
- Have a personal history of breast cancer. Note: A family history of breast cancer is not a reason to avoid the birth control pill. Studies show the birth control pill is not likely to increase your risk of breast cancer even if you have inherited a gene for breast cancer such as BRCA 1 or BRCA 2. I encourage you to review your individual risk with your doctor.

For most nonsmokers, the birth control pill is an appealing option. It may help regulate irregular or heavy menstrual periods. The estrogen in the pill may also alleviate hot flashes. It produces regular, light cycles that many women appreciate. Be sure to take folate, a type of B vitamin, while you are on oral contraceptives. It is important to have adequate levels of folate in your system to lower the risk of birth defects in the brain and spine of the developing fetus if you choose to conceive later.

A common question I'm asked is, "If I'm on 'the pill,' how will I know when I'm in post menopause?" The answer? It's tricky. Taking oral contraceptives can mask the exact timing of menopause. Sometimes, taking oral contraceptives during perimenopause can spur bleeding cycles when a woman may otherwise have stopped bleeding on her own. There is no single agreed-upon strategy to determine the onset of post menopause while taking oral contraceptives. Your doctor will advise you of the best strategy for your individual situation.

> **DID YOU KNOW?**
> It is not safe to assume that you are postmenopausal if you stop bleeding while you are on oral contraceptives.

Sometimes oral contraceptives cause you to stop bleeding due to a thin uterine lining, but it is not due to post menopause and permanent cessation of estrogen production in your ovaries. On the other hand, it is not accurate to assume that you are still perimenopausal if you continue to bleed on oral contraceptives. That is because oral contraceptives can cause cyclic bleeding even during post menopause because of the way the hormones are sequenced over the course of the month. The oral contraceptive cannot prevent sexually transmitted diseases. If you have more than one sexual partner—or your partner has other sexual partners—condoms will lower your risk of getting a sexually transmitted disease.

> DID YOU KNOW?
> The birth control pill, including low-dose birth control, lowers your risk of ovarian cancer by 50 percent. Low-dose birth control also lowers your risk of uterine (endometrial) cancer and typically eliminates hot flashes and night sweats. Consider Zakiya's story.

Zakiya's Story
HOT FLASHES AND THE PILL

I began having irregular menstrual periods three years ago when I was 46. I would skip a period every three or four months. I was also experiencing debilitating hot flashes that were extremely difficult to cope with in my job as a flight attendant, especially during long flights. I'd always had an erratic sleep routine with my unpredictable work schedule and layovers in different time zones. Once I began having night sweats, I got even less sleep. I tried different herbs with no relief. A friend suggested I try evening primrose oil, but I didn't see a difference. Eventually, I consulted my gynecologist. Because I'm a nonsmoker, they suggested I try a low-dose oral contraceptive. The pill they prescribed drastically reduced the number and severity of hot flashes, and it also gave me shorter, lighter, and more regular menstrual periods.

CONTRACEPTIVE SKIN PATCHES

A low-dose birth control patch (i.e., Ortho Evra) was a brand of contraceptive skin patch marketed in the United States that was taken off the market. It is now available in generic form as Xulane. The Xulane patch releases hormones slowly through the skin directly into the bloodstream 24 hours a day, seven days a week. A new patch is placed on the skin once a week for three consecutive weeks, followed by a patch-free week. You can expect to have a menstrual period during the patch-free week. It is best to place the patch below the waist on the abdomen or buttocks. The patch stays on during baths, showers, and swimming but may be less effective after prolonged time in the water.

Xulane releases more estrogen into the blood than most low-dose contraceptives that contain estrogen. Due to its higher estrogen levels, Xulane may not be the best choice for you if you are over 40 since it is likely to increase your risk of blood clots, stroke, and heart attack. Do not consider using the Xulane patch if you are over 35 years old and smoke cigarettes or vape.

> **DID YOU KNOW?**
>
> Contraceptive patches such as Xulane do not work well in women with a body mass index (BMI) over 30 and are less effective in women with a BMI between 25 and 30.

A new low-dose contraceptive patch with levonorgestrel and ethinyl estradiol (Twirla) was released in 2021. Twirla has a lower dose of estrogen, 30 mcg, comparable to many low-dose estrogen birth control pills, and its estrogen ethinyl estradiol is plant derived, as is its progesterone, levonorgestrel. Twirla is a safe choice for perimenopausal women over 35 who do not smoke and have no personal history of heart attack, stroke, or deep vein clots.

VAGINAL CONTRACEPTIVE RINGS

Vaginal contraceptive rings are small, soft, flexible rings inserted into the vagina. They do not require fitting. You will leave the contraceptive ring in the vagina for three consecutive weeks, including during intercourse. Then you will remove it for one week, during which you'll likely have a menstrual period. After the ring-free week, you will insert a new ring or reinsert the original ring, depending on which specific contraceptive ring you use.

There are two vaginal contraceptive rings available to consider: a ring with etonogestrel/ethinyl estradiol (i.e., NuvaRing) and ring with segesterone acetate and ethinyl estradiol vaginal system (i.e., Annovera), both of which release plant-based estrogen and progesterone into the bloodstream through the vaginal walls.

Vaginal contraceptive rings eliminate the need to take hormones by mouth daily. With a vaginal contraceptive ring, minimal estrogen is processed through the liver. Estrogen enters the blood through the vaginal walls, not the digestive system.

Vaginal contraceptive rings such as those described above may also ease hot flashes and night sweats in perimenopause. They are designed to achieve blood levels of estrogen and progesterone that prevent pregnancy. These blood levels are also high enough to help alleviate perimenopausal symptoms.

> DID YOU KNOW?
> Not all vaginal rings are contraceptives. Noncontraceptive vaginal rings have lower doses of estrogen. Postmenopausal women may use these rings to ease vaginal dryness and/or hot flashes. To learn more about noncontraceptive vaginal rings, be sure to read chapter 4.

FEMALE STERILIZATION

Female sterilization is an outpatient surgery during which your surgeon clips or ties your fallopian tubes, preventing eggs from reaching the uterus lining and meeting up with sperm. This procedure, also referred to as tubal ligation or permanent sterilization, is highly effective (usually 99 percent). Tubal ligation may be done at the time of a cesarean section after a vaginal birth through a small incision or at any other time using a laparoscope. While a tubal ligation can be reversed surgically, it should be considered a permanent procedure to prevent pregnancy, as reversal is not always successful.

> **DID YOU KNOW?**
>
> A tubal ligation lowers the risk of ovarian cancer by up to 50 percent, even in women who have inherited risk of ovarian cancer. Why? Researchers suspect that after a tubal ligation, certain environmental toxins may no longer be able to reach the ovaries and therefore cannot influence the ovaries to develop cancer.

One common myth about tubal ligations is that they cause abnormal, heavy, or irregular menstrual periods. Research has shown, however, that having a tubal ligation will not alter your menstrual cycles.

MALE STERILIZATION

Male sterilization, also known as vasectomy, is performed by a urologist, a surgical specialist knowledgeable about the male urinary system, kidneys, and reproductive system. It is done in the doctor's office using a sterile technique. During this minor surgical procedure, the urologist ties off the vas deferens, resulting in permanent sterilization. This procedure is analogous to a tubal ligation in a woman.

After the procedure, the urologist rechecks the sperm count to confirm that the procedure was effective. Although some refer to vasectomies as a nonpermanent form of birth control, it is important to note that procedures to reverse vasectomy are not always successful. Research is underway to find new birth control methods for men, including a birth control pill.

SPECIAL CONSIDERATIONS

For individuals who are transgender or nonbinary, the hormones you may be taking are different from birth control and will not prevent pregnancy. Speak to your health care clinician about options to consider that will prevent pregnancy if you are not trying to conceive.

FUTURE DEVELOPMENTS: ESTETROL

Estetrol is a type of estrogen naturally produced by the fetal liver only during pregnancy. The properties of estetrol look promising as a key ingredient in future contraception pills as well as future hormone replacement preparations. In preliminary research studies, estetrol does not cause blood clots and does not promote uterus lining growth or thickening. Estetrol may prove even safer for breast tissue than current oral contraceptives. At present, it looks beneficial for maintaining bone strength. It may also be linked with better control of menstrual bleeding. Estetrol does not appear to increase cholesterol or other lipid levels and may not affect carbohydrate metabolism. More research is needed to confirm these benefits and establish any other side effects or concerns in humans.[4]

IMPORTANT TAKEAWAYS

In summary:

- Even if you are in perimenopause, it's important to consider options for contraception if you don't want to become pregnant.
- The health risk of using contraception is much lower than the health risk of an unplanned pregnancy.

- Women have several contraception options to consider, some of which can also help with symptoms of perimenopause and menopause. Your doctor can help you choose the method that's best for you.

QUESTIONS FOR YOUR DOCTOR

1. If I want to get pregnant, what are my personal health risks? What immunizations do you recommend? Is it safe to take my current medications and supplements during pregnancy?
2. If I do not want to be pregnant currently, what are my options if I prefer not to use a hormonal method of birth control?
3. What contraception will also control my heavy, prolonged, or irregular menstrual periods?
4. What contraception method will also relieve my hot flashes and night sweats?
5. For long-term or permanent contraception, what do you recommend I consider?

RESOURCES

www.ACOG.org—The American College of Obstetricians and Gynecologists (ACOG) has different pamphlets that discuss types of contraception, including hormonal contraception, emergency contraception, natural family planning, barrier methods, sterilization procedures, and more. Many of these pamphlets are also available in Spanish. You may be able to obtain a free copy of up to five different printed pamphlets, or you can request those that interest you from your gynecologist.

www.CDC.gov/reproductivehealth/contracception

The above two sites give accurate, up-to-date information about contraception options.

CHAPTER 9

MOODS, MEMORY, AND MENTAL HEALTH

For some, menopause is a joyful time. For others, it's just the opposite. Here's what can happen and how you can cope.

FOR MANY WOMEN, menopause is a time of intense change: cyclic mood changes, memory loss, depression, anxiety, and more. It can feel overwhelming at times, but it's important to remember that talking about these changes can help you get the right care. In this chapter, I'll help you understand complex changes that may occur during menopause and how you can cope effectively. I'll answer these questions and more:

- What factors affect my mood, memory, and mental health during menopause?
- How can I treat premenstrual syndrome (PMS) and premenstrual dysphoric disorder (PMDD) effectively?
- How do I know whether I'm depressed? If I am depressed, what are some of my treatment options?
- How might cognitive behavioral therapy (CBT) help me?
- How do I know whether I'm experiencing memory loss or cognitive decline, and is there anything I can do about it?

UNDERSTANDING COMPLEX CHANGES

Women of all ages are susceptible to changes in their moods, memory, and mental health. As you enter perimenopause and post menopause, however, you may experience even more changes. One difficulty in understanding these changes is that each of you has your own individual biology and temperament. You also have your own physical health and psychological factors that affect your mood, memory, and mental health.

Until now, shifts in the emotional outlook or mental function of women over the age of 40 were attributed to hot flashes, night sweats, lack of sleep, or other life changes. While these are all legitimate sources of stress, researchers are developing a more complex picture that better describes how biological, hormonal, genetic, and social changes also influence our mood, memory, and mental health.

Before delving into information on worsening depression or anxiety during perimenopause, I'd like to emphasize that this chapter may not resonate with everyone. In fact, some of you may find yourself pleased with the new opportunities that emerge during this stage of life. You may further your education, develop new interests, plan a new career, or pursue an established career more vigorously. You may also enjoy more time on your own. Or you may enjoy time in a special relationship or with friends, family, children, or grandchildren. Even if the information in this chapter doesn't apply to you, it could pertain to someone you know and love.

CHANGES THAT MAY OCCUR DURING PERIMENOPAUSE

Even though perimenopause is a normal phase of life, you may experience changes that you didn't anticipate. For example, if you have a history of depression in the past, during your teens, twenties, or thirties, you are at higher risk of developing depression in your perimenopausal years. If you have experienced postpartum depression in the past, you are also more vulnerable to a recurrence of depression in your perimenopausal years.

Similarly, depression may also surface unexpectedly during the perimenopausal years, even if you never encountered it in your earlier years. In addition, anxiety, irritability, and difficulty sleeping are common. A panic attack may be difficult to distinguish from a hot flash. Finally, minor health problems may surface, even if you have enjoyed exceptionally good health throughout your life. All of these factors can affect your mood, memory, and mental health.

CHANGES THAT MAY OCCUR DURING POST MENOPAUSE

When post menopause arrives, you have passed the milestone of 12 consecutive months with no menstrual period, and you no longer ovulate. After a medical confirmation of post menopause, you may be relieved that you are no longer at risk for an unplanned pregnancy. You may also be free from experiencing erratic hormone fluctuations. Hot flashes and night sweats may resolve or linger before becoming milder. The stable hormones of post menopause contribute to greater mental resilience against stress and depression.

In post menopause, the heightened differences between the sexes start to diminish, and there are fewer gender differences in brain function. When you reach post menopause, you are less susceptible to depression caused by erratic estrogen levels. That's because your estrogen levels are low but constant. During post menopause, however, you are more likely to have a major health issue or become more socially isolated, have financial difficulties, or experience a lack of resources. These challenges can contribute to depression in their own right.

OTHER CHANGES YOU MAY EXPERIENCE

Perimenopause and post menopause are normal phases of life, not illnesses. But even today, you may hear that your hormones need to be "fixed" because you lack estrogen or notice you are more forgetful or sadder. Rather than feeling broken or needing to be fixed, you deserve to know that this may be a vulnerable time for your mental and physical health. You are at higher risk for problems with your memory, depression, susceptibility to stress, trouble with sleep, and worsening of premenstrual syndrome (PMS). Specifically, you will experience changes in:

- Hormone secretion. The hormonal peaks and valleys of perimenopause cause more than hot flashes and mood swings; they may be associated with depression that hormones will not alleviate. In post menopause, hormones are stable but at lower levels. Dealing with physical illness or social isolation may increase the risk of depression.
- Reproductive status. In perimenopause, fertility is ending. In post menopause, having more children spontaneously is typically impossible. This is not just a physical change. If your life has been defined by childrearing, you may feel a terrible sense of loss and confusion. On the other hand, you may feel emancipated.
- Appearance. Our culture does not value natural aging. You may feel the need to go to great lengths to continue looking as young as possible. The concept of growing old gracefully is no longer popular, making it difficult for those of us in our 40s, 50s, 60s, and beyond to feel confident.
- Sexuality. You do not have to stop having sex in perimenopause or post menopause. If you encounter challenges, there are strategies to consider. See chapter 7 for more information.
- Social context. More than our male counterparts, you may find yourself defined by your roles: partner or spouse, daughter, mother, sister, and/or member of a professional group. Your roles are likely to grow or change. Sometimes the change originating within you radiates outward. Other times, shifts are forced on you by circumstances you don't choose. For example, having an "empty nest" after decades of childrearing may come as a shock. Your relationship with your partner may change due to their health or work

circumstances or your own, or both. You may be in a relationship where one of you wants to retire and move to a new community while the other does not. You may be surrounded by loving family and grandchildren, or you may be isolated and alone.

HORMONES AND MOOD DURING MENOPAUSE

When trying to understand depression in menopausal women, scientists started by exploring the effect of hormones. Focusing exclusively on hormones, though, is like cropping a digital photo of an entire extended family to include only one person's face. The big picture of menopause includes genetic components, social context, and much more. For each woman, there is a complex relationship between the physical, mental, and emotional shifts that occur with each stage of menopause. Your lifestyle choices and social context also play a role. When women compare notes, they can be fooled into thinking they have the same problem because their cluster of concerns is so similar. In reality, the cause and the treatment may be very different for each one. Consider Jhumpa's story, which includes a hormonal component.

Jhumpa's Story
THYROID AND MOOD

I own a small boutique and employ three part-time sales associates. I enjoy selecting new fashions for my customers because it is a creative outlet for me. Since I can't stock too many items, I need to be strategic in my choices. Lately, it all seems like too much. I feel sluggish, have put on 10 pounds in the last two months, sleep poorly, and have less energy for my boyfriend, my customers, and my sales staff. My friends tell me it is perimenopause. "Welcome to the club," they say. "Expect to gain weight in your midsection weight and feel worse." Since I still exercise regularly and haven't changed what I eat, I made an appointment to see my doctor. They checked my thyroid blood test.

I have hypothyroidism. My thyroid function is sluggish. This slows my metabolism, adds to the weight gain I could get in perimenopause, and dampens my moods and energy. After taking thyroid medication for two months, I feel like myself again.

Today, the genetic underpinnings of mood changes, depression, and even susceptibility to hot flashes have been partially unearthed. As mentioned above, a woman who has had postpartum depression is at higher risk for depression during perimenopause. Other perimenopausal women at high risk for depression include those who experience more volatile hormone peaks and troughs, particularly if they occur over longer periods of time.

Estrogen affects mood by influencing neurotransmitters in the brain. Estrogen increases serotonin levels. Serotonin is associated with positive feelings and has a calming effect. Low levels of estrogen will result in diminished serotonin levels and worse moods. There are also other ways that low serotonin can occur, such as problems with the receptor for serotonin or inadequate serotonin production.

Receptors enable the body to capture specific hormones and lock them into place. But everyone's receptors act differently, and what works for one person may not work for another. It is like having your own personal prescription for eyeglasses or contacts. Although the prescription helps you, it may not help someone else. With hormone receptors, the fit is even more precise. Picture a jigsaw puzzle piece fitting exactly into the opening of the master puzzle. That is how a hormone fits into its specific receptor. The color, contour, size, and orientation must match exactly for the right fit.

Estrogen receptors occur in many cells of the body, but they are particularly prominent in the brain, the breasts, and the genital system. Estrogen receptors, however, are also prevalent in the hippocampus and other areas of the brain that are important for emotions. Researchers are currently studying these receptors, which suggests we'll be learning more about emotional changes associated with menopause. We already know that some women are particularly sensitive to estrogen changes during perimenopause and may experience changes in mood because of it.

Researchers have now linked sensitivity to stress, "blue moods," and depression with intermittent low estrogen levels. During the reproductive years, the pattern of low estrogen occurs monthly at specific predictable times during the menstrual cycle. In perimenopause, however, low estrogen levels are irregular and unpredictable, making it challenging to predict and manage changes in mood and memory as well as depression.

The hypothalamus also has progesterone receptors. Progesterone can decrease anxiety and produce a hypnotic effect. At times, however, it can also worsen mood or cause irritability. Some forms of progesterone are helpful in controlling moods, especially when there is too little progesterone during perimenopause.

Genetics also play a role, and some women are more sensitive to hormones than others. Genetic research points to differences in how an individual's receptors function. A woman who inherits weak or ineffective receptors for a specific hormone is unable to use that hormone effectively. For example, if you have weak or ineffective receptors for serotonin, a "feel-good" hormone, you will be more prone to depression. Even if you have enough serotonin, it will not produce the desired calming effect because it is not able to bind to a defective receptor.

Biological differences between women in perimenopause and post menopause also determine how susceptible they are to stress or depression. If you do not manufacture enough serotonin due to a biological processing problem, you will be prone to anxiety and depression even if your serotonin receptors are normal.

The debate over whether you should take hormones during perimenopause or post menopause cannot overshadow other aspects of your health and well-being. While hormones are certainly an important issue, other aspects of your health also merit attention.

CORRECTING LOW HORMONE LEVELS: SHOULD YOU DO IT?

Perimenopause and post menopause are normal phases of life that present unique opportunities for preventing disease and enhancing health. At least two polarized views about mental health and menopause crop up perennially. Neither view serves women well.

One view rationalizes that perimenopause and post menopause are healthy phases, not diseases, and therefore do not warrant diagnosis or treatment. Women should simply weather the changes as a side effect of menopause. But this view shortchanges women who develop a treatable mental condition.

The other view is that hormones are always warranted to preserve sanity and mental acuity (in addition to youth, long-term health, and sexual function). This view shortchanges a woman by advising hormones without discerning whether the benefit to her is greater than the risk at any particular time.

Here's the balanced view: menopause is a healthy state in which women are at risk for certain physical and psychological problems. First, you and your doctor must identify your specific vulnerabilities based on your lifestyle, current health, and personal and family history. Then, prevention and treatment efforts can be tailored to you—first in perimenopause, with its changing landscape of hormones, and then in post menopause.

Hormones are trees in the forest of menopause research. In the realm of mental health, we have been losing the forest for the trees.

TEND AND BEFRIEND: THE UNIQUE BIOLOGY OF FEMALE STRESS

Gender differences exist in mental health and in how men and women respond to stress. These differences are not fixed, though, and can vary with a woman's individual biology and her phase of menopause. Gender differences also change with age. For example, a perimenopausal woman reacts to stress differently than a man her age (she is more vulnerable). In post menopause, her reaction morphs, and her stress response becomes more robust and more similar to that of her male counterpart.

Our understanding of women's response to stress has changed dramatically in the past few years. "Fight or flight" (i.e., the instinctive physiological response to a threatening situation where an individual chooses to use force to resist a threat or runs away from it) is the traditional understanding of human response to stress; however, it is not an accurate description. For men and women, there are actually three stages of response to stress:

1. Alert (alarm) phase. During this phase, you feel disrupted.
2. Resistance phase. During this phase, you make biological and behavioral attempts to adapt to the stressor or eliminate it completely.
3. Exhaustion (decompensation) phase. During this phase, your coping skills deteriorate if you cannot successfully deal with the stressor.

Notice that the second phase is neither "fight" nor "flight." The female stress response is more accurately described as "tend and befriend." Tend involves nurturing activities that protect a woman and her offspring. These activities promote safety and reduce distress. Befriend involves creating and maintaining social networks that aid in the process of tending.

Gender studies provide a new lens through which to view how differently women and men deal with stressors. In one study, researchers looked at how men and women responded to the stress of being diagnosed with cancer. Men who were diagnosed with prostate cancer avoided disclosing the diagnosis to others. In contrast, most women diagnosed with breast cancer sought opportunities to discuss it with others and to share their emotional reaction to the diagnosis. Women used more "tend-and-befriend" mechanisms to deal with the cancer diagnosis than their male counterparts. When researchers looked at men's and women's reaction to losing a partner—which is, of course, associated with very high stress levels—women sought more social contact. Men avoided social contact and distracted themselves with activities such as drinking more.

There are sex differences in the psychiatric realm as well. More women get depressed than men, and they report more stressors. Women are also more likely to experience posttraumatic stress disorder (PTSD). Both men and women report less stress as they age, but elderly women still report more than their male counterparts. In general, women recall more details of negative life events than men do. Women also have a greater subjective response and more behavioral changes to stress than men. Women's increased susceptibility begins in childhood, when the changes of puberty amplify their sensitivity to stress. Although women have a more pronounced psychological reaction to stress than men, they have less of a physical reaction to it than men.[1] Consider Zelda's story.

Zelda's Story
WITNESS TO A CAR ACCIDENT

My husband and I are both 73 years old. We're in good mental and physical health. We witnessed a fatal car accident involving an acquaintance. Afterward, I developed what my doctor called posttraumatic stress disorder. My husband did not. I continually recalled details of the accident, and since then I have refused to drive. My husband is still comfortable driving.

THE STRESS RESPONSE IN MEN AND WOMEN

Other gender differences have emerged while examining how men and women respond to stress. Researchers are scratching the surface of a very interesting phenomenon: the connection between stress and values and how it differs for men and women.

More specifically, men and women differ in their response to stress on four levels:

1. Subjective or psychological reaction. In general, women tend to recall and share information about negative experiences and emotions. Women tend to express both positive and negative emotions more often and more intensely than men.
2. Biological responses. This includes measuring the blood level of cortisol, a stress hormone. In tests, men had cortisol responses to the cognitive challenges. Women had greater cortisol responses to social rejection. Other studies have shown that epinephrine (another indicator of stress that mediates the nervous system) increases in response to an intellectual challenge more in men than in women.
3. Behavioral responses. These are influenced by culture and family.
4. Mental and physical health consequences. Examples include changes in blood pressure and pulse as well as heart attacks, depression, anxiety, and PTSD. These consequences are not distributed evenly. As you read earlier in this book, heart attacks are more difficult to diagnose in women. Depression and anxiety are more readily diagnosed in women, as they are more likely to talk about it. More data is needed.

> DID YOU KNOW?
>
> In some ways, women are more vulnerable to stress than men. In others, they are more resilient. It's important to note that gender differences regarding stress response are not consistent, and they also vary over time. In post menopause, women tend to behave more like men in terms of their response to stress.

WOMEN AND OXYTOCIN

Oxytocin is a hormone secreted by the pituitary gland in the brain. It is secreted by men and women in response to many types of events, including stress. It also regulates and dampens other neurologic systems activated by stress. When oxytocin is released, there is a sedative effect. It produces relaxation and more maternal and caretaking behavior.

Androgens—male hormones—block oxytocin from being released. In contrast, estrogen enhances oxytocin release. Women have a greater release of oxytocin in response to stress. When estrogen wanes, women release less oxytocin and experience less of its sedative effect, less relaxation, and less friend-seeking and maternal behavior. As a result, postmenopausal women move more in the direction of the "fight-or-flight" stress response that males have throughout their lifetime.

Women have long reported that spending time with friends offers unique stress reduction benefits. Now there is a scientific basis for this. Oxytocin is released when women are stressed. Oxytocin release encourages a woman to gather with other women and tend to her children. Once she "tends and befriends," more oxytocin hormone is released, which dilutes the stress and calms her. Oxytocin is also high during labor and when a woman nurses her infant.

Numerous studies have found that social ties lower the risk of heart disease by lowering blood pressure, heart rate, and cholesterol. Those with the most friends over a nine-year period cut their risk of death by more than 60 percent.

Research has shown that women were less likely to develop physical impairments while aging if they had more friends. They were also more likely to be happy. The magnitude of the effect was so significant that the study determined not having close friends or confidantes was as damaging to one's health as smoking or being overweight.

In the book *Best Friends: The Pleasures and Perils of Girls' and Women's Friendships*, coauthor Ruthellen Josselson, PhD, noted that women frequently let go of their friendships with other women as soon as they get overly busy with work and family. By setting friendships aside, they deprive themselves of sources of strength and nurturing.

DID YOU KNOW?
Women outlive men in North America, on average, by 10 years or more.

Women's friendships are key to their enjoyment and health. Jean Baker Miller, a researcher who studied positive relationships between women, found that friendships between women generate the following five benefits:

- Desire for more connection
- Increased mental clarity
- Productivity/creativity
- Sense of worth
- Sense of zest

Women grow through connection. Relationships also influence psychological resilience. When we receive and provide support for each other, we become more resilient.

DID YOU KNOW?
There is biological proof that friendships are an important part of weathering perimenopause and post menopause.

PREMENSTRUAL SYNDROME (PMS)

PMS differs from illnesses such as chronic fatigue syndrome or depression. With PMS, a woman feels well and functions normally for the first half of her cycle. Then, for one or two weeks before her menstrual period, she has mood changes along with physical changes that make her uncomfortable. Women with chronic illnesses that coexist with PMS do not get a reprieve every month, although they may find that their symptoms worsen before a menstrual period. These subtleties can make PMS difficult to identify. A correct diagnosis is important because treatments differ depending on a woman's unique clinical circumstances.

> DID YOU KNOW?
> PMS may worsen in perimenopause. PMS cannot take place in post menopause when the menstrual cycles are no longer present.

Several medical problems imitate PMS. Thyroid disease is one of them. If a woman has PMS symptoms, it's important to check the thyroid function using a blood test. The blood test shows whether the thyroid is over- or underactive. Once the thyroid is normal after treatment, there may or may not be residual PMS symptoms. If there are no residual symptoms, thyroid disease was the sole cause of the PMS. If there are residual symptoms, thyroid is one contributing factor but not the only one. In addition to thyroid disease, depression, anxiety disorders, and perimenopause may also mimic PMS. Other medical conditions with similar features include migraine headaches and irritable bowel syndrome.

The exact causes of PMS are unknown; however, there is likely a chemical basis for it. In addition, the hormonal effect of transient low estrogen may also foster the development of PMS. Ovarian hormones interact with serotonin, the neurotransmitter that promotes feeling good and calm feelings. A woman with PMS may have lower blood serotonin levels in the second half of her menstrual cycle. This chemical imbalance could prevent her from feeling good and staying calm, but she will improve with medications that increase serotonin. Other women who are prone to PMS may lack tryptophan, an amino acid needed to synthesize serotonin.

> DID YOU KNOW?
> PMS is common, affecting up to 30 percent of women with regular menstrual cycles.

The presence and severity of PMS may be influenced by:

- Culture
- Diet
- Exercise
- Family example (i.e., your mother's premenstrual behavior)
- Genetics
- Individual biology (i.e., you may metabolize or process estrogen too quickly)

The symptoms of PMS include:

- Abdominal bloating
- Anger
- Breast tenderness
- Crying easily
- Difficulty concentrating
- Dizziness
- Extreme fatigue
- Forgetfulness
- Gastrointestinal upset
- Headaches
- Heart palpitations
- Hot flashes
- Increased appetite
- Mood changes

PMS is limited to the second half of the menstrual cycle. Your menstrual cycle officially begins with the first day of bleeding. Therefore, the second half of your cycle occurs immediately before the bleeding starts. PMS symptoms resolve within two days of when the menstrual bleeding itself begins. To help your doctor correctly diagnose PMS, it's helpful for you to keep a diary of PMS symptoms and their timing throughout the month for at least two menstrual cycles. Include daily ratings of your physical symptoms, moods, and feelings as well as their intensity. These ratings include the timing and severity of bloating, headaches, mood changes, anxiety, and other features in relation to the timing of your menstrual bleeding.

New and more effective treatments for PMS are needed. Some women benefit from oral contraceptives that include low-dose estrogen and progestin. These are prescribed to be taken to allow for a monthly menstrual period or every three weeks to override the PMS and menstrual bleeding. Another approach is to try a progesterone-only low-dose oral contraceptive (such as Camila, Slynd, or Nor QD) that supplies more progesterone and may ease PMS symptoms. Another approach is to take a selective serotonin uptake inhibitor (SSRI) antidepressant medication either daily or before the menstrual period each month to ease PMS symptoms.[3] Evening primrose oil is a natural remedy available over the counter that has been studied and found to ease breast tenderness associated with PMS.[4] Other remedies, including acupuncture and acupressure, are being studied.[2]

A diary of symptoms is the only way your doctor can accurately diagnose PMS. A retrospective recall of symptoms is not accurate enough. The timing of the symptoms must be precisely recorded in relation to the menstrual bleeding. Symptoms that spill over into the first half of the menstrual cycle or that persist throughout the cycle are not characteristic of PMS. Consider Gaye's story.

Gaye's Story
THYROID VS. PMS IN PERIMENOPAUSE

I am a 49-year-old woman with a history of depression. My depression has been well controlled on medication for the last five years until three months ago. Now, my moods are worse prior to my menstrual periods. The moods remain worse while I am bleeding. Despite taking antidepressant medication, I feel more depressed all the time. My partner is older than I am and very supportive. She wondered if I have PMS since I'm perimenopausal. She had worse PMS during her perimenopause. My life circumstances have not changed with the exception that I no longer exercise regularly. I am tired when I wake up, even after a full night's sleep. I've always been appreciated at work. However, my boss recently asked me if everything was okay. I seemed depressed to her and was curt with her and my coworkers. My doctor screened me for depression and found my depression had worsened. She also did a blood test for thyroid. The test showed I have a sluggish thyroid. Within two months after starting thyroid medication, my moods returned to normal. In my case, the worsening of my depression was from a sluggish thyroid, not PMS alone in perimenopause.

During the second half of the cycle, your body produces estrogen and progesterone. When estrogen and progesterone levels fall, the menstrual period starts. The low estrogen and progesterone levels can set off PMS in some women.

As you read earlier in this chapter, women are more sensitive to stress when estrogen is intermittently low. Estrogen levels drop during the second half of each menstrual cycle and intermittently during perimenopause as well. Both are times when women are more vulnerable to stress. A woman with PMS may shrug off a stressful situation that occurs during the first half of her menstrual cycle. When the same woman experiences the same stressful situation during the second half of her cycle, it causes considerable distress. One way to view PMS is as a heightened sensitivity to stress.

A woman is more likely to express her anger, unhappiness, or anxiety during the week before her period. At this time, low estrogen renders her more emotionally fragile. Our society does not tolerate women's feelings of anger or unhappiness, even when they are justified.

Women deserve societal tolerance of PMS-related moods. Society's tendency to dismiss women's negative feelings does not serve women or society well. In fact, this dismissal actually denigrates a woman's negative thoughts and feelings. Remember that adage, "If you do not have something nice to say, say nothing at all"? While women feel more intense anger premenstrually and are more likely to express it, they are seldom validated and heard. Consider Davida's story.

Davida's Story
NOT JUST PMS

I'm 45, have two teenagers at home, and am in a happy, stable marriage. My husband has been saying lately, though, that during the latter half of my menstrual cycle, I'm extremely anxious. He notices that the two weeks before my period, I'm intolerant of the kids and impatient with him. He always liked the fact that I've been level-headed and says that now, he only sees that side of me for two weeks a month. The change in my moods has compromised the relationship I have with my children, my husband, my coworkers, and my boss. I feel depressed for the two weeks each month before my period. I also have had little energy to do normal things like make dinner. In the daytime, during this part of my cycle, I avoid business meetings that I'm expected to attend. My office has an open-door policy, but I keep my door shut for those two weeks. Recently, my husband and coworkers encouraged me to see my doctor about it. I decided to take their advice. My doctor took a detailed history and ordered a thyroid blood test. The thyroid test was normal. She also asked me questions about my moods. Because I function so well for two weeks of the month preceding my period, and my mood changes so drastically during the second two weeks, she suspected I have premenstrual dysphoric disorder (PMDD), a more severe form of PMS. She asked me to keep a chart for the next two months and record my moods and the timing of my menstrual cycle. She also advised increasing my calcium intake to 600 milligrams twice a day over this time period. In addition, because my PMDD is more severe, I will be taking a prescription medication to manage it.

PREMENSTRUAL DYSPHORIC DISORDER (PMDD)

Premenstrual dysphoric disorder, or PMDD, is a more severe form of PMS that compromises the way a woman functions socially and at work. The timing of PMDD symptoms is the same as those of PMS. In other words, PMDD symptoms disappear when the menstrual period begins. The severity of the symptoms and the degree to which they impact a woman's functioning are what differentiates PMDD from PMS.

Criteria for PMDD include:

- Irritability
- Marked anger
- Marked anxiety
- More frequent and severe interpersonal conflicts
- Worse or more mercurial moods

A woman with PMDD must have at least one of the above criteria as well as four or more additional features, such as:

- Appetite changes
- Decreased interest in usual activities
- Fatigue
- Feeling out of control
- Physical symptoms
- Poor concentration
- Substantially depressed mood (for two weeks or less)

Unlike PMS, PMDD dramatically compromises a woman's ability to function well at work, home, or school and in social interactions during the second half of her cycle.

Problems with concentration and memory occur in women with PMDD as well as those with major depression. The difference is that the concentration and memory problems in women with PMDD are restricted to the second half of the menstrual cycle. A woman has more pronounced mental changes with PMDD, even if she has no physical symptoms.

> **DID YOU KNOW?**
> PMS is 10 times more common than PMDD.

Researchers recently discovered the biology underlying PMDD. More specifically, they found that women with PMDD do not bind serotonin normally. This means serotonin cannot act as effectively to improve their mood. This makes them susceptible to problems during the second half of the cycle. Anxiety is the most specific emotion a woman with PMDD experiences during the second half of her cycle. This makes sense biologically because she cannot effectively bind and use serotonin, which is the calming neurotransmitter.

NATURAL TREATMENTS FOR PMS AND PMDD

There are several ways to address PMS and PMDD naturally. For example, lifestyle changes that provide relief from PMS symptoms include:

- Increasing daily exercise
- Limiting daily caffeine intake. Caffeine aggravates PMS. Staying away from coffee, tea, sodas, and chocolate helps decrease PMS severity.
- Limiting daily salt intake
- Additional remedies include:
- Calcium. Get 600 milligrams in your food twice a day to ease PMS symptoms.
- Cognitive behavioral therapy (CBT). CBT is a helpful counseling approach that provides tools to blunt the sharp increases in mood changes and anxiety.
- Evening primrose oil. This natural remedy has been used for years to enhance mood for those with PMS.[4]
- A low-fat vegan diet. This diet decreases symptoms of PMS and PMDD by reducing the amount of estrogen in the

blood. A high-fiber diet and roughage help carry estrogens out of the body through the bile duct and the liver. This helps the body soak up estrogen and stabilize estrogen levels. Note: To reduce PMS symptoms by following a strict low-fat vegan diet, it must be followed for the entire month, not just before the menstrual period. It includes avoiding oily salad dressings, French fries, potato chips, butter, margarine, cooking oils, and shortening in most cookies and pastries. It may take one to two months to notice the benefits. Other benefits may include loss of excess weight and a reduction in the number and severity of migraines.[5]

- Fruit of vitex agnus-castus. This fruit from the chasteberry tree is an herbal remedy that may treat PMS. It is available as vitex or chasteberry or agnus-castus fruit extract. It may help treat the symptoms of PMS by antagonizing prolactin. In one study of 170 women with PMS, it decreased irritability, anger, and breast fullness. Vitex or chasteberry may be effective, but it may have unwanted effects as well. Chasteberry is reported to lower sex drive (I don't know if that is why "chaste" is in the name). Extensive studies of vitex or chasteberry have not been done, and the US Food and Drug Administration (FDA) does not regulate this substance.
- Magnesium. Take 200 milligrams three times a day.
- Vitamin B6. Take fewer than 100 milligrams per day to avoid nerve damage from excess B6.
- Vitamin D. Take 800 international units daily for PMS.

PRESCRIPTION TREATMENTS FOR PMS AND PMDD

In the past few years, a low-dose oral contraceptive (brand name Yaz) has been approved to treat PMDD and PMS. It also includes a diuretic ingredient that decreases bloating by promoting water excretion.

Prescription treatment of PMDD may include cyclic administration of certain antidepressant medications that control serotonin (i.e., selective serotonin reuptake inhibitors, or SSRIs). SSRI antidepressant medications may also be given daily for the entire cycle to assist with regulating mood, anger, and other signs of PMDD. SSRIs are very effective because they allow more serotonin to stay in the body. Prescription treatments for PMS symptoms, however, may not be effective when underlying medical or psychological disorders are not identified and addressed.

It may be helpful to try exercise, relaxation techniques (e.g., stretching, yoga, or hot bath), and vitamin and mineral supplements to treat PMS before taking prescription medication. These approaches can also be effective for PMDD, although PMDD will often require a prescription for an SSRI.[3]

ANXIETY

Women are more prone to anxiety than men, and this vulnerability is magnified during perimenopause. Excessive worry and anxiety that are difficult to control can cause distress and impair the quality of a woman's daily life. When worry and anxiety occur more often than not for at least six months, it is considered a generalized anxiety disorder.

As with PMS and PMDD, your doctor may offer you prescription medications for anxiety. There are many natural remedies to consider, however. For example, Cognitive Behavioral Therapy, or CBT, may provide you with tools to help you cope with the challenges you face. It can also help soften the anxiety to a manageable level.

Newer research indicates that relaxation breathing can offer you relief in the short term at no cost, even during a stressful or anxiety-provoking circumstance.

Finally, meditation is emerging as an excellent practice to manage anxiety. If you have debilitating anxiety, you may wish to pursue meditation under the supervision of a health care clinician. Keep in mind that you may choose to not treat your anxiety if it is not debilitating. Alternatively, you may choose to take prescription medication to improve your anxiety. Prescription medication can be helpful if you have a demanding schedule, have no time for CBT, and are not opposed to trying medication.

CBT is effective for treating anxiety. Some studies have found it to be effective for up to 84 months after completing the therapy. CBT is ideal for women who have time to pursue it on a regular basis with a therapist, as well as those who prefer to avoid medication. You can also use it in conjunction with medication for anxiety. For example, SSRIs are a type of prescription medication that can help with anxiety because they enhance levels of serotonin. Selective norepinephrine reuptake inhibitors (SNRIs) are another good choice because they increase levels of norepinephrine, another "feel-good" hormone.

In addition to medication and/or CBT, aerobic exercise—particularly high-intensity exercise—plays an important role in lowering anxiety. Mindfulness-based stress reduction and yoga may also help.

DEPRESSION

In addition to your own feelings about menopause and aging, you will be influenced by the views of your friends, family, coworkers, and our society. Consciously or not, you may ask yourself: What lies ahead after perimenopause? What can I look forward to?

The answer to these questions is highly dependent on the culture you live in. For example, Japanese society honors women as they mature. Women entering post menopause garner increasing respect and authority. In contrast, the youth-centered culture in North America has many women lamenting the fact that they no longer attract men's attention. There are negative connotations for women as they age, gain weight, or acquire wrinkles. Therefore, it's not surprising that aging women in North American are more likely to be depressed than those in Japan.

Culture counts. Societies that respect women recognize that a woman's intellectual and social expertise increases with her age and experience. As a woman, you have more to offer as you age, and the value of your experience increases over time. When society mirrors this type of respect, women tend to have smoother perimenopause transitions. For example, more than one study has shown that if you are depressed during perimenopause, you are more likely to be disrupted by hot flashes when compared with women who aren't depressed. Hot flashes can cause insomnia, and the resulting sleep deprivation can cause mood swings and memory issues, all of which are associated with high levels of depression.

> **DID YOU KNOW?**
>
> Before puberty, the prevalence of depression is the same in girls and boys. As females mature, however, anxiety disorders occur twice as often in women than men. Major depression is three times more common in women than men.

During the reproductive years, women are two times more likely to be depressed than men. They are also more likely to have seasonal affective disorder (i.e., a disorder in which individuals feel depressed during shorter, darker winter days). Throughout the world, depression is more common in women than men. It is unclear how much this is due to women's willingness to talk about their feelings or their readiness to seek help. Anxiety disorders are also more common in women. This includes phobias, such as agoraphobia, as well as panic disorders that are twice as common in women.

Women are more likely to be sexually abused as children. Abused children are more likely to suffer depression as adults. Women's higher rate of victimization also makes them prime candidates for depression.

Role overload is another contributor. More than 50 percent of women who work full-time still perform 70 percent of the housework and child care. It's safe to assume that role overload contributes to their sense of exhaustion, a factor for depression. Those with young children who work outside the home may also experience role conflict that occurs when women who work outside the home feel they should be at home with their children or loved one. They are pulled in two directions simultaneously due to competing demands.

Married men are less likely to be depressed than single men. In contrast, married women are more likely to be depressed than married men or single women. Married men, in general, have fewer demands on them than when they were single. For women, demands on their time increase with marriage. Women's socialization involves looking after others and minimizing their own needs or even dismissing them entirely.

Financial stability also plays a role. More specifically, women who are financially disadvantaged are more likely to be depressed.

FREQUENCY OF DEPRESSION IN PERIMENOPAUSE

For women in perimenopause, risk factors for depression include:

- Current alcohol or substance abuse
- Gender
- History of depression in a first-degree relative (i.e., a parent, sibling, or child)
- Lack of social supports
- Prior episode of major depression
- Significant stressful life events

Depression is also more likely to occur in perimenopausal women with a history of PMS, PMDD, or postpartum depression. Early perimenopause (before age 40) and surgical menopause (i.e., when both ovaries are removed, and estrogen stops abruptly) at an early age can also lead to depression. The same is true for a short perimenopausal transition that can occur with surgery, chemotherapy, or radiation. A typical transition from premenopause with regular menstruation and no erratic changes in estrogen levels to post menopause takes more than seven years. Those with a short perimenopausal transition who have only a few months between premenopause, perimenopause, and post menopause are more prone to depression. And the short transition may also lead to depression. Women with these conditions have hormone shifts that are more dramatic and sudden, and there is less time to adjust to the low estrogen levels.

For perimenopausal and postmenopausal women, there also may be a link between depression and smoking. Cigarette smoking hastens post menopause by one to two years.

While early perimenopause is a risk factor for depression, the reverse may also be true. A few studies even suggest the possibility that depressed women may have an earlier perimenopause. Their follicle-stimulating hormone levels rise sooner than in other women.[6]

FREQUENCY OF DEPRESSION IN POST MENOPAUSE

Based on her biology, a postmenopausal woman more than five years from her final menstrual period is less susceptible to depression than when she was perimenopausal because her low estrogen levels are stable and steady. She has adapted to them.[7,8]

Although postmenopausal women are biologically more resistant to depression, they are also more likely to have major health issues, financial difficulties, lack of access to medical care, or social isolation. The pressures of society may be more potent. Postmenopausal women are more likely to lose a partner to death, become impoverished, or lack adequate physical activity and intellectual stimulation as they age. Risk factors for late-life depression include:

- Being widowed, divorced, or separated
- Chronic or uncontrolled pain
- Compromise in mental functioning
- Limited finances
- Insomnia
- One or more serious medical conditions

SOCIAL ISOLATION

If you have been diagnosed with depression, please talk to your doctor about treatment options. Depression lowers your quality of life and impacts other medical conditions. Although the prevalence of depression is higher in women than men across all age groups, the difference is not as marked in elderly women. This is good news in terms of the passage into post menopause.

ASSESSING DEPRESSION

Major depression means suffering from at least five of the following nine symptoms:

- Being in a depressed mood or losing interest or pleasure in normal activities for most of the day nearly every day for a minimum of two consecutive weeks
- Change in sleep (i.e., you sleep too much or too little)
- Excess appetite or loss of appetite
- Weight gain or weight loss
- Change in psychomotor activity (i.e., increased nervous energy or lethargy)
- Loss of energy
- Trouble concentrating
- Thoughts of worthlessness or guilt
- Thoughts about death or suicide

The following two-question screen for depression has been proposed by the US Preventive Services Task Force:

1. Over the past two weeks, have you felt down, depressed, or hopeless?
2. Over the past two weeks, have you felt little interest or pleasure in doing things?

Any individual with a positive response to either question deserves a formal evaluation for depression. Depression must be diagnosed by a trained physician, social worker, or therapist. More than 90 percent of all depressed patients also have anxiety. An anxiety disorder itself can also put a woman at higher risk for major depression. Your doctor must diagnose anxiety. They can also prescribe antidepressant medications that have anti-anxiety features. CBT is also helpful. The same is true for general stress reduction techniques such as slow, deep breathing, meditation, and other relaxation techniques.

You may not meet the criteria for major depression, but you could have symptoms of mild or moderate depression, both of which can impact your ability to function in your usual manner. Mild or moderate depression is even more prevalent than major depression.

FACTORS THAT CAN AFFECT DEPRESSION

Depression is not a normal consequence of aging. What are some causes of depression? Consider the following:

- Genetics. A family history of depression means your risk of depression increases by 70 percent. The underlying basis of this may be an inherited sensitivity to stressful life events.
- History of breast cancer or other cancers
- History of stroke and brain injury
- Medical problems. This includes severe anemia, multiple sclerosis, Parkinson's disease, and Alzheimer's disease.
- Medications. This includes beta-blockers, a type of blood pressure medication, such as propranolol or atenolol. Steroids can also cause depression, as can chemotherapy.
- Thyroid disease. Stress-induced subclinical hypothyroidism can cause depression and should be evaluated with a thyroid blood test.

ARE YOU DEPRESSED?

The Geriatric Depression Scale is a questionnaire used to identify depression specifically in older patients. Questions include:

1. Are you basically satisfied with your life?
2. Do you often get bored?
3. Do you often feel helpless?
4. Do you prefer to stay at home rather than going out and doing new things?
5. Do you feel worthless the way you are now?

A single point is given for a "no" response to item 1. A single point is given to a "yes" response to each of items 2–5. A score of 2 points or higher is a positive screen for depression.

Sadness and grief are a normal response to life events such as the death of a loved one or the changes in social status that may come with retirement. Depression can also result after transitioning from independent living to assisted or residential care or after losing physical function after an illness. Despite the increasing frequency of these types of losses with age, healthy elderly individuals who live independently in the community have a lower prevalence of clinical depression than the general adult community. Those older individuals who have medical illnesses may have higher rates of depression.

> DID YOU KNOW?
> Thirty percent of elderly hospitalized patients are depressed. Forty percent of elderly hospitalized patients who have had a stroke, heart attack, or cancer have depression.

TREATMENT OPTIONS FOR DEPRESSION

The good news is that doctors are beginning to become more aware of depression and make more effort to identify and treat it. As the stigma recedes, women who are depressed may be more receptive to acknowledging their depression and participating in treatment. Consider Dahlia's story.

> **DID YOU KNOW?**
> Only 33 percent of women with depression receive treatment.

Dahlia's Story
"EMPTY NEST" OR DEPRESSED?

About a year ago, when I entered post menopause, I stopped participating in several activities I used to enjoy. For two years, I just haven't felt the same enthusiasm for life in general. I'm now 53 years old, and I thought this was just part of life and the "empty nest syndrome." I used to volunteer five days a week teaching English as a second language and also worked for my congressman, but I gave that up. I've stopped writing letters to my daughter in college, an activity I used to enjoy every week. My husband and friends are concerned that something has changed, and they have encouraged me to see my doctor about it. When I saw my doctor, our conversation brought up the fact that I remembered my mother feeling blue when I left home to go away to college. I had to admit I hadn't felt this much hopelessness since the birth of my daughter, when I was diagnosed with postpartum depression.

My doctor used a screening tool to assess me for depression, saying that my lack of motivation and withdrawal from activities also pointed to depression. They recommended CBT and counseling. I felt better after starting these, but I also needed a prescription for an antidepressant to feel like myself again. It's been over a year now and I do feel like myself again. Eventually, after I felt like myself for six months, I was able to taper off the antidepressant medication under my doctor's supervision.

Treatment may include an over-the-counter remedy, prescribed medication for depression, and counseling/psychotherapy. Exercise has a therapeutic benefit as well; it can prevent or decrease depression.

OVER-THE-COUNTER REMEDY FOR DEPRESSION: ST. JOHN'S WORT

St. John's wort is a natural remedy that affects levels of neurochemicals in the brain and is somewhat effective against depression. Its long-term effectiveness (i.e., beyond six months), however, is not known. Also of concern: Because it is not approved by the FDA, we don't know a lot of about potential interactions between St. John's wort and medications you may already be taking. Lastly, manufacturing standards may vary greatly. This means the St. John's wort you purchase may have too little of the active ingredient (i.e., hyperforin). Also consider the following other important details about St. John's wort[20]:

- St. John's wort interacts with oral contraceptive birth control pills and compromises their effectiveness.
- St. John's wort reduces the effectiveness of medications used to treat HIV and cancer.
- St. John's wort interacts with digoxin, a common heart medication.
- St. John's wort interacts with statin medications given to lower cholesterol.[9]
- Some pills of St. John's wort contain an excessive amount of the active ingredient that could be toxic or harmful to some individuals.
- Potential side effects of St. John's wort include gastrointestinal symptoms, dizziness/confusion, tiredness/sedation, photosensitivity (including reports of second-degree burns from sunlight), dry mouth, urinary frequency, anorgasmia, and swelling.[10]
- St. John's wort should be stopped before surgery due to potential interactions with medications and anesthesia.

This does not mean that St. John's wort is not effective. Nor does it mean that you should avoid it. Just be forewarned that if you decide to try it, you're technically taking a substance that has not been manufactured and marketed to a high-quality standard. It should never be taken with prescription antidepressant medication due to a potentially toxic reaction called serotonin syndrome.

If you choose to try taking St. John's wort, you should purchase a product that has a seal of approval from one of these independent organizations offering quality testing:

1. US Pharmacopeia
2. ConsumerLab.com
3. NSF International

This tells you the product adheres to their manufacturing standard, but it does not ensure it is effective or safe for you or another individual.

PRESCRIPTION MEDICATIONS FOR DEPRESSION

Currently, there is a trend to prescribe medication for depression. Medications such as bupropion (Wellbutrin), fluoxetine (Prozac), paroxetine (Paxil), venlafaxine (Effexor), escitalopram (Lexapro), or duloxetine (Cymbalta) are usually effective. Fluoxetine and paroxetine are selective serotonin reuptake inhibitors (SSRIs) that help maintain blood levels of serotonin (the feel-good hormone) in the blood by lowering reabsorption. Venlafaxine, escitalopram, and duloxetine are selective norepinephrine reuptake inhibitors (SNRIs). They lower resorption and help maintain blood levels of norepinephrine as well as serotonin. Smaller doses are often needed for those over the age of 70 years because these individuals may be more sensitive to medication. Normally, medications for depression can take six weeks to be effective. In those over the age of 70, the complete response may not occur until 12 or 16 weeks after beginning treatment.[6,8]

Antidepressant medications influence the brain and modulate neurotransmitters. In women, SSRIs are especially effective because they act on the neurotransmitter serotonin. As you read earlier in this chapter, serotonin is key to a woman's sense of wellbeing. For those who also have anxiety, some combination of counseling, CBT, and/or medication to reduce anxiety may also be helpful.

COUNSELING/PSYCHOTHERAPY FOR DEPRESSION

During the past decade, counseling has been a secondary approach to treat depression. Today, it is common for doctors to rely on prescription medications alone. This is unfortunate. Counseling offers critical tools and approaches to difficult situations women face on multiple fronts. Providing a woman with different ways to frame her situation and address her challenges is invaluable and empowering. Counseling can treat general depression. I find it fascinating that psychotherapy itself changes brain chemistry in a different way than antidepressant medications do. This means the advantages of therapy are distinctly different from those of an antidepressant. Many individuals benefit from both medication and counseling.

When considering therapy, two approaches may serve you well in different ways. Research has shown that both approaches (i.e., CBT and interpersonal psychotherapy [IPT]) are effective.

CBT focuses on the relationships between your thoughts, behaviors, and emotions. The goal is to help you understand and change patterns of thinking and behaviors that contribute to negative feelings. CBT uses strategies to cope with anxiety. It can help you handle provoking situations and avoid patterns that make you more discouraged. Cognitive restructuring helps identify and alter automatic negative thoughts that go along with depression and anxiety.

IPT, on the other hand, focuses on life stress and mood. It identifies and addresses interpersonal issues that are associated with current symptoms. Four interpersonal areas are typically addressed:

1. Role disputes (disagreements in key relationships)
2. Role transitions (life events or role changes)
3. Grief (complicated bereavement)
4. Interpersonal difficulties (chronic relationship difficulties or dissatisfactions)

IPT may be particularly relevant to midlife women. In midlife, you are biologically vulnerable to anxiety and depression. You're also saddled with more life stress, such as caregiving for ailing parents and partners, adult children, and grandchildren, often while simultaneously juggling work demands. It's no wonder women are at risk for anxiety and depression at this time of life.

In addition to mitigating depression and anxiety in perimenopause, there is also an opportunity to build on your strengths, positive emotions, coping skills, and sources of resiliency. If you are not depressed, this can help prevent depressive episodes if you have a history of depression. You can use both CBT and IPT to support your mental health. Our society in the United States has strong gender socialization messaging that encourages us to focus on the needs of others while neglecting our own. When this occurs midlife, it is heightened when caregiving demands escalate.[11]

Older postmenopausal patients who are depressed may benefit greatly from individual psychotherapy. Couples or family therapy may also be helpful. You can undergo CBT or problem-solving therapy over two to four months, and it can produce significant results in older postmenopausal patients.

In perimenopause, volatile hormones increase vulnerability to stress during a time when the number, type, and severity of stressful events multiply. In post menopause, the hormone storm quiets, but social stressors increase. Ideally, each woman would have access to a trained social worker or psychologist to provide fresh perspective, tools, and support for dealing with the multiple challenges she faces at this time. Researchers have demonstrated that counseling is particularly effective in postmenopausal women.

EXERCISE TO TREAT DEPRESSION

Exercise can alleviate depression; however, it may take longer to notice its effects when compared with antidepressant drugs. One study showed that 16 weeks of exercise provided the same relief from depression as an SSRI prescription. Note that it typically takes six to eight weeks before you can assess the efficacy of an SSRI. Exercise can be difficult to start or maintain when one is depressed. Nevertheless, it can be a very important intervention for those who are depressed. More importantly, it can help ward off future episodes of depression.

USING ESTROGEN TO TREAT DEPRESSION

Some perimenopausal women who are depressed may improve with estrogen treatment; however, this treatment is controversial. Treating depression with counseling and/or antidepressant medication is the well-established approach. This approach also applies in post menopause. Rarely, after treatment with antidepressants or counseling or both, low-dose estrogen may provide additional relief.

NEW AND EMERGING TREATMENTS FOR DEPRESSION

Interesting research is emerging on psilocybin, the psychedelic compound in mushrooms. This compound may rewire the brain to ease depression and anxiety. Trials are being conducted in a few academic centers nationwide, including centers in Baltimore and Chicago. When administered in a therapeutic setting, the exposure to psilocybin may instill dramatic and long-lasting changes in women and men with resistant major depressive disorder that does not respond to traditional antidepressants.

Here's how it works: The psilocybin enters the brain the same way as lysergic acid diethylamide (commonly known as LSD) or serotonin, meaning it interacts with the proteins on the surface of the brain, where serotonin receptors are located. Within 30 minutes, scientists see changes in brain neuron connectivity. It also changes connections between areas of the brain and restructures them. An individual's thinking can become more flexible with the increased growth of neurons.

When taking psilocybin, it's important to work with someone who has experience with this treatment method to minimize negative side effects and maximize benefits. Still, some people taking psilocybin report increases in blood pressure, heart rate, and body temperature. A word of caution: Be sure to stop SSRIs before psilocybin treatment or it will not work. If you have a personal history of bipolar disorder, schizophrenia, or a family history of psychosis, you should not consider this treatment because it could unmask a psychosis or lead to a psychotic event where you lose touch with reality in an unhealthy way.[12]

BRAIN FOG IN PERIMENOPAUSE

During the perimenopause transition, many women report they have "brain fog." Pauline Maki, PhD, a prominent researcher in menopausal psychology, provides this definition in her review on brain fog: the constellation of cognitive symptoms experienced by women around menopause, which most frequently manifest in memory and attention difficulties and involve such symptoms as difficulty encoding and recalling words, names, stories, or numbers; difficulty maintaining a train of thought; distractibility; forgetting intentions (reason for coming into a specific room); and difficulty switching between tasks.[14]

Before discussing brain fog with your doctor, consider whether you may be depressed (discussed earlier in this chapter) or have sleep issues (including waking up tired after a full night's sleep or difficulty falling or staying asleep, discussed in chapter 10), are experiencing a high level of stress, or meeting demands from many areas (partner, parents, work, children, grandchildren, friends, volunteer activities, maintenance of house/apartment). If so, consider including this information when you discuss causes of brain fog with your clinician.

Hormone therapy is not currently recommended at any age to treat "brain fog" or cognitive concerns or to prevent dementia. Using menopausal hormone therapy early in post menopause (within 10 years of the final menstrual period) or under age 60 appears safe for cognitive function. For most women in perimenopause, the cognitive changes you may experience are mild and resolve in post menopause.[14]

During perimenopause, I found, as many of my patients and colleagues have, that multitasking is no longer practical. While multitasking, individuals rapidly change from one task to another. In perimenopause, many individuals will benefit from modifying or altering their approach and strategizing to focus on one task at a time before changing to another, as the ability to "multitask" often diminishes at this time.

MENTAL DECLINE IN POST MENOPAUSE

Cognition embodies many aspects of your thinking. It includes mental processes such as reasoning, thinking, evaluating, remembering, perception, and problem-solving. It is separate from emotional reactions to events or automatic responses. It is the core of your most sophisticated and creative thinking, as well as your ability to analyze and plan.

Perimenopause and post menopause are often associated with poor memory or more sluggish thinking. In one study, more than 62 percent of women reported their memory had worsened during perimenopause and early post menopause. It is difficult to sort out the reasons for this shift in memory and mental processing because many factors could be responsible.

I often hear women in perimenopause talking about the fear of "losing their mind." This fear can be set off by losing keys or glasses, representing forgetfulness or short-term memory problems. Other triggers may include difficulty retrieving a person's name, difficulty finding the right words, an inability to focus or sustain attention, or becoming more distractible. Consider Nadia's story.

Nadia's Story
I'M LOSING MY MIND

I'm 58, and I had my last menstrual period six months ago. Although I no longer have hot flashes, I am concerned about my memory. It has definitely worsened over the past three years. I've always been organized. My memory lapses were previously associated with episodes of hot flashes, or my menstrual cycle. I was especially forgetful the week before my period. Now I'm even more frustrated and forgetful. I forget my keys, lose my glasses, and cannot remember appointments I've made. I have difficulty retrieving names of people I know. These episodes of forgetfulness are more noticeable in some months than others. I've begun to fear that I'm developing early Alzheimer's disease.

I've spoken with my doctor about these concerns. Now that I no longer menstruate, the memory lapses are more random. They don't follow a cycle. My doctor said they are most likely related to the periodic low estrogen levels I still experience. They also wanted to review the number of things I try to track. For example, I keep a mental list of my priorities. Recently, I have taken on additional responsibilities at home and at work. This has increased the number of people to whom I'm accountable and the number of projects I need to monitor and complete. According to my doctor, the number of tasks is too great. I have information overload, and multitasking is making my memory problems worse. My doctor suggested I dedicate myself to one project or task at a time and to keep written lists of my priorities to decrease my mental load and improve my memory.

Nadia is an example of a healthy perimenopausal woman who is overextended, stressed, and multitasking. The multitasking further taxes her memory and compromises her ability to think clearly. Once she narrows her focus and stops stretching herself too thin, she can function well again. For Nadia, as for many of us, focusing on one thing at a time and keeping written records of commitments may free up our brains to function more as we wish they would.

MEMORY LOSS IN PERIMENOPAUSE

My patients frequently ask me: "Is this a normal memory lapse or cognitive decline/early dementia?" For some, perimenopause is commonly accompanied by poorer sleep quality, depression, and a disrupted sense of well-being. Eighty percent of women also experience disruptive hot flashes or night sweats. All of these changes may contribute to poorer memory. The memory lapses that are common during perimenopause and in midlife do not usually signal cognitive decline, dementia or Alzheimers. Memory lapses that are common in perimenopause are typically short term or transient. For example, it may take you longer to remember the name of a colleague you have not seen or spoken to in a year. This type of delayed recall is not typical of cognitive decline. In contrast, if you put your keys in the refrigerator or forget how to drive home from work, you should be evaluated for early cognitive decline. Forgetting where you parked your car is usually not indicative of cognitive decline.

If you nurture your mental health and stay physically active, you can establish a mental reserve to draw upon as you age. Think of it as mental horsepower that keeps your cognition running strongly.

Permanent memory difficulties do not wax and wane. If your memory worsens with your hot flashes, PMS, or PMDD—and then resolves or improves at other times—you are not likely to be experiencing a cognitive disorder. If there is any doubt, a neurologist, neuropsychologist, or other specialist can perform a formal assessment for memory impairment. For example, a neuropsychologist may administer specific tests to determine whether your memory problem is due to normal aging, dementia, brain injury, stress, anxiety or depression, attention disorder, or excess alcohol. If the diagnosis confirms a thought process problem, memory deficit, or other compromise in cognitive function, there are tools a specialist can provide to help you manage these difficulties.

Years ago, at a postgraduate course, I met an intelligent woman with a PhD who fell off a horse and suffered a serious brain injury. She was able to function professionally using the tools provided by a neuropsychologist that included organizational and memory aids as well as regular notetaking. She confided that she felt she was an even better professional than before her accident because her notes were more specific and detailed.

In an age of social connectedness, we all interact with more individuals than ever before. These interactions take place in person and remotely with people who could be down the hall or in another time zone. It's a lot to manage, and it may be different from the reality to which we're accustomed. For example, when I was single and working in obstetrics and gynecology, I could retain details of my schedule in my head for weeks on end. I could also remember what I needed to bring to each clinic and hospital. At that time, I could remember my social and on-call commitments also—all without difficulty. Once I married and had children, the ability to keep the schedules of colleagues, spouse, children, and employees diminished. It was also easier when I only had to check my phone messages and my beeper. Now, like many of you, I have an office phone and a cell phone. I am obliged to check multiple email accounts, snail mail, text messages, voicemails, and social media.

Today, there are so many ways to connect with others, but these tools generate overwhelming demands. Being available and accessible by cell phone and email 24/7 has not contributed to peace of mind, happiness, or satisfaction. These additional burdens flood our minds and cloud our thinking. It's no wonder we can't remember things as well.

In addition to the abundant, hectic distractions we have, other environmental and lifestyle choices can decrease memory and compromise cognition. Alcohol kills brain cells, dulls thinking (when consumed in excess), and disrupts deep sleep. Lack of physical activity will also decrease cognition, as will lack of mental stimulation.

DEMENTIA AND ALZHEIMER'S DISEASE: WHO GETS IT AND WHY?

Dementia is characterized by impairment of memory and at least one other cognitive domain such as aphasia (inability to speak), apraxia (inability to move), and agnosia (inability to think, reason, or remember). Dementia represents a decline from previous function severe enough to interfere with daily function and independence.

> DID YOU KNOW?
> The strongest risk factor for dementia is age. This is particularly true for Alzheimer's disease.

In addition to age, family history can also be a risk factor for developing Alzheimer's disease. Those with a first-degree relative with dementia have a 10 to 30 percent increased risk of developing it.

Vascular dementia—disease of the blood vessels in the brain—is another risk factor for dementia and Alzheimer's disease. Still, other risks that can increase the chance of getting Alzheimer's disease include diabetes, high blood pressure, heart disease, and smoking. High blood cholesterol also increases the risk of dementia in some studies. Diabetes has been associated with a 50 to 100 percent increase in the risk of Alzheimer's disease and dementia, as well as a 100 to 150 percent increase of vascular dementia. It's possible that diabetes impairs cognitive status mainly in those over the age of 70. The relationship between diabetes and the increased risk of dementia is not well understood and is being explored.

STAYING SHARP

Three lifestyle components help ward off dementia and Alzheimer's disease[17,18,19]:

1. An active social life. Social interactions boost one's resistance to dementia and Alzheimer's disease. Emotional and intellectual interactions with others stimulate brain function differently than solitary intellectual pursuits. Relating to different people challenges our social skills and forces the brain to read cues from people's expressions. One theory suggests that mental activity, learning, and social interaction prevent or reduce cognitive deficits by activating brain plasticity (flexibility) and enhancing synaptogenesis and neurogenesis (good communication in the nervous system).

2. Mental challenges. Intellectual stimulation can include activities such as learning a new language or reading about an area of interest such as history or literature. Doing puzzles (crossword puzzles, number puzzles, or jigsaw puzzles) also challenges the brain, as does learning or practicing a musical instrument. Higher levels of education are associated with a reduced risk of Alzheimer's disease. There is more developed brain capacity, and thus the reserve brain function is more generous. Even in the face of some loss of brain function with age, there is plenty of mental capacity left to function well.

3. Regular physical activity. Physical activity, including both exercise and daily activities, correlates with good cognition. Physical activity increases blood flow to the brain as well as the rest of the body. It enhances vascular and non-neuronal brain components that support neurons. When someone exercises regularly, the blood flow to the brain is better, and the nerve centers are healthier.

4. Maintain adequate hearing. A review of 11 large studies shows that impaired hearing or hearing loss is a risk factor for dementia and Alzheimer's. Get hearing aids if you need them![20]
5. There are other theories as well. For example, the vascular hypothesis suggests that social, mental, and physical activity prevents or reduces dementia and Alzheimer's disease through reduction of heart disease and stroke. These types of activities increase blood supply to the heart and brain.

The stress hypothesis suggests that active individuals maintain a more positive emotional state. Reduced stress leads to a lower susceptibility to Alzheimer's disease. In contrast, increased stress changes the feedback to the adrenal glands, a stress hormone center. The adrenal glands interact with cortisol stress receptors in the brain. As the imbalance worsens, the stress receptors in the hippocampus portion of the brain are affected, and this part of the brain atrophies and shrinks. In turn, this impairs mental function, including reasoning, memory, and judgment.

There are difficulties in studying the impact of lifestyle and activity on dementia, however. One is the fact that those with higher cognitive activity and functioning have higher baseline intellectual function. Even after being diagnosed with Alzheimer's disease, these individuals are still left with adequate cognitive skills to avoid the diagnosis of dementia.[15,16]

DID YOU KNOW?

Becoming and remaining intellectually active lessens the effect of dementia if it does occur.

MINDFULNESS MEDITATION

"Mindfulness is purposely paying attention to experiences in the present, moment in a non-judgmental way."
—Kabat-Zinn (1990)

Mindfulness meditation and paying attention to the present moment using sustained attention not only decreases anxiety and depression but may also stave off Alzheimer's disease. Training your brain to stay focused while monitoring for the presence of random thoughts leads to meta-awareness (i.e., observing your thoughts, emotions, and feelings as being separate from yourself) that you can further develop with mental training. The beauty of mental training is that you can practice mindfulness anytime and anywhere.

Mindfulness is now scientifically validated to lower stress and proven to lower the stress hormone cortisol. It has also been proven to decrease the symptoms associated with depression, anxiety, pain, and insomnia. Mental training for mindfulness will also increase satisfaction with work, family, and health.

Beyond these desirable benefits, scientists have discovered that mental training improves cognition in several ways. Consider the following:

- Episodic memory of past events improves in contrast to the memory loss that is specific with advancing age.
- Working memory improves as the ability to take information and use it to solve problems increases.
- Mental flexibility is increased as the ability to understand different points of view increases.

There is even more encouraging news: Meditation changes brain activity and structure. Those who meditate have more gray matter in the brain.[13] Researchers have found that individuals who meditate can better integrate their thoughts, senses, emotions, and awareness of their body, including heart rate, breathing rate, and hunger. Meditators also have more fluid intelligence. The fluid memory is involved in thinking and figuring things out.

The front half of the brain is what we use for cognition and reasoning. It's also the part of the brain that shrinks with age. The cerebral cortex peaks in your early 20s. Those who meditate are able to better able to preserve cortical thickness with aging.

Meditators also notice a change in their perceived stress after eight weeks of yoga or meditation. Researchers have discovered that gray matter can also change with yoga or meditation after eight weeks.[15]

Mind wandering is associated with Alzheimer's disease. After receiving eight weeks of meditation training, the regions of your brain associated with mind wandering would be "turned off" while meditating. The result? Decreased depression and PTSD along with fewer signs of Alzheimer's disease.

After eight weeks of meditation, neuroscience researchers now know that the hippocampus can remodel synapses and communicate more effectively between synapses while simultaneously generating new neurons. Meditation also assists with enhanced emotional regulation as well as learning and memory.

Sara Lazar, PhD, and her colleagues studied whether mindfulness late in life helps cognition. They looked at 120 healthy adults ages 65–80 with no dementia. All adults had normal cognition. The adults chosen for the study had not meditated or done yoga or tai chi in the past. The researchers studied the brains of adults who learned mindful meditation and compared them to the brains of adults who played daily brain games such as Sudoku or crossword puzzles.

The adults who did 40 minutes of mindful meditation daily were tested at baseline and at the end of the program eight weeks later. They were also tested 12 months and 24 months after the program. The results? The mindfulness group continued to improve while the group playing brain games reverted to baseline brain function.[16]

Lastly, researchers looked at sustained attention over 16 minutes and how well adults could focus on a task. The mindful group continued to improve, maintained attention span at the end of 16 minutes, and remained better than baseline. In contrast, the control group who did puzzles returned to baseline. The mindful group had better recall and specificity. This counteracted age-related changes that often occur when losing details of something new. For example, consider two 65-year-old adults, only one of whom meditates regularly. When shown two photos of two different-colored lunch boxes and then asked to recall the colors five minutes later, those who meditate regularly are more likely to discern the difference.

At this time, there are no established guidelines for guided versus self-guided meditation. The same is true for frequency or duration of meditation, but meditating 20–40 minutes five days a week has many advantages. For those who would like to try a guided meditation, there are resources found on Headspace. If you are new to guided meditation, it is OK to start with five minutes daily. If you have anxiety or depression, it is best if you work with a meditation teacher.

> **TOOLBOX**
> Consider a free meditation app such as:
> - Headspace

Just as positive interactions and activities stimulate the brain, there are activities and other factors that compromise brain function. These include stress, poor-quality sleep or inadequate amount of sleep, and alcohol consumption that destroys brain cells. Consider Esther's story.

Esther's Story
MAKING THE MOVE TO ASSISTED LIVING

I'm 68 years old, and I have lived alone for years with no problems. My closest family member is 45 minutes away. I have a bad hip that has limited my activity, so I no longer go to my stretching class at the YMCA three times a week. Since my hip has become painful, I have trouble getting in and out of the car and have not gone to lunch with my friends. I've had trouble paying my bills, and I make more mistakes doing the arithmetic. Plus, I've been misplacing the bills and forgetting to pay them. Occasionally, I forget to call to have my groceries delivered. My daughter visited and noticed there was no food in the refrigerator, and she found unpaid bills in unusual places in the apartment. She was alarmed and scheduled a medical evaluation for me. A neurologist diagnosed me with early dementia after performing a history and physical exam. Testing showed that I previously had a transient ischemic attack, or "mini stroke." I agreed to move to an assisted living community and build regular activity back into my schedule. Since walking is difficult for me, I agreed to do aqua jogging. This did not put pressure on my hip joint. Even though I don't swim, I've been able to participate in this activity that involves wearing a float around my waist and moving my legs in the water to music. The doctor says the physical activity has improved my mental and physical health. The increased social interaction in the assisted living community has also been beneficial.

ESTROGEN AND COGNITION

The Women's Health Initiative Memory Study (otherwise known as WHIMS) was part of the Women's Health Initiative (WHI). (For more background information about WHI in general, see chapter 3.) In this portion of the WHI study, 4,000 postmenopausal women with no dementia at the start of the study were followed on a combination of estrogen and progesterone. Postmenopausal women ages 65 and older were at higher risk for dementia after taking estrogen and progesterone for four years. Hormone treatment did not prevent mild cognitive impairment in these women.

Another large study in the United Kingdom, the Women's International Study of Long Duration Oestrogen after Menopause (otherwise known as WISDOM), was also stopped due to concerns about estrogen promoting dementia in older women.

It has become clear that estrogen does not benefit women over 65 years old who had their final menstrual period more than 10 years ago. It will not help their memory at this age and stage of menopause.

Neither of these studies refutes the benefit of prescribing estrogen for younger women (i.e., those under age 60) or in perimenopause or early post menopause who have had their final menstrual period within the last 10 years. In this group of women, estrogen has not increased the risk of dementia. At this time, there is no clear research to support that estrogen lowers the risk of dementia. For these women, doctors prescribe estrogen to relieve debilitating hot flashes. If a younger woman with severe hot flashes meets criteria to take low-dose estrogen and wishes to take it, she will not increase her risk of dementia.

In contrast, starting or restarting systemic estrogen in a woman over 60 is not typically advisable. It may worsen her mental health.[17,18,19]

TESTING FOR EARLY SIGNS OF DEMENTIA OR ALZHEIMER'S

If you or a loved one has questions about early memory loss, Alzheimer's, or dementia, your doctor may offer a short office test to determine if there is early evidence of these changes. The St. Louis University Mental Status exam (SLUMS) is one tool to do this (www.slu.edu). It has questions about the day, year, and month for orientation and a short memory testing component as well as a clock drawing test. It is available free online.

IMPORTANT TAKEAWAYS

In summary:

- Women experience aging very differently. While some women experience menopause as a joyful time, others may struggle with mood, memory, and mental health.
- Although hormones play an important role during menopause, other factors such as genetics, culture, diet, exercise, and more can affect an individual's mood, memory, and mental health.

- There are many ways to address cognitive and mental health changes that occur during menopause, and not all of them require prescription medication. There are also lifestyle changes, natural remedies, mindfulness meditation, and counseling options to consider.
- Although the risk for dementia and Alzheimer's disease increases with age, there are ways to "stay sharp" and lessen the effects.

QUESTIONS FOR YOUR DOCTOR

1. I'm often in a bad mood. Am I depressed or just cranky?
2. I'm more irritable before a menstrual period. Do I have PMS? If so, what are my options to alleviate my symptoms?
3. I am more anxious in the past year. What treatment options are available? Do I have to take medication?
4. I can no longer multitask. I am more forgetful. Is this an early sign of dementia or Alzheimer's disease?
5. What can I do to lower my risk of dementia and stay sharp?

RESOURCES

AARP (www.aarp.org). You may be too young to join, but you are eligible for membership in this nonprofit when you turn 50. *AARP the Magazine* and the corresponding website cover wellness tips for mental and physical health in addition to a wide range of other topics that impact your quality of life.

www.Alz.org—Alzheimer Association

www.BetterHelp.com—remote access to cognitive behavioral therapy

www.SBM.org—Society for Behavioral Medicine

www.FisherWallace.com—offers at home technology for transcranial alternating current stimulation developed by Columbia University researchers

www.menopause.org/. See Mental Health, Memory and Cognition under Patient materials: Mental Health.

www.nia.nih.gov—Alzheimer Disease Research Centers from National Institute on Aging, including ongoing clinical trials

www.nytimes.com/2000/02/15/health/vital-signs-nutrition-for-some-vegan-diet-relieves-pms.html, "Vegan diet relieves PMS for some."

www.womenshealth.gov/menstrual-cycle/premenstrual-syndrome/premenstrual-dysphoric-disorder-pmdd

APPS

MoodKit: A CBT app. There are four main tools, including activities focused on coping (with domains for individual productivity, social relationships, physical activity, and healthy habits), a thought checker, a mood tracker, and a journal. It can be used as a self-help app.

MoodMission: Recommends strategies based on CBT for those with low moods or are feeling anxious. Five missions promote confidence to handle stressors. The MoodMission app molds to the user's style and frequency of use. There are motivating rewards included. This app is helpful to lift mood and decrease anxiety and depression (free in App Store and Google Play).

Moodnotes: Based on CBT and positive psychology. Helps recognize traps in thinking and healthier thinking habits. Helps avoid catastrophic thinking where someone thinks a small error will have disastrous results and mind-reading where a person assumes others are critical of them without evidence of this.

NOOM MOOD: A 16-week introduction to cognitive behavioral therapy with exercises to give you tools to think clearly and lower anxiety.

What's UP: Incorporates CBT and ACT (acceptance and commitment therapy for depression, a counseling approach). Identifies common negative thinking patterns. Methods to overcome these negative patterns include useful metaphors, a catastrophe scale, grounding techniques, and breathing exercises. Data is synced across multiple devices. Information is passcode protected. It can become active in support forums where others discuss similar feelings and useful strategies. Available free in the App Store and Google Play.

BOOKS

Brehony K. *Awakening at Midlife: Realizing Your Potential for Growth and Change*. Riverhead Books; 1996. This book captures the imagination and provokes you to think of new possibilities that will break you out of your current mold.

Cain S. *Bittersweet: How Sorrow and Longing Make Us Whole.* Crown; 2022.

Genova L. *Remember: The Science of Memory and The Art of Forgetting.* Penguin Random House; 2021.

Green SM, McCabe RE, Soares CN. *The Cognitive Behavioral Workbook for Menopause.* New Harbinger Publications; 2012. A self-paced CBT behavioral workbook geared to menopausal women.

Gupta S. *Keep Sharp: Build a Better Brain at Any Age.* Simon & Schuster; 2021.

Lembke A. *Dopamine Nation: Finding Balance in the Age of Indulgence.* Dutton; 2021.

Petersen A. *On Edge: A Journey Through Anxiety.* Crown; 2017.

Mosconi L. *The XX Brain: The Groundbreaking Science Empowering Women to Maximize Cognitive Health and Prevent Alzheimer's Disease.* Penguin Random House; 2020.

Mosconi L. *The Menopause Brain.* Avery Penguin Random House; 2024.

Smith J. *Why Has Nobody Told Me This Before? Everyday Tools for Life's Ups and Downs.* Harper One; 2022. There are also free YouTube videos with some of this content.

CHAPTER 10

SUCCESSFUL SLEEP

Proper "shut eye" affects weight, memory, mood, and more. Here's why ... and how to get it.

SLEEP PROBLEMS COMMONLY OCCUR IN midlife, even if you don't have hot flashes or night sweats. Some sleep disorders are specific to peri- or post menopause. Others are more common as you age. Patients often come to me with questions about the quality of their sleep, which is why I'm devoting a chapter to this topic. In this chapter, I'll answer the following questions:

- How much sleep do I need as I get older?
- What are the consequences of sleep deprivation?
- How are sleep and weight gain related?
- How do I know whether I have insomnia?
- How do I know whether I have sleep apnea, and what are the risks associated with it?
- What can I do to promote a good night's sleep?

WHY SLEEP IS IMPORTANT

Sleep is an activity both your brain and your body need to maintain the health of all your cells, tissues, and organs. Sleep sets the "internal clock" in all your cells and tissues. The internal clock tells the cells and tissues when to perform their functions in your body. This clock is integrated with your metabolism, immune system, and nerve pathways. Melatonin, the sleep-inducing hormone, also influences temperature regulation and incorporates information about whether your environment is light or dark. The influence of melatonin is found in different organs, including the liver, lung, and pancreas.[1]

There are other clocks in the gastrointestinal system, muscles, white blood cells, and kidneys. Sleep–wake disturbances and lack of adequate quality sleep disrupt health in many ways:

- Affect mood, alertness, and performance
- Alter the blood vessel lining (endothelium) to increase risk of heart disease
- Alter the central nervous system and the peripheral nerves
- Increase amyloid deposition, a precursor to Alzheimer's disease and dementia[2]
- Increase insulin resistance in the pancreas
- Increase risk of obesity and excess adipose tissue
- Increase the amount of inflammation
- Increase the risk of breast and colon cancer as well as diabetes
- Increase visceral fat, which is deep fat around internal organs
- Influence neurodegeneration that increases the risk of Alzheimer's disease
- Worsen insulin resistance in the muscle

> DID YOU KNOW?
> - If you spend four hours versus nine hours of time in bed over the course of 14 nights, you'll increase your calorie intake by 310 kcal/day?[3]
> - Sleep fragmentation is associated with a higher risk of Alzheimer's disease and cognitive decline.[2,4]

Before delving into the types of sleep issues and what you can do about them, here are some questions to identify whether you have a sleep issue:

- Do you get tired easily during the day even if you had enough sleep?

- Do you have unintentional leg movements before you fall asleep?
- Do you have trouble falling asleep (i.e., does it take you more than 30 minutes)?
- Do you have trouble staying asleep (i.e., do you wake up more than once a night)?
- Do you sleep fewer than six hours a night?
- If you get enough sleep, are you still tired when you wake up?

If you answered "yes" to any of these questions for more than three days a week, you may have a sleep problem.

If you've determined you might have a sleep problem, how long has it been happening? Have you had it for more than three months? If so, talk with your doctor—particularly if you have morning fatigue or fatigue during the day, brain fog, or any other issues with your sleep. It is helpful to keep a sleep diary and bring it to your doctor. They can help you identify strategies to improve your sleep quality or quantity. In addition, there are now free online tools proven to help with many of these issues.

POTENTIAL SLEEP PROBLEMS YOU MAY EXPERIENCE

Many women may experience one or more sleep problems during menopause.

INSOMNIA

Insomnia is the most common sleep disorder. More than one out of three women have insomnia. For women, the association between insomnia and depression, anxiety, and other psychological mood changes is very strong.

The risk of insomnia increases with age. Before age 40, men and women have similar experiences with insomnia. Once a woman is over 40, however, she has a much higher risk of insomnia than a man her age. Beginning with perimenopause, women also have a higher risk of insomnia, even without hot flashes or night sweats. As you read in the previous chapter, women have a higher risk of depression than their male counterparts. In women, depression itself contributes to the higher risk of insomnia. Finally, a woman over age 40 is much more likely to have a psychological cause for her insomnia, such as depression, than a man over age 40 with insomnia.[13]

Insomnia involves difficulty falling asleep and/or staying asleep. It is characterized by:

- Difficulty falling asleep
- Early waking or waking up before you planned to end your sleep period
- Feeling tired when you wake up
- Problems with concentration and memory as well as irritability
- Sleepiness during the day
- Waking frequently during the night and having trouble going back to sleep

You likely have insomnia if you:

- Can't sleep
- Can't sleep and wake at normal times
- Can't stay awake the next day
- Have unusual behaviors or sensations with sleep

DID YOU KNOW?
Sleep difficulties are a major symptom in 40 to 60 percent of peri- and postmenopausal women.

Insomnia increases the risks of:

- Cognitive decline
- Death

- Falls
- High blood pressure
- Obesity

Sleep problems typically begin or worsen during perimenopause and post menopause independent of age. Add to that the fact that aging itself also affects men's and women's ability to sleep. This places even more importance on improving sleep habits to avoid insomnia. For optimum mental and physical functioning, plan on seven or eight hours of good-quality sleep each night.

A National Sleep Foundation poll found that 70 percent of American women reported sleep problems some nights. Researchers looked at insomnia reported by different women who woke up not feeling refreshed as well as those who woke up too early or were unable to go back to sleep. While 33 percent of women ages 18 to 24 reported sleep problems, 48 percent of women ages 55 to 64 reported sleep problems—an increase of nearly 50 percent.[9,10]

Note that there are two types of insomnia:

1. Primary

    Primary insomnia is not related to a discernable cause.

2. Secondary

Secondary insomnia has an identified cause related to medications or illness. Insomnia can be a chronic/long-term issue or an acute/recent one. Chronic insomnia, lasting three months, is extremely common in women who are depressed or anxious. It can also occur if you experience chronic stress or have pain at night. Before identifying menopause as the cause of poor sleep, review your medical history and medications with your doctor to identify those that may be contributing to poor sleep.

Medications and substances that may contribute to insomnia include:

- Alcohol
- Antidepressants

- Asthma medications such as bronchodilators
- Blood pressure medication
- Cannabis
- Decongestants or medication for allergies or a cold
- Nicotine
- Steroids

Medical conditions that affect sleep quality include:

- Alzheimer's
- Anxiety
- Depression
- Diabetes
- Gastric reflux
- New physical discomfort (such as pain from an injury or arthritis)
- Parkinson's
- Sleep disorders such as insomnia or sleep apnea
- Substance abuse
- Thyroid disease (untreated, undertreated, or overtreated)

Life impact stressors affecting sleep include:

- Changing work shifts/schedule
- Death of a family member or close friend
- Jet lag
- New physical discomfort (pain from an injury or arthritis)
- Relationship stress
- Work-related stress

There are various recommended treatments for insomnia.[6,7] In this section, I'll dive into several of them.

The first is cognitive behavioral therapy for insomnia (CBT-I). Here are some facts about CBT-I:

- CBT-I is a short, structured, and evidence-based approach to combating insomnia by focusing on the connection between the way we think, the things we do, and how we

sleep. It includes strategies to optimize the sleep environment (e.g., creating a cool, dark, and quiet space). It also increases your body's natural drive for sleep by consolidating sleep time and reducing time in bed not sleeping.[13]
- CBT-I is the first-choice treatment for insomnia.
- CBT-I is recommended by the American College of Physicians and The Menopause Society.
- Note that CBT and CBT-I are two different therapies. Regular CBT has not been shown to improve sleep or insomnia.

Once sleep is efficient, a CBT-I coach or use of the CBT-I app can guide you to gradually increase your sleep time, so you sleep a healthy amount.

> DID YOU KNOW?
> Eighty percent of individuals benefit from CBT-I. The benefit of CBI-I is equal to acute treatment with hypnotic medications.

In addition to CBT-I, there are other options to consider when treating insomnia. Consider the following:

1. Estromineral Serena
   This supplement is a combination of isoflavones as well as magnolia extract and lactobacilli with magnesium, calcium, and vitamin D. Research has shown it improves hot flashes and night sweats as well as sleep over 24 weeks.[5]
2. High-Intensity Exercise (HIT)
   Subjective questionnaires indicate that HIT improves sleep.
3. Hypnosis
   After five weeks, subjective questionnaires indicate that hypnosis improves sleep.
4. Long-Acting Melatonin

This remedy was reported to help men and women over age 55 improve the quality of their sleep. A newer study suggests melatonin helps menopausal women with pain from migraine, fibromyalgia, and joint pain but is less helpful for insomnia in menopause.

5. Massage

    One hour of massage twice a week improved quality of sleep according to sleep diaries; however, this research shows no changes in sleep measurements.

6. Micronized Progesterone (such as Prometrium)

    This prescription hormone may also help with sleep/insomnia in menopause regardless of whether it is prescribed alone or with estrogen.

7. Mindfulness/Relaxation Training

    A large review of 19 articles from 16 randomized controlled trials of 2108 peri- and postmenopausal women indicates that mindfulness and relaxation training does improve sleep. Assessment included sleep questionnaires and objective sleep measurement studies.[6]

8. Phytofemale Complex

    Phytofemale Complex may be another option. Though evidence is limited, this remedy looks promising. Vasomotor symptoms and sleep quality improved in the 50 women studied.[5]

9. Pycnogenol

    Made from French maritime pine bark extract, this remedy has limited evidence of effectiveness but looks promising in a small study. Consider Pycnogenol if other treatments fail; 60 mg daily improved sleep in 170 women.[5]

10. Sleep Restriction Therapy (SRT)

    SRT is a beneficial component of CBT-I; however, it is unclear whether it benefits menopausal women as a stand-alone strategy. One feature of SRT is only using the bed for sleep and sex, as well as modifying behaviors over time to make the bed a more effective and efficient place for sleep. For example, if you lie in bed for 8 hours but only sleep for 6.5 of those hours, you will stay in bed only the 6.5 hours that you sleep and get out of bed when not sleeping.[13]

11. Valerian Root

    This remedy is suggested if CBT-I is not elected. In 100 perimenopausal women with chronic insomnia, 530 mg twice a day improved sleep.[5]

12. Walking and Other Physical Exercise

    This remedy likely promotes sleep through:
    - Changing nerve chemistry
    - Reducing anxiety and depression
    - Regulating temperature control
    - Shifting the body time clock in the circadian system

13. Yoga

    Yoga has mixed reviews in terms of improving sleep. Only subjective—not objective—questionnaires indicate it may be helpful.

DID YOU KNOW?

RECOMMENDED:

- Low-and moderate-intensity exercise improves sleep. This likely includes yoga, Pilates, moderate-intensity aerobic exercise, strength training, and walking. More data is needed on each type of exercise in the menopausal population.

NOT RECOMMENDED:

- Kampo is not recommended to treat insomnia. Three trials showed no improvement. AVOID Kampo.
- Acupuncture is not recommended to treat insomnia. Current sleep studies show that acupuncture does not lead to any improvement.

DID YOU KNOW?
Insomnia is not the same as sleep deprivation. Insomnia assumes you could sleep and are unable to fall or stay asleep. Going to bed late or deliberately waking up early deprives you of sleep. If you get six hours of sleep or less, you may still benefit from CBT-I or sleep hygiene measures designed to improve the amount of time you sleep. But if you only go to bed and set an alarm to wake up six (or fewer) hours later, that is not considered insomnia.[13]

SLEEP APNEA

Sleep apnea refers to disturbed breathing patterns that occur when there is an interruption in breathing during nighttime sleep. People stop breathing on multiple occasions during the night, sometimes as often as 300 times. In some cases, an obstruction in the upper airway prevents air from flowing freely into the lungs. When someone has sleep apnea, carbon monoxide can build up in the blood because it is not being properly oxygenated.

Sleep apnea is more common in postmenopausal women, even those who are slender. In post menopause, physical changes and hormone shifts affect muscle tone. Progesterone levels are lower in postmenopausal women and can affect muscle tone in the neck, compromising the airway and causing halted, inadequate breathing during sleep. This can affect your moods and energy level, contribute to weight gain, and even increase your risk of diabetes or cancer.

There are three types of sleep apnea:

1. Central sleep apnea (CSA) Normally, the brain automatically instructs the muscles involved in breathing to take a breath. Central sleep apnea occurs when the brain does not send the signal to the muscles to take a breath, and there is no muscular effort to do so. As a result, breathing stops.

2. Obstructive sleep apnea (OSA). OSA occurs when the brain sends the signal to the muscles, and the muscles try to take a breath, but the airway is blocked (obstructed), usually due to the collapse of soft tissue at the back of the throat.
3. Mixed sleep apnea. This is a combination of both CSA and OSA.

Sleep apnea is common in those who snore and are sleepy during the day. It is also more common in people with central obesity (weight centered in the abdominal area). Type 2 diabetes, insulin resistance, and polycystic ovarian disease are conditions also associated with a higher risk of sleep apnea. Early perimenopause and post menopause are risk factors for sleep apnea. Advancing age is a risk factor for sleep apnea, up to age 60.

Sleep apnea is associated with heart attacks, heart failure, stroke, obesity, depression and mood disorders, excess daytime sleepiness, injury from accidents, poor quality of life, and alterations in sex hormones. Blood pressure and sleep apnea are closely related. Their relationship is as perplexing as that of the old "chicken and egg" conundrum. High blood pressure is a major risk factor for sleep apnea, and sleep apnea exacerbates high blood pressure.

Sleep-disordered breathing becomes more common in midlife. With age, muscle tone in the neck weakens with loss of progesterone in menopause. This is more common in women who are overweight, but it also occurs in slender women.[13]

Sleep apnea is confirmed using specialized testing and evaluation by a sleep expert. The testing may include a formal sleep study done at a sleep center. During a sleep study, your breathing, body movements, heart rate, and oxygen levels are monitored. Sleep studies may also be conducted in your home where you sleep in your own bed.

If you snore or your bed partner tells you that you stop breathing during the night, consider trying an apnea strap that goes under your chin like a bike helmet. This may give you relief and more quality sleep while you are waiting for a formal sleep study.

There is relief for those with sleep apnea. Controlled positive airway pressure (CPAP) is a therapeutic technique where air pressure is used to keep the airway open at the back of the throat. A CPAP machine pumps slightly pressurized air into a face mask or nasal pillows that sit in your nostrils while you sleep, keeping air flowing into your lungs. There are a variety of masks and nasal devices available now to increase your comfort. The new CPAP machines are quieter than their older counterparts and are less disruptive to the person using them and their bed partner.

Apnea also decreases with weight loss and exercise. Apnea does not respond to hormone treatment. Consider Marla's story.

Marla's Story
SLEEP APNEA

Six months ago, I was diagnosed with obstructive sleep apnea at age 51. It's nice to have an explanation for why I was having trouble concentrating and why it is so hard for me to lose weight. I was 50 pounds over my ideal body weight even though I walked regularly and went to the gym twice a week. I had trouble sleeping. Unlike my friends, I have no night sweats. My wife tells me that I snore at night. During a recent physical examination, I learned I have high blood pressure, and my cholesterol is high now. My doctor asked if my family members have sleep apnea. My father does, and my brother is undergoing a sleep test next month. My sleep study showed I stopped breathing 30 times an hour. This compromised and interrupted my sleep. I saw a sleep specialist who examined my nose, throat, and lungs, and prescribed a CPAP mask that I wear to keep my airway open at night. After six months of using it, I've been able to lose weight! I have also successfully modified my portion sizes—something I always had trouble doing—and am continuing with regular physical activity. My mood and concentration have returned to normal since using CPAP for my sleep apnea.

DISCUSSING SLEEP PROBLEMS WITH YOUR DOCTOR

When preparing to discuss sleep issues with your doctor, remember that a sleep history involves a 24-hour history of sleepiness, behaviors, routines, and alertness. Consider keeping a sleep log or diary including these details:

- Activities prior to bed
- How long you are awake during the night
- How many times you wake up
- How you feel in the morning
- How you feel the next day and when fatigue sets
- Time you go to bed
- When you fall asleep
- When you last eat
- Whether you wake up early

THE BIOLOGY OF SLEEP

Two phases of sleep represent two distinct activity states.

Phase one is nonrapid eye movement (NREM) sleep. During the NREM sleep:

- Your body repairs tissues.
- You build bone and muscle.
- You strengthen your immune system.

Phase two is rapid eye movement (REM) sleep that usually begins 90 minutes after falling asleep. During REM sleep, dreams occur. The first period of REM is short, lasting 10 minutes. Each time you enter REM after that, the phase lasts longer, up to one hour.

Normally, your body cycles between NREM and REM sleep. As you age, deep sleep is less intense. Periods of deep sleep also become shorter. Adults spend 20 percent of their sleep in REM.

A popular strategy is to deprive yourself of sleep during the workweek and then try to make it up by sleeping in on weekends. Unfortunately, our bodies adapt poorly to missed sleep, and this strategy will not allow us to make up for the loss.

If you are sleep deprived, there is nothing else that can meet your body's needs. You can function on less sleep, for example, by drinking coffee or tea, or eating chocolate, but the caffeine will not address your body's need for sleep.

The quality of your sleep matters as much as the quantity of sleep you get on a regular basis. The question I ask my patients to tease this out is: If you get enough sleep, when you wake up in the morning, are you rested or tired? If you are tired even after getting enough sleep, the quality of your sleep is likely compromised. Quality sleep includes a certain amount of deep sleep. Both perimenopausal and postmenopausal women have problems with the quality of their sleep after they have fallen asleep.

DID YOU KNOW?

Sleep deprivation has many consequences. These include:

- Anger and crankiness
- Compromised immune system
- Decreased alertness
- Depression
- Difficulty thinking and processing information
- Impaired memory
- Impaired thought processes (brain fog)
- Worsened performance at work or home

Sleep deprivation will also magnify alcohol's effect on your body. If you're tired and sleep deprived—and you drink alcohol—you will be more impaired than if you are well rested.

Studies show that decreasing your sleep by one and a half hours for one night decreases your daytime alertness by one-third.

SLEEP AND SEX

Quality sleep in healthy amounts influences sex in menopausal women. The Data Registry on Experiences of Aging, Menopause and Sexuality (DREAMS) study used questionnaires to evaluate sleep and sex in menopausal women using questionnaires. They found:

- Overall, 54 percent of the women had female sexual disorder (i.e., distress over sexual functioning).[8]
- Overall, 75 percent of the menopausal women had poor sleep quality.
- Women in the study who were sexually active were more likely to report good sleep quality compared to those who were not sexually active.
- Women with poorer sleep quality had a higher risk of female sexual dysfunction.
- Women with shorter sleep duration (i.e., less than five hours a night) had a greater risk of female sexual dysfunction.

THEORIES OF MENOPAUSE AND SLEEP

The relationship between estrogen, serotonin, and sleep is being explored. So far, researchers have found that estrogen influences serotonin production. Serotonin is necessary to produce melatonin, the sleep hormone. Deficiencies in serotonin and/or melatonin disrupt the length, timing, and quality of sleep. Lack of melatonin and serotonin may also disrupt your body's circadian rhythm, its internal clock.

Estrogen influences how well your body's thermostat works. The thermostat is in the hypothalamus area of the brain. With estrogen loss in post menopause, the thermostat in the hypothalamus does not function as well, and temperature regulation may be poor. Temperature regulation is helpful for quality sleep.

Progesterone is made in the ovaries prior to menopause. After menopause, the lack of progesterone weakens the supporting muscles in the airway. This may make women susceptible to airway collapse from weak muscles, causing sleep apnea even in women who are not overweight.

SLEEP PATTERNS IN PERI- VERSUS POSTMENOPAUSAL WOMEN

A large Canadian study evaluated menopausal changes in women ages 45–60. Researchers studied 6,179 women to learn about the quality of their sleep.[9] Researchers examined:

- Age
- Blood pressure
- Body mass index (BMI)
- Daytime sleepiness (i.e., difficulty staying awake despite seven or more hours of nighttime sleep)
- Difficulty falling asleep
- Gender
- Neck circumference
- Observed apnea
- Rapid eye movement sleep behavior disorder (RBD)
- Restless leg syndrome
- Satisfaction with sleep
- Snoring (STOP BANG questionnaire)
- Tiredness
- Total hours of sleep
- Wake up after sleep onset (WASO) (hard to stay asleep, hard to fall asleep again)

They found the following results:

- Insomnia symptoms begin around the time of menopause.
- Obstructive sleep apnea increases with age, as does periodic limb movements (i.e., restless leg syndrome), rapid eye

movement sleep behavior disorder, and changes in the normal sleep cycle.
- Postmenopausal women are more likely to have obstructive sleep apnea.
- Postmenopausal women are more likely to have sleep-onset insomnia disorder.
- Postmenopausal women need 30 minutes or more to fall asleep.
- Satisfaction with sleep decreases through post menopause.
- Sleep apnea increases through post menopause.
- Sleep patterns change with age over time.

Limitations of the study include the following:

- All data are self-reported.
- Individuals may not be aware of their daytime sleepiness.
- No neck circumference measurements were available.
- The study does not include input from bed partners or doctors.

Strengths of the study:

- Comprehensive list of sleep symptoms and disorders
- Data to show an association of various sleep disorders with aging and different stages of menopause
- Large population-based study

SLEEP AND WEIGHT

Sleep loss leads to hunger. It affects metabolism in a way that makes it more difficult to lose or even maintain weight. Sleep loss affects the stress hormone cortisol. Cortisol plays a role in regulating appetite. If you are sleep-deprived, you will feel hungry even when you are full. In addition, when you are sleep-deprived, you will store more fat. Your body's ability to metabolize carbohydrates is compromised. Your body will store more body fat. The insulin you produce will not be as effective, and your body will not respond to it as it should. You may then develop insulin resistance.[12]

The hormones ghrelin and leptin work together to control appetite as well. Ghrelin, produced in the gastrointestinal tract, stimulates hunger. Leptin, produced in fat cells, decreases hunger. When you don't get enough sleep, your levels of leptin are lower, allowing your hunger to grow out of control. Your levels of ghrelin rise, stimulating hunger when you would usually feel satisfied. With sleep deprivation, high ghrelin and low leptin create the perfect scenario for overeating—and it occurs after as little as two nights of sleep deprivation. Those who sleep less than seven hours per night are more likely to be overweight.

Growth hormone is released during deep sleep. Growth hormone helps the body regulate its proportion of fat and muscle. Less sleep leads to less growth hormone release. All of this contributes to excess weight.

If you are at a healthy weight, you will sleep better than if you are overweight. Studies of women who have lost weight or had weight loss surgery show a dramatic improvement in the quality of their sleep after a significant weight loss. For example, 82 percent of obese patients snore, but only 14 percent snore after losing weight. While 33 percent of obese women have sleep apnea, only 2 percent of these women have sleep apnea after weight loss. Abnormal daytime sleepiness and poor sleep quality also resolve dramatically with weight loss.[10] Consider Isabelle's story.

Isabella's Story
BURNING THE CANDLE AT BOTH ENDS

I work full-time and care for my elderly parents. I've always heard that you need less sleep as you get older, and at age 54, I get by on a lot less sleep. To get everything done, I do chores until 11:00 p.m. and get up at 5:00 a.m. My large coffee at 3:00 p.m. gives me the energy to keep going. Dinner at 8:30 p.m. is my big meal of the day. Two glasses of wine with dinner help me relax after my long busy day. If I have any energy left, I do a few exercises in front of the TV at 9:30 p.m. I never feel rested, even if I sleep later on weekends.

At my annual physical, I mentioned I was exhausted. My blood pressure was normal, but I was still 15 pounds overweight. My doctor asked if I snored. I don't know since I don't have a current partner. My doctor recommended I taper my coffee consumption gradually and avoid backlit screen use for two hours prior to bedtime to improve the quality of my sleep. If I still wake up exhausted after making those changes, they will recommend a home sleep study. I learned that many of my routines put me at risk for insomnia.

HOW TO HAVE A GOOD NIGHT'S SLEEP

If you cannot fall asleep in 30 minutes, sleep experts recommend that you get out of bed and do something else. Avoid lying in bed worrying. It's best to go to a different room for a relaxing activity and return to bed when you feel you can go to sleep. This way, your body associates your bedroom with sleeping (or sex) instead of tossing and turning.

Sleep quality is influenced by sleep habits and routines (in medical lingo, "sleep hygiene"). Beneficial sleep routines are healthy measures you can try to improve the quality of sleep, especially if you turn them into habits. Healthy sleep habits help your body ritualize the pre-sleep preparation in anticipation of quality rest and adequate sleep. If you are experiencing sleep problems, try these measures first for a restful sleep. If you still wake up tired, your physician can determine what aspects of the sleep process are disturbed. Problems like difficulty falling asleep, difficulty staying asleep through the night, and waking up before you plan to do so are all likely to respond to improved sleep habits.

Following are some steps you may take to improve your sleep:

FOOD INTAKE

Avoid spicy foods for dinner and avoid eating within three hours of bedtime. If you have gastritis (or gastroesophageal reflux disease [GERD]), you are prone to acid reflux when you lie down. Avoid going to bed extremely hungry. If you do not have GERD, have a small snack that includes tryptophan, an amino acid that is sleep-inducing. Milk has tryptophan, as do bananas.

> **DID YOU KNOW?**
> Eating a small portion of a starchy carbohydrate four hours before bedtime may help you fall asleep faster. The carbohydrates increase tryptophan and serotonin.

Carbohydrate-rich snacks can also help. For example, consider a bowl of oatmeal, yogurt with a graham cracker, or an apple with some pretzels. Some people benefit from a cup of soothing herb tea. Avoid excess protein or a heavy meal at bedtime. Eating too much sugar at bedtime will spike your blood sugar before it plummets.

EXERCISE

Exercising regularly helps the quality of sleep. The timing of the exercise matters. Vigorous exercise within three hours of bedtime may compromise sleep quality. Exercise decreases stress, increases energy and overall well-being, and may help you to sleep well if you have not exercised too close to your bedtime.

CAFFEINE

Caffeine can make it hard to fall asleep even when 12 hours have elapsed since you've had it. That's because it takes six hours to clear half the caffeine you consume. Drinking large quantities of caffeine and/or consuming caffeine later in the day ensures that the caffeine will be in your system after you go to sleep. Large amounts of decaffeinated coffee may also compromise sleep due to the amount. Caffeine will increase the number of times you wake up at night and decrease the total amount of time you sleep. If you are sensitive to caffeine, avoid coffee, tea, chocolate, and soda. Green tea does not have as much caffeine as black tea; however, it is not caffeine-free. Try slowly cutting back on caffeine over time and see whether your sleep improves.[13] (See chapter 2 for tips about tapering your coffee consumption.)

FLUIDS

Dehydration is associated with insomnia, so make sure you stay hydrated during the day. Some people can wake up to go to the bathroom and go right back to sleep again while others never recover from the interruption. If nighttime urination is a problem for you, stop drinking fluids two to four hours before bedtime or finish drinking most of your fluids at dinner.

SMOKING/NICOTINE

Nicotine disrupts the quality of sleep. Although low doses of nicotine from smoking are relaxing and produce a mild sedative effect, high doses of nicotine have a stimulant effect in the bloodstream at night.

ALCOHOL

Initially, alcohol (beer, wine, or liquor) is calming, relaxing, and slightly sedating. As alcohol is metabolized or processed, however, withdrawal causes poor sleep quality and sleep disruption. Deep REM sleep is disrupted and compromised by alcohol. Even two to three hours after the alcohol is eliminated, there is an after-effect of sleep disruption and awakening.

CANNABIS

Cannabis does not improve sleep quality.

NAPS

A daytime nap can interfere with the quality of your overnight sleep. If you have trouble sleeping at night, avoid daytime naps. If a nap is unavoidable, it's helpful to limit it to 30 minutes or less. That way, you won't fall into a deep sleep, but you'll wake up refreshed.

PRE-SLEEP RITUALS

Destressing for 10 to 60 minutes before bed is helpful. Relaxing pre-sleep rituals cue the body that it's time to wind down. These could include a warm bath, light reading, relaxing, or meditating. Some people can fall asleep watching late-night TV, but most experts advise taking the television out of the bedroom. They also advise using the bed for sleep and sex alone. For those with sleep problems, training your body to associate the bed with sleep and sex alone helps ingrain good sleep habits. Avoid stimulating or disturbing practices such as reading online or a back-lit screen, viewing upsetting news, having stressful discussions with family members, or doing demanding work. If you prefer to relax before bed by reading on an electronic device, consider using blue light filtering glasses, apps, or settings. Some experts advise not using any type of electronics, such as working on your computer, and avoiding TV for an hour before bedtime because computer use and TV watching stimulate the brain and keep it from unwinding. Falling asleep is associated with a drop in body temperature. If you take a warm—not hot—shower or bath, you can hasten this process.

Decreasing bright light and backlit screens for two to three hours before bedtime is more important than ever, according to new research.[11] Light at night in older age is associated with an increased risk of:

- Diabetes
- Hypertension
- Obesity

MAKING A SCHEDULE AND STICKING TO IT

Select a regular time to go to bed and a regular time to wake up seven days a week. Yes, even on weekends. This helps your body habituate to a healthy sleep routine and gets it accustomed to having enough sleep beginning at a particular time.

SLEEP ENVIRONMENT

Make sure your bed and pillow are comfortable. Open the window for some fresh air. Turn down the thermostat because it's easier to sleep in a cool room. Use layers to adjust to the room temperature so you're comfortable. For some, this will mean no night clothes and only a light blanket. For others, this may mean breathable night clothes and a sheet or an electric blanket that regulates your part of the bed. A pleasant sleep environment is dark and quiet. Darkness not only hides distractions but is also essential for your body to make melatonin. Liquid crystal displays on alarm clocks or other electronics should be covered or turned away from you. Room-darkening shades may be helpful. Eye masks may help. Ear plugs may help in more active households. Use a small night light if necessary.

Some women have their sleep disrupted by restless leg syndrome (their legs move uncontrollably during sleep). This can be associated with iron deficiency and can be diagnosed with a sleep study.

Certain medications, such as steroid medications or over-the-counter cold remedies or allergy remedies, can disrupt sleep. Untreated or undertreated thyroid disease can also decrease sleep quality.

Pets should probably not join you in bed unless you find them soothing. They move about, and allergies to pets may influence the quality of your sleep.

IMPORTANT TAKEAWAYS

In summary:

- Estrogen used to treat night sweats may improve the quality of sleep in perimenopausal women but not in women who have been postmenopausal for more than a few years.
- If you think you could have sleep apnea, it's important for your doctor to evaluate you. That's because sleep apnea is associated with heart attacks, heart failure, stroke, obesity, depression and mood disorders, excess daytime sleepiness, injury from accidents, poor quality of life, and alterations in sex hormones.
- Insomnia is the most common sleep disorder, and your risk of developing it increases with age.
- Sleep affects metabolism in a way that makes it more difficult to lose or even maintain weight. Several factors can affect sleep quality, including food intake, exercise, caffeine, sleep rituals, sleep environment, and more.
- Sleep patterns change with age, but quality sleep is critical to maintaining optimal health.
- Too little sleep will impair your memory and thought processes. It may also make you depressed, and it will compromise your immune system.

QUESTIONS FOR YOUR DOCTOR

1. I'm not sure whether I'm getting enough sleep. How much sleep do I need each night?
2. If I don't get enough sleep each night, what might I expect in terms of mental and physical health consequences?
3. I've noticed my hunger has been more pronounced. Could sleep loss be one reason why?

4. Based on my symptoms, I think I have insomnia. If you agree, what causes it, and what nonprescription treatment options should I consider?
5. How can I identify and address potential sleep apnea?
6. Might estrogen be beneficial in terms of improving my sleep quality?
7. What other steps can I take to improve sleep quality?
8. I've always been rested after eight hours of sleep. Now after eight hours of sleep, I wake up tired. What's going on and how do I feel rested again?

RESOURCES

American Sleep Apnea Association (www.sleepapnea.org)

Medline Plus; Sleep Disorders (www.nlm.nih.gov/medlineplus/sleepdisorders). This site is sponsored by the US National Library of Medicine and the National Institutes of Health. It is a comprehensive site that has a great deal of information about various sleep disorders as well as links to additional resources. It is available in 12 languages.

National Sleep Foundation (www.sleepfoundation.org)

Pathway to Better Sleep and automated six-week online CBT-I program (www.veterantraining.va.gov/insomnia/) or CBT-I Coach in the app store

Society of Behavioral Sleep Medicine (www.worldsleepsociety.org) to help identify experts in behavioral sleep medicine

BOOKS

Edelman JS. *Successful Sleep Strategies for Women*. Harvard Health Publications; 2012. Includes sleep strategies and review of research on women's sleep issues.

Prather AA. *The Sleep Prescription*. Penguin Life; 2022. A current review of sleep strategies and the rationale behind them.

CHAPTER 11

BETTER BONES

Be Aware of Silent, Invisible Changes That Affect Your Bone Health, and Act Now

IF YOU'RE A PHYSICALLY ACTIVE woman with no bone pain, you probably assume your bones are healthy and strong. You may be right. If you are in post menopause, you may be seriously mistaken. Post menopause sets silent, invisible changes into motion that weaken bones over time. This is true even if you continue to look strong and healthy. To some degree, these silent changes take place in every postmenopausal woman.

In this chapter, I'll answer the following questions:

- Why are healthy bones essential to physical health and well-being?
- Why are osteoporosis and low bone mass dangerous, and who is most at risk?
- What are the two major types of bone in the body, and how does each respond to post menopause differently?
- What tests are currently available to identify women who have thin bones who are at risk for a fragility fracture?
- What are the most helpful strategies to promote bone health?

BONE THINNING: IS THERE ANYTHING YOU CAN DO?

Many women I see in my medical practice assume they have no bone thinning if they have no joint pain or bone pain, but osteoporosis is typically silent.

The good news? It is possible to prevent excess bone thinning through lifestyle choices and getting adequate amounts of calcium and vitamin D. If you already have osteoporosis or had a fragility fracture (a fracture that occurs without a fall or injury), you can strengthen your bones and lower your risk of fracture by taking a prescription medication. The goal is to work with your doctor to prevent the first fracture.

> DID YOU KNOW?
> - Fifty-five percent of North American women over age 50 are living with osteoporosis or are at risk for osteoporosis.[1]
> - One in two women over 50 years old will break a bone due to osteoporosis at some point during their life.[1]

WHY SHOULD I WORRY ABOUT MY BONES?

For your grandmother or great-grandmother, bone strength was not a big concern. That's because they lived shorter lives and spent less time in post menopause, the period when bone loss accelerates. Today, women spend at least one third of their adult lives in post menopause. For postmenopausal women, bone health is a major issue.

Healthy bones are essential to your physical health and your ability to be independent and self-sufficient. Bone health impacts the quality of life you will enjoy from the time of your final menstrual period until the end of your life.

OSTEOPOROSIS: THE SCARY STATISTICS

Osteoporosis, a condition of weak bones or having bones so thin they are at high risk of breaking, is increasingly common. According to the National Osteoporosis Foundation, half of all women over 50 will have an osteoporosis-related fracture regardless of whether they are actually diagnosed with osteoporosis.

DID YOU KNOW?
Your risk of hip fracture is equal to your combined risk of breast, uterine, and ovarian cancer.[1]

In 2010, a National Health and Nutrition Examination Survey (NHANES) estimated that 10.2 million older Americans had osteoporosis (severe bone thinning with a high risk of fracture), and 43.4 million additional older Americans had low bone mass (with a lower risk of fracture). Two million osteoporotic fractures occur each year in the United States, and 7 out of 10 of those fractures occur in women.[1]

If you have mild bone thinning, now called low bone mass (formerly called osteopenia), lifestyle modifications and prevention measures are still important for your general health. Most fractures occur in women with low bone mass (osteopenia), not osteoporosis.

IMPORTANCE OF BONE HEALTH

Whether you are perimenopausal or postmenopausal, embrace prevention strategies for bone health. Carefully consider prescription treatment if you need it. Bone health is key to your longevity and quality of life.

Just how important is bone health? Consider the following:

- Half of the women over age 70 who have an osteoporotic hip fracture never regain the degree of function they enjoyed before the fracture.
- Once you break a bone in your hip or spine, you are likely to lose your mobility and independence, severely compromising your quality of life.
- One in five women who walk around with no restrictions before breaking a hip require long-term care after their hip fracture.
- Six months after a hip fracture, only 15 of 100 women with a hip fracture can walk across a room unaided.

- Women who do not regain their pre-fracture level of functioning need outside assistance in their home or require nursing home care.

In addition, osteoporosis can be life-threatening. Consider the following:

- After getting an osteoporotic fracture, you may die prematurely from complications.
- Once bedridden, the risk of developing other medical problems (e.g., pneumonia or a blood clot) is high. This is particularly true as you age.
- One out of every four women ages 50 and older who have a hip fracture die in the year following their fracture. Two out of every five women ages 70 and older die the year following their fracture.
- Some complications of osteoporotic fracture are related to being bedridden.

It is tempting to rationalize that these numbers do not apply to you personally. Neither my female colleagues, my patients, nor I envision becoming victims of osteoporosis. Statistics show, however, that 50 percent of us go on to develop the disease. In addition, 50 percent of us will experience an osteoporotic fracture.[1]

LOW BONE MASS (FORMERLY OSTEOPENIA)

Bone quality and bone density both contribute to bone strength. At present, the dual-energy X-ray absorptiometry (DXA) test allows us to measure bone density. It is a simple test with minimal radiation. Avoid wearing any metal and you won't even have to change your clothes and put on a hospital johnny! This test is key to screening for weak bones.

Low bone mass (formerly called osteopenia) is the term for low bone mass that may progress to osteoporosis. Low bone mass is a diagnosis made from measuring bone thickness on a DXA.

Typically, if you have a mild degree of bone thinning or low bone mass, lifestyle modifications may improve your bone strength. But if you are over age 60 or have other risk factors for thin bones or a fracture, lifestyle modifications alone will not prevent fractures, and you may be offered medication to lower your risk of fracture. If you already have severe bone thinning or osteoporosis, you'll need a prescription medication. Lifestyle modifications prevent fractures and enhance bone health in a different way than medications, providing a unique benefit to your health or enhancing improving results from medication.

OSTEOPOROTIC FRACTURES: A SILENT PROBLEM

An osteoporotic fracture occurs due to weak bones, often without warning. The fragile state of the thinner, weaker bones is usually invisible to you and your doctor. You do not have to fall or experience physical trauma such as a car accident to get an osteoporotic fracture.

> DID YOU KNOW?
> Weak bones in the spine or hip may break even in the absence of a fall or injury.

If you fall from a standing position and break a bone, you have a fragility fracture. If your bones were not weak, a fall from standing would not cause a break. If you have a fragility fracture in your spine, hip, or arm, you are diagnosed with osteoporosis. The diagnosis of osteoporosis holds even if you have not had a DXA measurement or your DXA does not show osteoporosis.

Most women never realize they have critically thin bones until they get an osteoporotic fracture. That's because osteoporosis is typically painless. Osteoporotic spine fractures can cause height loss and, in severe cases, may compromise lung capacity. If you lose more than 1.5 inches of height, ask your doctor to order a spine X-ray to determine whether you had a fragility fracture. If you did, your doctor may initiate treatment to prevent other fractures.

> **DID YOU KNOW?**
> Your likelihood of getting an additional fracture is especially high during the first two years after a fracture.

NATURAL BONE FORMATION

There are two major types of bone in the body: trabecular bone and cortical bone. These two types of bone respond differently to post menopause.

Trabecular bone, a more porous bone like a spider web, is found in the central core of a bone. It is the central inner marrow you see when you break a chicken bone in half. Trabecular bone weakens with the loss of connections, just as a spider web weakens when it is torn or broken.

Cortical bone is the hard, smooth, compact layer of bone that covers the outer surface. Muscle strain affects cortical bone, as do changes in blood supply, nerve connections, and vitamin D levels.

Bone is restored by a process called remodeling. Just as skin replenishes itself throughout a lifetime, older bone is resorbed or dissolved as newer bone is laid down. Cortical and trabecular bones remodel differently. Trabecular bone remodels quickly, showing 25 percent turnover within a year, while cortical bone changes slowly at 2 percent. In trabecular bone, the rapid changes may produce loss of struts and connections, weakening the structure and compromising bone strength.

DID YOU KNOW?
Even after you reach adulthood, your bones continue to change. After you reach your adult height, your bones continue to form, dissolve, and reform throughout your lifetime.

Two kinds of cells are involved in bone renewal. Osteoblasts build new bone, and osteoclasts are responsible for resorption or clearing and removing old bone. Both osteoblasts and osteoclasts engage in remodeling. Bone formation and bone removal are part of the remodeling process.

Early in life, bone formation is rapid and exceeds the amount of bone that dissolves. During the teenage years, bone builds quickly and then stabilizes. In your twenties, bones form and dissolve at roughly the same rate. Bones are in balance so that women in their twenties do not build extra bone as they did during their teen years, nor do they lose bone as they will later in life. During the mid-to-late thirties, the balance begins to shift. Closer to post menopause, the osteoclast cells dissolve bone faster than bone is formed. Then there is more bone dissolving than bone forming.

BONE THINNING

Aging is associated with a slow process of bone thinning. Both men and women experience slow bone thinning as a gradual process that starts around age 35. Postmenopausal women, unlike men, experience a second type of bone loss that is more rapid and occurs at the beginning of post menopause. Due to low estrogen, a rapid decline in bone strength and thickness occurs during the first five years after the final menstrual period (or after both ovaries stop making estrogen or are removed).

> **DID YOU KNOW?**
> You can lose up to 20 percent of your bone mass during the first five to seven years of post menopause.

In addition to these two bone-thinning processes encountered by all postmenopausal women, you may have other risk factors that will make your bones thinner compared to those of your peers.

The rapid bone loss seen in early post menopause affects trabecular bone first. The early vulnerability of trabecular bone explains why women commonly fracture a vertebra in their spine long before men do. Vertebrae are mostly trabecular bone and are most sensitive to estrogen loss in early post menopause. Stress fractures of the vertebrae in the spine and radius bone of the forearm are the first to occur.

After the initial rapid weakening of the bone, a slower decrease in bone density and strength continues for the remainder of your life. This slow, age-related bone thinning in men and women is called type 2 or senile osteoporosis. Age-related bone thinning affects both trabecular bones and cortical bones equally. Female anatomy puts women at greater risk of fracture than men. Women's lighter, more delicate skeletons are more vulnerable to damage and breakage than the heavier, more robust male skeleton.

Bone loss occurs in the early postmenopausal period because the rate of remodeling or bone turnover increases by 300 to 400 percent. This high turnover compromises bone quality on a microscopic level. It decreases bone mass, so the bone becomes lighter even when it remains the same size. It also disrupts the trabecular cross-struts that provide strength throughout the bone. Finally, it decreases the amount of calcium and other minerals in the bone, making the bone more porous inside.

After age 50, your cortical bone, the outer bone surface, becomes weaker and more porous. Researchers theorize that the cortical bone recedes from the inside during post menopause and beyond, meaning it thins from the inside out. If you put a heated stick into an ice pop, the inner core becomes a larger cavity while the outer portion of the ice pop stays frozen. The overall thickness of the ice pop decreases as it melts from the inside out. This is analogous to cortical bone becoming hollowed and weakened from the inside. It decreases in diameter, thickness, and strength. In addition, it becomes more porous, further decreasing its strength. When the normally solid cortical bone suffers from thinning and becomes more porous, it starts to look more like trabecular bone. If cortical bones become even slightly more porous, bone strength dramatically decreases.

If healthy bones look like cheddar cheese, osteoporotic bones look like Swiss cheese. They are no longer solid, strong, or thick. Another way to think of the difference in bone quality is by imagining two hand-knit sweaters of the same size. The first sweater, knitted with fine yarn, small needles, and tight stitches, represents strong bones that are less likely to tear or unravel. Their architecture is robust. The second sweater, knitted loosely with large, loopy stitches and lots of spaces, has more holes and will likely tear or unravel sooner. The loopy sweater is more fragile. Similarly, weaker bones have a weaker architecture and greater susceptibility to fracture.

In addition to the poorer, less robust quality of the bone itself that comes with age, other circumstances increase the risk of falls. With age, eyesight worsens, and it becomes more difficult to negotiate stairs and uneven terrain. Coordination becomes compromised. Muscle strength weakens. Balance is worse. Brain processing and signals are slower. Over time, the risk of falling increases as the bone becomes more fragile, increasing the likelihood of a fracture—which is why prevention of bone thinning and fall prevention are vital.

WHO IS AT RISK FOR OSTEOPOROSIS?

If you are a woman over the age of 50 or have entered post menopause, your bone health is important to your overall health. Most women are not aware that they might be at increased risk for developing osteoporosis. Their doctors may not be aware either.

GENERAL RISK FACTORS FOR OSTEOPOROSIS

Several risk factors affect all women. These include the following:

- Age. The older you get, the greater your risk for developing osteoporosis.
- Alcohol. The exact threshold of alcohol consumption to produce bone thinning is unclear, but it may be as little as one drink a day.
- Anorexia or bulimia (past or current)
- Being small-boned and thin. Slender individuals weighing less than 127 pounds are at higher risk of osteoporosis. Similarly, a woman whose weight falls in the lowest 25th percentile for her height is at higher risk for fragility fractures. A woman who is underweight should be followed closely and assessed for her risk of osteoporosis. On the other hand, being "big boned" does not protect against osteoporosis.
- Caffeine: Excess caffeine is an insult to healthy bones.
- Certain hormones. Depo Provera (a long-acting progesterone injection for contraception), especially when used in late perimenopause.
- Certain medical conditions: Consider the following:
  1. Any disorder or procedure that affects the ability to absorb calcium adds to the risk of developing osteoporosis, such as weight loss surgery or digestive disorders that impair the ability to absorb calcium.
  2. Certain types of anemia, including sickle cell anemia, are associated with a higher risk of osteoporosis.
  3. Diabetes and hyperthyroidism are associated with a higher risk of osteoporosis.
  4. Inflammatory bowel disease/syndrome, celiac sprue disease, and gastric bypass surgery are associated with a higher risk of osteoporosis.

5. Kidney disease is associated with a higher risk of osteoporosis.
6. Rheumatoid arthritis is associated with a higher risk of osteoporosis.
- Certain medications. Consider the following:
    1. Antidepressants. This includes the SSRIs (see chapter 9).
    2. Anti-estrogen medications. The long-term use (beyond six months) of Lupron or other anti-estrogen medications will produce osteoporosis. These anti-estrogen medications are used to treat fibroids and endometriosis.
    3. Chemotherapy. This includes aromatase inhibitors used to treat breast cancer, such as letrozole or anastrozole, which are anti-estrogen medications.
    4. Glucocorticoids (steroids). Over time, when given by mouth, injected, or inhaled, these medications can increase the risk of osteoporosis.
    5. Lithium. This medication, used to treat those with bipolar disease, can increase the risk of osteoporosis.
    6. Long-term use of heparin. This blood thinner can increase the risk of developing osteoporosis.
    7. Proton pump inhibitors. These medications, used to treat those with ulcers or gastroesophageal reflux disease, can increase the risk of osteoporosis.
    8. Seizure medications. Depakote or Dilantin can increase the risk of osteoporosis.
- Family history of osteoporosis. Note that the absence of a family history of osteoporosis should not be interpreted as immunity, particularly when there is a family history of broken bones. It is common for a woman to have osteoporosis, even if there is no family history: that is why it is important for your doctor to evaluate you to determine your risk.

- High-protein diet or high-protein weight loss diet. Excess protein alters kidney function and increases calcium loss from bone.
- Low calcium intake. Low intake increases a woman's risk of developing osteoporosis, so vitamin supplements or dietary changes may be necessary.
- Low estrogen levels. Low levels increase a woman's risk of developing osteoporosis.
- Low vitamin D intake. Low vitamin D intake increases the risk of developing osteoporosis. Vitamin D supplements and dietary changes are often advised.
- Missed periods. Otherwise known as amenorrhea, this risk factor is associated with lower estrogen, which can lead to osteoporosis.
- Salty foods. Foods with high sodium or salt content thin bones by leaching out calcium and decreasing bone strength.
- Sedentary lifestyle. With a sedentary lifestyle or lengthy periods of inactivity, weaker bones develop. Consider the following:
  1. Bones become thinner and weaker when not exercised. The same is true for muscles that don't work against gravity.
  2. Less physical activity weakens muscles and bones.
  3. The type of exercise, how often it is done, and the number of years of exercising all influence your bone strength.
  4. Weight-bearing exercise maintains bone health.
- Smoking. Cigarette smokers have weaker and thinner bones, although the reason for this association isn't exactly clear.
- Soda. Soda weakens bones in different ways. The high phosphorous content increases calcium loss from bones and

weakens them. This is true regardless of whether the soda is diet or regular, with or without caffeine. All types of soda also have a high sodium content that decreases bone strength.
- Vitamin A. When taken in excess, vitamin A can increase the risk of developing osteoporosis.

PERSONAL RISK FACTORS FOR OSTEOPOROSIS

An individual's personal medical history may harbor clues that predict an increased risk of osteoporosis independent of laboratory testing or bone measurements. These include the following:

- Breaking a bone. This may be a sign of osteoporosis, even if it occurs with a fall.
- Ethnicity. Asians have weaker bones than Caucasians, but both Asians and Caucasians are at higher risk for osteoporosis than African Americans. Even with stronger bones, one in four African American women still gets osteoporosis.
- Height loss of more than one inch may signal the presence of osteoporosis in the spine or a spinal fracture.
- History of fragility fracture, such as a vertebral spine fracture or a hip fracture. A personal history of a fracture, particularly after age 50, increases the risk of osteoporosis and future fractures.
- Never achieving your peak bone mass. Normally this is achieved in your twenties.
- Poor nutrition. This could be past or present, including a history of anorexia or bulimia.
- Untreated depression. This is particularly true when depression persists long term.

Consider Padma's story, highlighting the risk of developing osteoporosis.

Padma's Story
HISTORY OF STEROID MEDICATIONS

I've been taking steroid medication for severe asthma for many years. That, plus my slender build, sedentary lifestyle, and family history of osteoporosis, put me at risk for compression fractures. My doctor suggested improving my calcium intake with calcium-rich foods and calcium supplements to reach a total of 1,200 milligrams of calcium a day. They advised me to get most of the calcium from food, if possible, and to avoid consuming more than 600 milligrams of a calcium supplement at once. They told me about common "bone robbers" that could speed up bone loss and sabotage my efforts to strengthen my bones, including soda, cigarettes, alcohol, coffee, and high-sodium foods. Although I've never smoked, I do drink a lot of soda. They also recommended that I begin bone-building exercises, particularly for my spine. Without these interventions, they told me that my bone thinning would progress to a severe level, leading to fractures in my spine. I followed their advice, and five years later, I'm still fracture-free.

MEASURING BONE HEALTH

DXA

The gold standard for assessing whether you have osteoporosis or low bone mass is the dual-energy X-ray absorptiometry (DXA) test. Other tests, such as an X-ray, can identify whether a fracture has already occurred in the spine or hip, but the DXA bone density test is different. The DXA test detects other aspects of bone health.

Currently, DXA is the test of choice to diagnose osteoporosis as well as its precursor, low bone mass (formerly osteopenia). It does this by measuring bone mineral density (BMD), an indicator of bone strength. Bone mineral density looks at how much bone material is present in that area of bone. Is it porous like Swiss cheese or solid like cheddar cheese?

The DXA scan is a painless test using low-dose X-rays. DXA assesses bone mass by measuring the amount of low-dose radiation passing through the tissue. It is a precise measure of bone thickness at the hip and the spine. Ideally, the same facility (and same machine) will measure the bone densities of one individual over time so their doctor can easily compare results to that individual's baseline evaluation. This minimizes differences between machines and technicians. The machine does not touch the body. Wearing clothes and undergarments with no metal hooks, snaps, or zippers, typically means you can remain clothed during the test.

The National Osteoporosis Foundation recommends a baseline DXA at age 65 and sooner when there is a family history of osteoporosis or other risk factors such as hyperthyroidism, a malabsorption disorder, corticosteroid use, seizure medications, prior anorexia, or bulimia. Reliable DXA data for premenopausal women is not yet available. The good news is that a healthy woman under age 50 is extremely unlikely to have a hip or spine fracture unless they have an unusual medical history.

To plan treatment and prevention strategies for thin bones, a postmenopausal woman and their doctor need to know the degree of bone thinning present and the location of the weakest bone. The treatment may include lifestyle modifications and/or medication.

Following are three questions to ask your doctor:

1. Do my bones show early mild thinning, allowing time for preventive measures?
2. Is my bone thinning severe enough that my weakened bones may fracture without warning?
3. What are my T scores? A T score compares your current bone density to your bone density at age 28, assuming you were the same height and weight with strong bones. If you have strong bones, your T score will be zero or a positive number. If your bones have started thinning, you will have a negative T score.

DXA accuracy depends on entering your precise height and weight to adjust the calculations.[2]

DXA: MORE ABOUT T SCORES

Consider the following when interpreting T scores:

- A positive T score indicates your bones are not thinning. But if you have arthritis, it may mask the thinning. If you have arthritis, ask your doctor to check your radius arm bone on the next DXA. This area may show osteoporosis when arthritis masks bone thinning elsewhere.
- A T score of negative 2.5 or below indicates osteoporosis.
- If your T score is zero to negative 1.4, you have minimal thinning.
- If your T score is between negative 1.5 and negative 2.5, you have low bone mass or mild thinning.

A T score showing osteoporosis indicates the BMD is more than 2.5 standard deviations below that of a healthy 28-year-old, and indicates the individual is at high risk of a fragility fracture.[2]

> DID YOU KNOW?
> Even if the average T score is normal, that person may still have early osteoporosis in an individual vertebra or specific location in the hip.

Averaging a weak bone density in one area with stronger densities elsewhere may mask the presence of the weaker area. To prevent fractures, treatment is based on "the weakest link," meaning the worst or thinnest of the individual measurements.

The average T score may be falsely reassuring. If you have had a bone density test and your doctor is deciding whether you need treatment for thin bones, consider asking these questions:

- What is the lowest T score on my DXA?
- Where is the weakest area on the DXA (e.g., spine or right or left hip)?
- What are the pros and cons of treatment based on the weakest bone measurement in my DXA study? Ask this question if you have a T score below –2.5 anywhere on your DXA report, even when your average bone density is within normal range. For example, if one of the vertebrae in your spine shows osteoporosis with a T score of –2.7, but the other measurements in your spine are reassuring, the average T score for your spine may be in the low bone mass range of –1.2. But you may still benefit from treatment because one vertebra shows osteoporosis at a T score of –2.7. It is also possible that arthritis with bone spurs is causing the other vertebrae in your spine to appear denser or stronger than they really are.

Earlier in my career, I prescribed treatment for a postmenopausal woman with a T score of –2.9 in one vertebra. Her average T score for all the vertebrae was not in the osteoporosis range. A colleague called me up and asked me why I was prescribing medication to our mutual patient with a normal T score. They had read the first page summary of the DXA report, indicating an overall normal T score for the entire spine, not the individual measurement of the weakest vertebrae in the spine affected by osteoporosis. The weakest vertebra was at high risk for a fragility fracture.

DID YOU KNOW?

Vulnerability to fracture increases with age, even with the same T score. For example, a T score of –1.5 in a 55-year-old woman indicates osteopenia or mild thinning. A 70-year-old woman with a T score of –1.5 has an elevated risk of developing an osteoporotic fracture in the next 10 years based on her age.[2,3]

Strengthening the bone at that point will decrease your risk of fracture there, even if your DXA measurement stays the same after treatment. If you focus your interventions on the most negative T score, you will have the best outcome. Often, a woman hears that her average T score is close to normal or in the osteopenia range. She feels relieved. In reality, there may be an area of osteoporosis in her hip or spine that needs more aggressive management. She may not be receptive to her doctor's advice to take medication because she is not convinced of the severity of the bone thinning. She is falsely reassured by the average value. Is your weakest T score measurement in your hip or spine, or are they both equally affected by thin bones? Certain medications are more effective in targeting the spine, while others are more effective in strengthening hip bones. Some are appropriate for both. Consider Cameron's story.

Cameron's Story
FOCAL OSTEOPOROSIS OF THE SPINE

I'm 54 and have been postmenopausal for five years. I'm lactose intolerant and do not drink milk or other dairy products. I only recently started to drink calcium-fortified cashew milk and calcium-fortified orange juice. I was not enthusiastic about taking calcium pills and rarely took them. My DXA showed a T score of −2.9 for the L4 vertebra (the fourth lumbar bone in my lower back) in my spine. The average T score for my spine, compared to that of other women my age, is only −1.2. I concluded that my −1.2 score was only osteopenia, but my doctor had a different perspective. They were concerned about the −2.9 measurement at L4. They explained that treatment is based on the weakest bones that are measured, not just the average. Part of my spine had already progressed to osteoporosis. Treatment would prevent me from suffering a fracture or break of the vertebral bone in my spine. I asked my doctor if I could correct the thin area in the spine by being more consistent in taking calcium and vitamin D supplements as well as exercising. They told me that taking calcium and vitamin D would certainly help in preventing further thinning, but it would not address the severe thinning that had already taken place. I thought more about their advice after an older neighbor had a fracture in her spine. The neighbor went from walking daily to a rehabilitation facility to a nursing home because she was bedridden. I got enough calcium in my foods, took vitamin D, did Miriam Nelson's weight-bearing exercises three times a week at home, and started the prescription for alendronate that my doctor advised. Five years later, my osteoporosis is in remission and my bones are stronger. I'll need lifetime monitoring, but my risk of fracture is much lower now since the medication and lifestyle modifications.

CLINICAL DIAGNOSIS OF OSTEOPOROSIS AND NEED FOR MEDICAL TREATMENT

- A T score of −2.5 or below in the spine, hip, or radius arm bone means you need to seek medical treatment.
- Low-trauma spine or hip fracture, regardless of bone mineral density, requires medical intervention.
- A T score between −1.0 and −2.5 and a fragility fracture of the proximal humerus, pelvis, or distal forearm require medical treatment.
- A T score between −1.0 and −2.5 and a high fracture risk assessment tool (FRAX) score to estimate fracture risk require medical treatment.[5]

ADVANTAGES OF THE DXA

One strength of the DXA test is that it provides information about the amount of bone you have as well as your bone strength. But the DXA test cannot provide information about the number and type of trabecular connections or properties of your cortical bones. Picture a broken ladder that is missing rungs. It becomes unstable and unsuitable for weight bearing. Trabecular bone that is missing connections or struts will not provide adequate support. In women, loss of trabecular connections causes bone fractures more frequently than decreases in bone mineral density as identified by DXA studies. As researchers and clinicians can monitor the loss of trabecular connections more closely, they can assess whether individual medications can stop the loss of trabecular connections and treat osteoporosis more effectively.

At present, it is not possible to monitor the loss of trabecular connections closely or to evaluate the effects of various medical treatments. Fortunately, researchers are developing technology to assess these factors. The goal? To establish a range of values (other than DXA and FRAX) for healthy bones versus osteoporotic ones.

LIMITATIONS OF DXA

One limitation of DXA is that it uses an algorithm or formula that does not take age into consideration. Age is an independent risk factor for fracturing a hip, distinct from BMD. In addition to not accounting for age, DXA does not account for other risk factors that increase fracture risk.

Increased risk factors for fracture not reflected on DXA include the following:

- Arthritis in the hip or spine
- Family history of osteoporosis or fracture
- Long-term steroid treatment
- Prior fracture. This puts you at high risk of another fracture.
- Weakened bones from illness or medications. Illness or medication may change the quality or architecture of the bone before altering the actual bone density.

The gold standard for predicting your risk of fracturing a bone in your spine or hip in the next 10 years is the fracture risk assessment tool (FRAX). Your risk will be underestimated, however, if you do not discuss your medical history, family history, and medications with your doctor. Your doctor needs to include this information when estimating your risk of fracture.

DXA AND Z SCORES

The Z score is also reported on DXA studies. The Z score tells a woman how her bone density compares to that of other women her age, but the Z score is not an accurate indicator of fracture risk. Women with a normal Z score may still be at high risk of a fracture. After all, half of women over age 50 have an osteoporotic fracture in their lifetime. Therefore, medical treatment should not be based solely on a Z score.[5]

BMD: WHAT YOU NEED TO KNOW

BMD may also mislead you because it can underestimate your risk of a fracture. Why? Because arthritic changes or scarring from a previous fracture can cloud the results. For instance, if you have arthritis, you may have thickening or spurs in bones that create a falsely elevated bone density and do not actually show the quality and strength of the bone. This means you may be at risk of fracture even though you have a reassuring T score on DXA.

Researchers have learned more about bone properties. Bone thickness is still important to assess bone health. Mineral content is also critical to bone health. For example, even if the bone is thick enough on a measurement, it will fracture if there is not enough calcium or vitamin D in it. Bone thickness and mineral content do not completely explain how bone behaves. Bone architecture, or microscopic internal structure, is important but difficult to measure.

THE FRAX TOOL

In February 2008, the World Health Organization (WHO) published an interactive tool called the FRAX to help predict a woman's personal fracture risk for the next 10 years. This is a more comprehensive approach to managing fracture risk than the DXA alone. The DXA result is still helpful, and physicians may include it in the FRAX algorithm to predict fracture risk. FRAX is the most comprehensive assessment tool to date. That's because it considers the following variables:

- Age
- BMD
- Family history
- Family or personal history of fractures over age 50
- History of rheumatoid arthritis
- Personal history of hip fracture
- Smoking status
- Steroid use for more than three months

The FRAX tool also considers ethnic differences in bone fragility and fracture risk. These differences are based on specific epidemiology that includes statistics about illness and mortality for different groups. This information increases the accuracy of the fracture risk predictions. The predictions will be more accurate for African American, Hispanic/Latinx, Asian, and Caucasian men and women. These additional factors allow more accurate predictions of your fracture risk over the next 10 years. This tool may be accessed online at www.shef.ac.uk/FRAX/ (click on Calculation Tool). Here are some additional facts about the FRAX tool:

- FRAX is designed to predict fracture risk for the next 10 years only for patients who have not been treated for thin bones before and who have never had a fracture.
- FRAX is most accurate in predicting fracture risk for the hip. There is no entry for vertebral score for the spine bone density.
- When bone thinning occurs in your spine, your doctor may use the T scores from your DXA scan and the clinical assessment to make treatment recommendations but cannot use FRAX to assess your risk of spine fracture.[2,3,5]

PROMOTING BONE HEALTH

Today, maintaining bone health includes these strategies:

- Avoid "bone robbers," such as excess alcohol, cigarette smoking (active or passive), high salt consumption, soda, caffeine, excess vitamin A, and aluminum (found, for example, in antacids).
- Get adequate calcium intake daily in food and, if necessary, divided doses of supplements.
- Minimize your risk of falling. Minimizing the risk of falls, particularly as age increases and eyesight and coordination decrease, requires you to use good lighting, ensure walking paths inside and outside the home are free of obstacles, avoid loose throw rugs, and avoid slippery outdoor conditions whenever possible. Improving your balance through specific exercises also helps.
- Take calcium supplements if you had gastric bypass surgery or have trouble absorbing calcium-rich foods. Participate regularly in weight-bearing and muscle-strengthening exercises.
- Take adequate vitamin D daily.
- Talk to your doctor about bone health. This includes when to have a bone density test and whether you would benefit from prescription medication to prevent or reverse osteoporosis.

CALCIUM BENEFITS AND GUIDELINES

Your skeleton contains 99 percent of your body's calcium reserves. If you do not consume enough calcium daily, especially after age 50, your bones will leach out calcium to keep the calcium level in your blood at a healthy level. Consider the following important facts about calcium.[4]

- A normal blood calcium level does not always correlate with strong bones.

- Avoid taking more than the standard dose (600 mg of calcium) at once because your body will not absorb the excess. Instead, try 600 mg of dietary calcium twice a day at least four hours apart.
- Calcium carbonate and calcium citrate are the two most common calcium supplements; see below for the best ways to absorb each.
- Calcium in foods does not increase the risk of kidney stones.
- Calcium-fortified milk may have 450 mg of calcium per cup.
- Canned salmon with bones and sardines are both excellent sources of calcium.
- Cheese typically has more protein than calcium. Check the label.
- Dairy milk (i.e., skim, 1 percent, 2 percent, or whole) has 300 mg of calcium per cup.
- Drink 10 oz of fortified milk. Options include calcium-fortified Lactaid milk (if you are lactose intolerant or like it), Fair Life milk available in a variety of fat contents (also lactose free), fortified almond milk, and fortified cashew milk. If you do not like drinking nondairy milk or don't prefer to drink milk twice a day, consider making a shake with frozen unsweetened berries, spinach, and pea protein powder or peanut butter powder.
- If calcium bothers your stomach, try Tums.
- Inulin is a type of fiber that your body can absorb well with calcium.
- Perimenopausal women under age 50 typically need 1,000 mg of calcium daily, divided.
- Postmenopausal women or those over age 50 need 1,200 mg of calcium daily, divided.
- The body does not absorb calcium and iron well when taken together, so it's best to avoid combining them. The same is true for calcium and fiber.
- To estimate calcium from foods, check the label. Thirty percent of the daily calcium requirement per serving

equates to 300 mg. Simply add a zero to the daily requirement per serving to calculate the total milligrams of calcium per service.
- Unless you have had gastric bypass surgery, your best option is to get most of your calcium from your food to lower the risk of kidney stones. If you had gastric bypass surgery, take supplements as directed, no more than 600 mg of calcium at one sitting, so you can absorb all of it.
- Vegetable sources of calcium such as beans, spinach, and kale add a modest amount of calcium to the diet (i.e., 40 mg of calcium per serving).
- Women over age 70 tolerate calcium citrate better than calcium carbonate.
- Your body absorbs calcium carbonate better with food.
- Your body absorbs calcium citrate well on an empty stomach.

Other benefits of calcium include the following:

- Calcium improves blood pressure.
- Calcium decreases the risk of getting colon and rectal cancer.
- Preliminary research shows that calcium may decrease the risk of obesity.

Consider Amanda's story, which highlights the importance of sufficient calcium.

Amanda's Story
LOW CALCIUM INTAKE

I am 55 and lactose-intolerant. I recently started drinking calcium-fortified soy milk after a lifetime of avoiding dairy products. I swim once every week. My first bone density test was done two years ago, and the result showed a T score of -1.5 in the hip and spine. I was placed on calcium supplements and vitamin D, but I often forget to take them. Two years later, my T score on a repeat DXA test was -2.5.

My risk of fracture had doubled in two years! At this time, my doctor prescribed alendronate (Fosamax) and emphasized the need for calcium and vitamin D daily. They plan to recheck my bone density and evaluate my progress in two years. They encouraged me to continue swimming since I enjoy it and it is great for heart health. However, swimming will not count as weight bearing exercise. They recommended starting a strength-training program either at a gym or on my own at home using Miriam Nelson's book Strong Women, Strong Bones. This program improves bone strength and balance. A friend and I did the program faithfully for two years and each of our doctors noticed better T scores on our DXA studies.

VITAMIN D: WHAT WE NOW KNOW

Research has shown that achieving and maintaining normal blood levels of vitamin D is essential to strong bones and muscles. It also decreases the risk of falls. Vitamin D is produced in human skin and then transformed into its active form by the liver and kidneys. Here are a few more facts about vitamin D:

- Desirable blood levels of vitamin D are between 30 nanograms per milliliter to 60 ng/mL.
- If your blood level of vitamin D is low, your doctor may recommend 4,000 or 5,000 IU of vitamin D daily until your blood level of vitamin D is in the normal range.
- More vitamin D is not always better. Toxic levels of vitamin D may cause loss of appetite, vomiting, and muscle weakness.
- Muscles have vitamin D receptors. With adequate vitamin D levels, muscles are stronger.
- Perimenopausal women and those under age 50 typically need 1,000 international units (IU) of vitamin D daily.
- Postmenopausal women and those over age 50 typically need 2,000 IU of vitamin D daily.

- Take your daily vitamin D supplement all at once. There's no need to divide the dose.
- Vitamin D is made in the skin. Sun exposure supplies minimal vitamin D and sunscreen blocks vitamin D absorption.
- Vitamin D may lower blood pressure in postmenopausal women.
- Vitamin D in the Women's Health Initiative Study was associated with a lower risk of colon cancer.[4]

WEIGHT-BEARING EXERCISE

In addition to adequate calcium and vitamin D intake, healthy bones require regular weight-bearing exercise. Weight-bearing exercises (e.g., walking and weight-lifting) defy gravity. Weight-bearing exercises also help maintain and restore bone strength.

Researchers found that even inactive women in their eighties and nineties living in nursing homes were able to improve bone strength through weight-bearing exercise. These women were given adequate calcium and vitamin D and started on an exercise program with weights. The program was designed to target major muscle groups in the upper and lower body that support the spine and hip to improve bone strength. Even the octogenarians improved their bone strength with this program. (Modifications are included for wheelchair-bound participants.) These results demonstrate it is never too late to begin an exercise program.

Women also lose their balance as they age. Loss of balance increases the likelihood of falling, which is associated with bone fracture. Miriam Nelson, PhD, author of *Strong Women Stay Young* (as well as two other books: *Strong Women Stay Slim* and *Strong Women, Strong Bones*), has done the most thorough research in this area. The exercises she studied increased bone strength in women who did them three times a week.

> **DID YOU KNOW?**
>
> "Bone robbers" weaken bones and should be avoided. These include the following:
> - Drinking soda (phosphorous leaches out calcium from bones)
> - Salt in the diet
> - Sedentary lifestyle
> - Smoking
> - Two or more servings of alcohol a day

MEDICATIONS FOR BONE HEALTH

You may be able to prevent fractures and keep your bones healthy with the lifestyle modifications reviewed above as well as by avoiding bone robbers, getting enough calcium and vitamin D, and participating in regular weight-bearing activity that targets your hips and spine.

Additional intervention may be required for those who do get thin bones due to heredity, medical conditions, medications, or other causes. This includes different types of medication that lower the risk of fracture and restore bone health.

Shared decision-making is critical to the successful improvement of thin bones. You and your doctor must work together to choose the best medicine for you. Consider asking your doctor the following questions:

- Why do I need this medication?
- Does my personal medical history, family history, or lifestyle make me vulnerable to thin bones or a silent fracture?
- What can I expect if I try adequate daily calcium, adequate daily vitamin D, and lifestyle modifications and decline to take a medication at this time?
- What are the side effects and precautions of taking the medication you recommend?
- What are the risks of taking the medication?

- Is the risk of taking the medication less than the risk of not taking it?
- Where is the most bone thinning on my DXA, and how severe is the bone thinning?
- What is my risk of fracture in the next 10 years?
- How does my risk of fracture compare to the baseline risk?
- My older sister is getting injections with a bone builder. Why are you only recommending a medication that blocks bone dissolving for me?

Consider Abigail's story.

Abigail's Story
ABIGAIL, AN ACTIVE 66-YEAR-OLD WITH HEIGHT LOSS

At 68, I am an active woman who has always taken charge of my health. I've always walked daily. I am a vegetarian. I maintain my weight within a 10-pound range of my ideal body weight. Because I was active, I did not suspect that I had early signs of bone thinning. When measured at my doctor's office, I learned I was 1.5 inches shorter than my previously measured adult height. They ordered a DXA bone density test. My T scores were −2.1 for the hip and −2.3 for the spine, both showing low bone mass (osteopenia). The doctor encouraged me to take a prescription bone builder to treat the changes, but I wasn't receptive. Instead, I agreed to try exercises specifically designed to strengthen my bones. I committed to doing them two times a week for 20 minutes each session. I also agreed to take calcium supplements with vitamin D to boost my daily calcium intake. After two years of this new regimen, the DXA showed my bones were no worse, but they did not improve. I have agreed to continue the exercises and calcium supplements but also added a prescription bone builder to increase my bone strength. Now, two years later at age 70, my DXA test shows that my bone density is closer to the normal range, and my bones are stronger. I still have osteopenia, but my fracture risk is lower.

LOOKING AT TREATMENT OPTIONS THROUGH THE LENS OF RISK

Evaluating your risk of fracture requires your doctor to review the following information:

- Alcohol consumption
- Anorexia or bulimia, past or present
- Athletic activities in your past that stopped your menstrual periods
- Current medications
- Exercise, including type and frequency
- Family history of osteoporosis
- Fracturing a bone in the past
- Height loss of 1.5 inches or more
- Most concerning T score on DXA
- Smoking status (smokers have thinner bones)

The above aspects of your health, along with your age and T score on DXA, will determine your risk of fracture soon or in the next 10 years. This information also frames the discussion you have with your doctor about what medication to consider and why.

LOW RISK OF FRACTURE

The following factors put you at low risk of a fracture:

- Age under 70
- FRAX risk of less than 3 percent for hip fracture
- FRAX risk of major fracture less than 20 percent in 10 years
- No prior fracture
- T scores of –1 or better
- Lifestyle modifications, adequate calcium and vitamin D intake, and normal vitamin D levels all help maintain bone strength. The same is true for avoiding bone robbers. You may not need medication.

MODERATE RISK OF FRACTURE

The following factors put you at moderate risk of a fracture:

- No prior fracture
- T score between –1 and –2.5
- FRAX risk of less than 20 percent for major fracture
- FRAX risk of less than 3 percent for hip fracture

A few other helpful pointers:

- Systemic estrogen also helps prevent further bone thinning.
- Consider raloxifene if you have spine thinning and are between 50 and 69 years old.
- Bisphosphonates such as Alendronate (Fosamax) in your mid or late 60s or earlier might be helpful.

HIGH RISK OF FRACTURE

The following factors put you at high risk of a fracture:

- Older single prior fracture (more than two years prior)
- T score more concerning than –2.5 or worse
- T score better than –2.5 with FRAX showing 20 percent or more risk of major fracture
- T score better than –2.5 and FRAX showing 3 percent or higher risk of hip fracture

Consider a bisphosphonate or denosumab (Prolia) and potentially estrogen or raloxifene if you are under age 59 and have a low spine T score. These may also be options if you are younger, typically under age 60, and have a low spine T score.

VERY HIGH RISK OF FRACTURE

The following factors put you at very high risk of a fracture in the near future:

- History of multiple fractures
- Over 30 percent risk of major fracture on DXA
- Over 4.5 percent risk of hip fracture on DXA
- Recent fracture in last one to two years
- T score less than −3.0
- Very high fracture risk by FRAX

For women at very high fracture risk, the goal is to lower the risk of fracture quickly and improve BMD as fast as possible. Target is a T score better than −2.5.

In this case, bone health experts recommend starting with a bone builder or anabolic treatment. Anabolic agents build bone quickly to lower fracture risk. Examples of anabolic agents are teriparatide (Forteo) and romosozumab (Evenity). These agents are typically prescribed for 12 months, and then it is critical to take a different medication to slow bone resorption or dissolving such as alendronate (Fosamax), denosumab (Prolia), or zoledronic acid (Reclast) to maintain the new bone and prevent it from dissolving rapidly. Anabolic agents are best prescribed by experts in bone health, typically an endocrinologist or rheumatologist or another certified specialist.

Now that you have a framework for fracture risk, I will provide additional information about the types of medications for each risk group.[2,3,5]

BISPHOSPHONATES

Bisphosphonate medications slow the process of bone dissolving during remodeling. Examples of bisphosphonates include the following:

- Alendronate (Fosamax). Take once a week by mouth on an empty stomach with plain water and stay upright (sit/stand/walk for 30–45 minutes). This medication is prescribed for postmenopausal women only.
- Ibandronate (Boniva). Take this medication by mouth once a month. Note this medication only helps the vertebral spine, not the hips.

- Risedronate (Actonel). Take this medication just as you would take alendronate.
- Zoledronate (Reclast). This medication is given by intravenous (IV) injection once a year.

More about bisphosphonates:

- Bisphosphonates are not hormones. They do not affect estrogen levels, breast cancer risk, or the frequency and severity of hot flashes.
- Bisphosphonates decrease bone loss so bone can build with less dissolving.
- Some bisphosphonates can be prescribed for preventing osteoporosis or treating it. Other bisphosphonates are cleared only for treatment.

EFFICACY OF MEDICATIONS AND WHAT YOU CAN EXPECT

DID YOU KNOW?
Osteoporosis is a lifelong condition. Treatment lowers your risk of fracture and strengthens bone. Long-term monitoring is key to maintaining improvements.

- Alendronate decreases the number of spine, hip, and wrist fractures by 50 percent over three years in those who have already had a previous spine fracture. It lowers the risk of spine fractures by 48 percent over three years for those with no previous spine fracture.
- Bisphosphonate treatment strengthens your bones and lowers your risk of fracture while you take the medication (and at times for an additional two years or more).
- Bisphosphonates stay in your skeleton due to a long half-life and are not advised for premenopausal women or when pregnancy is possible.

- Bone strength and DXA scores increase after taking bisphosphonate for three to five years.
- Ibandronate (Boniva) is a long-acting bisphosphonate. You can take it by mouth once a month or administer it every three months by IV injection. The oral form can be given for prevention or treatment. Ibandronate targets only the spine and reduces the risk of spine fractures by 50 percent over three years. If you take it by mouth, follow the same precautions as for alendronate (above).
- If your bones are stronger, and your DXA score improves, you still have osteoporosis.
- Risedronate (Actonel) lowers the chance of spine fractures by 41 to 49 percent and other fractures by 36 percent over three years in those who have had a previous spine fracture.
- With osteoporosis, you benefit from treatment and continue to have medical care and follow-ups throughout your remaining life.
- Zoledronate (Reclast) is given once a year by IV infusion over a 15-minute period and is approved by the US Food and Drug Administration (FDA) to treat osteoporosis in postmenopausal women. Zoledronate lowers the incidence of spine fractures by 70 percent. It lowers hip fractures by 41 percent over three years.

> DID YOU KNOW?
> Bisphosphonates and other medications are not a cure for osteoporosis.

POTENTIAL SIDE EFFECTS OF BISPHOSPHONATES

Osteonecrosis in bone ends the bone's ability to self-repair. Osteonecrosis of the jaw is a rare condition seen in patients with cancer getting IV chemotherapy and high doses of IV alendronate. Even in this rare circumstance, the risk of osteonecrosis of the jaw while taking alendronate is less than 1 in 200,000. It is even rarer in individuals taking a regular oral dose of alendronate for fewer than five years. Consider Fiona's story.

Fiona's Story
POOR HEALING AFTER A BROKEN HIP

By the time I was 58, I already had a hip fracture that I attributed to being clumsy. I later learned that my hip "gave out" prior to my fall. I was hospitalized for a week after the hip surgery. My rehabilitation was difficult, and physical therapy was a struggle. The hip did not heal rapidly. My doctors were concerned that I was not active enough after the surgery. When the hip pain worsened with walking, I spent more time in bed. I even started to use a walker. While I was bedridden, I got a pulmonary embolus, a clot that formed in the blood vessels near my hip and migrated to my lungs, where it caused a blockage. I had to go on blood thinners for six months after I had additional surgery to prevent future blood clot formation.

It's two years later, and I still walk with a cane. When I saw my gynecologist, I still hadn't had an evaluation for osteoporosis. When a DXA scan revealed osteoporosis, I learned that this was most likely the cause of my hip fracture—not my clumsiness as I had previously thought. I fell after my hip broke. Osteoporosis ravaged my hip bone, and the break was from a fragility fracture.

I had a habit of drinking three glasses of milk a day and assumed I was staying healthy. Reviewing my medical history and lifestyle in more detail made me realize that I normally drank eight cups of coffee a day. Each mug I used was 16 ounces, so each cup was really two cups. I also enjoyed diet soda—up to four cans a day. I am a former smoker: two packs of cigarettes a day for 20 years. My evening routine to unwind from a day's work included two glasses of wine while preparing dinner. I was unaware that adequate calcium intake alone would not protect me from getting osteoporosis. I also didn't know that the high amounts of phosphorous in my soda prevented my bones from absorbing the calcium I took in with food. In addition, the wine I enjoyed while preparing dinner thinned my bones further. I didn't *know alcohol thins bones and promotes osteoporosis. When I committed to improving my bone health, I tapered off soda, cut back on alcohol, and now enjoy one glass two or three times a week instead of daily. I also enjoy one cup of coffee instead of eight but tapered slowly to avoid headaches.*

DENOSUMAB (PROLIA) FOR LONG-TERM OSTEOPOROSIS TREATMENT

Consider the following facts about denosumab:

- After stopping denosumab, a bisphosphonate is often prescribed to preserve bone strength.
- Atypical femur fracture is rare at 0.8 cases in 10,000 patient-years.
- BMD of the spine and hip continue to increase over time.
- Denosumab and bisphosphonates are the most common treatments for osteoporosis.
- Denosumab improves strength and BMD in the hip and spine. Fracture protection occurs within the first 12 months of taking denosumab.
- Denosumab blocks receptor activation of nuclear factor kappa B ligand (RANKL inhibitor) that's needed by osteoclasts to clear away bone. Blocking bone resorption allows more bone formation with less bone dissolving.
- Denosumab is given as a subcutaneous injection (under the skin) every six months.
- Denosumab, like bisphosphonates, can be used for long-term treatment.
- Drug holidays are not advised with denosumab.
- If you stop taking denosumab, you'll need to take another medication to maintain your bone strength.
- Osteonecrosis of the jaw is extremely rare at 5.2 cases in 10,000 patient-years.

- Side effects do not increase over time for up to 10 years of treatment.
- Strength improves in both cortical and trabecular bone types.[2,3,5]

ESTROGEN AND COMBINED HORMONE THERAPY

Systemic estrogen and estrogen/progesterone combinations are approved by the FDA for preventing osteoporosis but not for osteoporosis treatment. The Women's Health Initiative found five years of Prempro (synthetic estrogen and progesterone) lowered the risk of clinical spine fractures and hip fractures by 34 percent. Estrogen or estrogen and progestin may be given to healthy younger women (who have been in post menopause fewer than 10 years or who are under age 60) to control debilitating hot flashes or night sweats.

SELECTIVE ESTROGEN RECEPTOR MODULATORS

Selective estrogen receptor modulators (SERMs) are modified estrogen hormones. Tamoxifen is the most well-known SERM. Tamoxifen is chemically made by modifying estrogen so it prevents breast cancer. Like tamoxifen, SERMs lower the risk of breast cancer. SERMs act like estrogen in some ways and act opposite to estrogen's normal behavior in other parts of the body.

Raloxifene (Evista) is an example of a SERM that increases bone strength in the spine and, like its cousin tamoxifen, decreases the risk of breast cancer. One drawback is that it may worsen hot flashes to a small degree in some women. Raloxifene does not improve or worsen vaginal dryness. Raloxifene does not cause uterine cancer or change the uterine lining. Here are some other details about raloxifene:

- An active woman is less likely to get a clot. After taking raloxifene for a year, the risk of developing a blood clot is even lower.

- Raloxifene is associated with a higher risk of deep vein clot formation, also called deep vein thrombosis.
- Raloxifene lowers the risk of spine fracture by 30 percent in those with a prior spine fracture.
- Raloxifene lowers the risk of spine fracture by 55 percent in those without a prior spine fracture.
- Take raloxifene by mouth once a day, with or without food. For thinning in the vertebral spine and no hip bone thinning, it may be an excellent choice.
- The risk of deep vein thrombosis is small but significant. Out of every 10,000 women taking raloxifene, three additional women will develop deep vein clots.

BONE BUILDERS AND ANABOLIC MEDICATIONS

Teriparatide (Forteo), a parathyroid hormone (PTH), promotes bone growth by stimulating osteoblast activity. Teriparatide is reserved for high-risk individuals with severe osteoporosis who do not respond to other medications or who cannot tolerate them. It is given as a daily subcutaneous (under the skin) injection. In individuals with osteoporosis, Teriperatide decreases the risk of spine fractures by 65 percent and non-spine fractures by 53 percent after approximately 18 months of treatment. Teriparatide provides a large and rapid increase in BMD and reduces the risk of fracture quickly. Another parathyroid hormone analog, abaloparatide, has similar properties.

Romosozumab is a bone builder that works by blocking sclerostin, a substance required for bone resorption. Romosozumab (Evenity) works in two ways to strengthen bone: It increases bone formation and also decreases bone resorption. It is given once a month for 12 months. Its use is geared toward women with a high risk of fracture or a recent fracture who need to build bone quickly and reduce fracture risk in the short term before another fracture occurs. Long-term safety is not well established. After 12 months of romosozumab, another medication such as alendronate or denosumab is introduced to maintain gains in bone strength.

If you are at high risk for a fracture or you had a fracture recently and require an anabolic medication, it is typically best to consult a bone specialist. Many bone specialists are endocrinologists or rheumatologists with additional expertise in osteoporosis.[6,7,8]

Consider Wilma's story to learn more about an initial diagnosis of osteoporosis and how to respond appropriately.

Wilma's Story
HEALTHY, ACTIVE 74-YEAR-OLD WITH NEWLY DIAGNOSED OSTEOPOROSIS

At age 74, everyone who knows me is impressed by my vigor. I walk three miles a day at a brisk pace and maintain a normal healthy weight. I feel healthy. When my doctor advised me to have a test to check my bone density, I bristled. I told him, "But I walk three miles a day. My bones must be very strong." Unfortunately, the DXA revealed I had moderate osteoporosis and was at high risk for a hip fracture or spine fracture even if I didn't fall. At first, I took the news very poorly. I was crestfallen that my lifelong rigorous fitness routine had not produced strong bones. When the disbelief and disappointment faded, I was ready to consider my options. In the past, my treatment options would have been limited, but I found I had several alternatives, a few of which were acceptable to me.

Since my osteoporosis is severe, my bone loss is already substantial. I wanted to try taking more calcium, without additional medication, to improve my bone strength. My doctor was concerned about my high risk of bone breakage since my bones were already very weak. Just taking calcium and vitamin D would leave me vulnerable to further bone loss and a high risk of fracture. I needed medication to build bone quickly and lower my high risk of fracture. I reviewed the side effects and effectiveness of these medications: Fosamax (alendronate), a bone builder that works through the calcium system, and Evista (raloxifene), a modified synthetic hormone that does not cause any vaginal bleeding or breast tissue changes. I settled on trying alendronate.

I initially thought I did not have to change my diet if I took the medication. My doctor advised me to increase the daily calcium intake in my food and use calcium supplements. This would provide enough calcium for the medicine to help improve my osteoporosis. I was encouraged and surprised that I could actually improve my severe bone loss and attain strong bones again even at my age. I hadn't realized that the new medications could reverse bone loss and allow a return to normal bone strength over time. Today, after two years of medication and conscientious daily intake of calcium, I have made substantial progress. A subsequent DXA scan shows that my bone mass is closer to normal. I committed to continuing the Alendronate for five years since I tolerate it well. My doctor said osteoporosis is a chronic condition. Even though my bones are stronger, and my osteoporosis can go into remission, it can resurface. I will need to be monitored for bone strength throughout my life to stay healthy.

ONGOING REASSESSMENT

DXA is used to assess the impact of treatment on bone strength. Depending on the severity of the osteoporosis and the type of medication prescribed, the interval for performing another DXA may be one to three years.

> **DID YOU KNOW?**
> Your medication may be working even if your DXA has not yet improved. Taking osteoporosis medications lowers your risk of fracture as long as you have adequate calcium intake and normal vitamin D levels. The DXA results may not always reflect the lower risk of fracture. This may be because the medication is improving other features of the bone that the DXA cannot measure.

Once you have been treated for thin bones, the average T score for your spine or hip is more helpful. More than four individual T score measurements make up the spine T score, and several hip measurements make up the hip T score. Before treatment, the lowest T score in the group is used to determine the need for treatment as it is the most vulnerable area. Once treatment is started, the average T score for that area is more helpful to gauge treatment efficacy.

New studies are underway to identify what supplements, lifestyle modifications, exercises, and medications are most effective to strengthen bones. After updating your medical history and reviewing current medications and supplements with your doctor, plan to discuss your bone health. Do this annually. Consider Maya's story.

Maya's Story
WHICH MEDICATION IS BEST?

I'm 60 years old and travel extensively for my job. I've been postmenopausal for eight years since age 52. Because of my schedule, my last gynecology visit was more than three years ago. When I finally made the time, my doctor ordered a DXA scan. It showed thinning in my hip that was severe enough to meet the criteria for osteoporosis on one measurement. The average measurement of the hip was not as alarming, and the spine bone strength was normal. My doctor was concerned. One of my favorite actresses was in an advertisement for Boniva, the bisphosphonate that can be taken once a month. I asked for that medication. My doctor explained that my severe bone thinning was in my hip and that Boniva only lowers the risk of spine fractures. They advised I take alendronate, a bisphosphonate, once a week by mouth. It has a strong track record for restoring hip strength as well as strength in the spine. I took the alendronate once a week as directed and tolerated it well. Two years later, I had another DXA, and it showed that my osteoporosis was improving. My bones were stronger, and my doctor assured me my risk of fracture was lower and would continue to improve as I finished a five-year course of the medication.

FUTURE TRENDS

Researchers are identifying changes in the porosity of cortical bone associated with post menopause. Cortical bone becomes weaker as its architecture is compromised. At present, no established clinical tools measure the strength of cortical bone. Researchers are analyzing the effect of various medications on the microscopic structure of the hip. Preventing cortical bone compromise in post menopause will involve stopping the cortical bone from becoming more porous and increasing its thickness. This will lower the number of hip fractures.

MORE ABOUT BONE QUALITY

In addition to maintaining bone density and strength, another treatment goal is to preserve bone quality. Measuring bone quality is challenging and is still in the research phase.

If the architecture of your bone structure is compromised, the bone will not be as robust and will not function as well. This is true even in the presence of a reassuring bone volume. Even if two women have the same the DXA as well as intact architecture, the fracture risk will be higher for the woman with the compromised architecture.

Consider Barbara's story about her experience with osteoporosis.

Barbara's Story
OSTEOPOROSIS AND A FAMILY HISTORY OF BREAST CANCER IN A 52-YEAR-OLD

I have avoided milk and other dairy products most of my life because I am lactose-intolerant. My mother developed breast cancer when she was 45 years old and died within two years of her diagnosis. I am now 52, an age I never expected to reach. In perimenopause, I had severe hot flashes but was reluctant to take any estro-

gen because of my family history of breast cancer. My gynecologist ordered a DXA bone density test that showed osteoporosis with enough thinning of the vertebral bones in my spine to predict that I might fracture my spine even if I did not trip or fall. My doctor was also concerned about my height loss that can be associated with osteoporosis. So even though I had taken good care of myself, felt well, and looked healthy, I was at high risk for a vertebral spine fracture. At my doctor's suggestion, I am taking a medication, raloxifen (Evista), to strengthen my bones and avoid a fracture. My gynecologist says I am greatly reducing my chances of a spine fracture and height loss with the medication, and I'm also lowering my risk of breast cancer.

IMPORTANT TAKEAWAYS

In summary:

- Even if you continue to look and feel healthy, post menopause is accompanied by silent, invisible changes that weaken bones over time.
- Osteoporosis can be prevented by getting adequate amounts of vitamins and minerals and making certain lifestyle choices.
- Osteoporosis can be life-threatening. It is painless until a fracture occurs.
- Our bones continue to form, dissolve, and rebuild throughout our lifetime.
- Some of the risk factors for developing osteoporosis include family history of the disease, being small-boned and thin, low calcium and vitamin D intake, sedentary lifestyle, certain medications, and more
- The gold standard for testing and assessing whether you have osteoporosis or significant bone thinning is a dual-energy x-ray absorptiometry scan.

- You can take steps to improve bone health, such as getting adequate calcium intake, participating in weight-bearing and muscle-strengthening exercises regularly, and avoiding bone robbers.

QUESTIONS FOR YOUR DOCTOR

1. What is my risk of developing osteoporosis? How do I know whether I might already have it?
2. I have no bone pain or joint pain. Could I still have osteoporosis?
3. What is my risk of having a fracture in the short and long term?
4. What are some strategies I can use to maintain good bone health?
5. What can I do to make sure I get enough calcium while also not taking too much?
6. What can I do to make sure I get enough vitamin D?
7. Should I consider any medications to prevent osteoporosis? If so, what are the pros and cons of each one?

RESOURCES

American College of Obstetrics and Gynecology (www.acog.org). This professional organization is dedicated to women's health across the life span. Its members are board-certified obstetricians and gynecologists who have been recommended for membership and attain a high standard of education, training, and practice by passing examinations and updating their credentials on a regular basis. They have excellent materials on most major topics in women's health that are updated frequently. Several booklets on bone health are available online or at your doctor's office.

International Osteoporosis Foundation (www.iofbonehealth.org). There is an interactive IOF One-Minute Osteoporosis Risk Test you can take online.

The Menopause Society (www.menopause.org). This association includes nurses, nurse practitioners, and physician assistants as well as medical researchers and pharmacists and those from other disciplines dedicated to menopausal health. They certify menopausal clinicians who have attained a certain level of expertise and require them to maintain the credential with regular educational updates. They have current information on osteoporosis.

National Osteoporosis Foundation (www.nof.org). In addition to their other resources, you can click on FRAX™ WHO Fracture Risk Assessment Tool and estimate your risk of breaking a bone in the next 10 years. After you pull up the FRAX WHO Fracture Risk Assessment Tool, click on Calculation Tool, then your country of origin, followed by your race or ethnicity, to get the most accurate estimate of your fracture risk. You will also need your DXA T scores to enter.

World Health Organization (www.who.org). The FRAX™ tool was developed by this organization. They post other helpful information about bone health.

BOOK

Nelson M, Wernick S. *Strong Women, Strong Bones: Everything You Need to Know to Prevent, Treat, and Beat Osteoporosis*. Perigee Books; 2006. Miriam Nelson is a PhD who did groundbreaking research on women in their seventies and eighties who strengthened their bones by doing the exercises in this book on a regular basis.

CHAPTER 12

LIFESTYLE CHOICES FOR LIVING LONGER

Living a healthier life is well within your reach. All you need to do is seize the opportunity.

AGE AND MENOPAUSE BOTH impact body composition and fat distribution. Even if you are lean and fit, you are likely to encounter challenges maintaining a healthy body in the absence of healthy nutrition and exercise. Genetics also plays a role. Even if your family history predisposes you to being overweight, research now shows that a healthy active lifestyle may dampen or even counteract the effect of those genes.

In this chapter, I will review new research on how to achieve and maintain a healthy body during menopause and beyond. While there are new insights, many factors that impact obesity have yet to be discovered. The nutritional and activity choices you make will influence how much independence you preserve and how much energy you will have to actively enjoy the rest of your life.

In this chapter, I'll answer the following questions:

- What medical conditions increase the risk of heart disease and stroke, and how can women lower their risk of developing these conditions?
- How fit should women be during menopause?
- Why is exercise so important, and what should women consider when choosing an activity?

- How can women promote optimal nutrition, and why is this so important as they age?
- What should women consider as they choose a healthy diet?
- What barriers could prevent a woman from losing weight?
- What are examples of best practice strategies for assessing progress?

While no one can guarantee you will avoid obesity, diabetes, metabolic syndrome, heart disease, or bone thinning, if you eat wisely and exercise regularly, you will be much less likely to visit your doctor for these medical problems. With regular physical activity and wise nutritional choices, you will also lower your risk of many types of cancer (see chapter 13 for more information).

MIDLIFE WEIGHT GAIN

Perimenopause heralds the initial changes: slower metabolism, diminishing muscle mass, and erratic hormones. Regardless of your starting weight when you enter perimenopause, you will see your body shape change, and you will put on some weight even if you still eat and exercise the same way.

How significant is this problem? Very. Consider the following:

- Two of three women over age 40 are at a weight that falls in the overweight or obese range.
- Three of four women over age 60 are at a weight that falls in the overweight or obese range.
- Midlife women gain more than 1.5 pounds per year.

DID YOU KNOW?
Weight gain or excess weight bothers women more than hot flashes and night sweats.

What causes midlife weight gain? The following changes occur more frequently as you age:

- Physical activity decreases. This may be subtle or even go unrecognized.
- You experience a decrease in resting and total energy expenditure.
- You experience an increase in adiposity (i.e., you'll see more fat deposits). This includes more subcutaneous fat deposits (i.e., fat deposits under the skin) as well as visceral fat deposits (i.e., deep fat around the internal organs), both of which lead to weight gain.
- You lose lean body mass. When this occurs, it's called sarcopenia.
- You spend less time in moderate- to high-intensity exercise.

ESTROGEN AND MIDLIFE WEIGHT GAIN

How does estrogen affect menopausal weight gain? In some ways, it mitigates weight gain. For example, it induces lipolysis (i.e., breaking down of fat) in visceral fat, but in other ways, it promotes weight gain. For example, it inhibits lipolysis in subcutaneous fat. In addition, loss of estrogen in menopause increases abdominal fat regardless of your age, total body fat, or level of physical activity.

Prior to perimenopause, estrogen promotes fat storage in the hips, thighs, and buttocks. Before perimenopause, estrogen enhances lipolysis (fat breakdown) in the abdominal region and lowers fat production in the deep visceral fat that surrounds the internal organs.

In perimenopause, loss of estrogen over time shifts fat storage to the abdominal area, increasing deep visceral fat around the internal organs and shifting the appearance to a more apple shape.

Estrogen loss is not directly responsible for significant weight gain beyond 3–5 pounds over three years, but it does influence where fat is stored.

Age, slower metabolism, and decreased activity influence weight gain more than estrogen alone.

Currently, most researchers believe that estrogen or menopause hormone therapy influence the distribution of weight but not weight gain or weight loss. Additional studies are needed to more fully understand the role of estrogen combined with weight loss medications such as GLP-1 agonists, discussed later in this chapter.

CHALLENGES THAT CAN CAUSE WEIGHT GAIN FOR MIDLIFE WOMEN[1]

There are many reasons why midlife women gain weight. Here are some of them:

- Decrease in lean body mass (muscle and bone)
- Increase in abdominal (visceral) fat even with no weight gain
- Increase in total body fat
- Increase in waist circumference even with a normal BMI (body mass index)
- Loss of estrogen allows more fat deposits in the abdomen even with no weight gain
- Mood changes and anxiety
- Musculoskeletal changes, arthritis, and fibromyalgia
- Sleep disruption
- Stress and a busy life (sandwich generation)
- Vasomotor symptoms (hot flashes and night sweats)

MENACING MEDICAL CONDITIONS

In North America, many medical conditions formerly attributed to aging are directly related to lack of activity and less-than-ideal nutrition. This tells us we can prevent the most common medical conditions with lifestyle strategies. If you are overweight, you are not alone. Sixty-five percent of North American women are overweight and at risk for metabolic syndrome, diabetes, cancer, heart disease, and even osteoarthritis due to the increased strain that excess weight places on joints. Even if you are lean or normal weight, your body composition may still put you at risk. Lean or normal-weight women may have excess abdominal fat that compromises their health.

DIABETES AND METABOLIC SYNDROME (SYNDROME X)

Being overweight or obese increases your risk of diabetes and metabolic syndrome (syndrome X). These two major medical conditions drastically increase the risk of heart disease and stroke as well as death from other complications. As I discuss in chapter 4, one out of two women over age 50 dies of heart disease. If you develop metabolic syndrome or diabetes, you will be in the high-risk group. Once you have either of these conditions, your health is compromised unless you develop new strategies to change your eating and exercise routines.

DIABETES MELLITUS

With diabetes or prediabetes, the body does not process carbohydrates and glucose effectively. This causes abnormal levels of glucose in the blood. Insulin, a hormone secreted by the pancreas, controls carbohydrate metabolism and sugar processing. Insulin does not function normally in diabetics. More specifically, when someone has diabetes, they may experience one or more of the following:

- Insulin resistance (i.e., the insulin doesn't work effectively)
- Lack of sufficient insulin production
- Timing of insulin release is delayed

> **DID YOU KNOW?**
> Getting older and gaining weight both increase the risk of acquiring diabetes.

Individuals with the poorest glucose control (i.e., those who have severe or advanced diabetes) are more likely to have heart attacks. Diabetics who have heart attacks are less likely to survive them. Individuals with long-standing or severe diabetes may also have trouble with their vision and their circulation. They may also lose sensation in their feet.

If you have diabetes and work closely with your doctor to keep your blood sugar in the normal range, you will lower your risk of heart attack, stroke, and blindness. New studies suggest that good glucose control and adequate exercise with healthy nutrition may lead to remission of your diabetes. When in remission, you enjoy normal blood glucose levels without medication.

METABOLIC SYNDROME (SYNDROME X)

Metabolic syndrome, or syndrome X, is a cluster of abnormalities related to obesity and high blood sugar that has grave consequences. No uniform definition of metabolic syndrome is universal. Key features of metabolic syndrome are:

- Abdominal obesity
- Abnormally high cholesterol or other lipids
- Heart disease
- High blood pressure
- Type 2 diabetes or high blood sugar

In 1998, the World Health Organization (WHO) diabetes group proposed criteria for metabolic syndrome. To be diagnosed with metabolic syndrome, a woman must have diabetes, high fasting glucose, or hyperinsulinemia (i.e., high insulin levels in the blood) as well as two of the three following characteristics:

1. Abdominal obesity with a waist-to-hip ratio of over 0.9, a body mass index (BMI) of 30 or more kilograms per meter squared, or a waist girth over 37 inches (94 centimeters)
2. Blood pressure of 140/90 millimeters of mercury or more or taking medication for high blood pressure
3. Dyslipidemia (i.e., abnormal lipids, including cholesterol) with a serum triglyceride of 150 milligrams per deciliter or more or a high-density lipoprotein (HDL) cholesterol ("good cholesterol") of fewer than 35 milligrams per deciliter

Important Facts About Metabolic Syndrome

Metabolic syndrome will:

- Double the risk of developing heart disease
- Increase the risk for type 2 diabetes by more than five times
- Increase the risk of heart disease, stroke, and diabetes more than obesity
- Increase the risk of stroke by 75 percent
- Increase inflammation in the body (thus increasing the risk for cancer)
- Increase the risk of blood clots (further increasing the risk for heart attack and stroke)

Risk Factors for Metabolic Syndrome

Risk factors for metabolic syndrome (syndrome X) include:

- Being postmenopausal
- Eating a high-carbohydrate diet
- Excess abdominal fat mass
- Leading a sedentary lifestyle

Having obesity often leads to insulin resistance. When this occurs, there is no response when insulin signals that glucose should be removed from the blood. Insulin resistance leads to excess insulin and excess blood glucose.

You do not have to be overweight to be at risk for metabolic syndrome. If you are a normal weight but carry extra fat in your abdomen, you can develop insulin resistance. Accumulating core fat around the internal organs such as the liver and intestines dramatically increases the risk of diabetes. Consequences of abdominal obesity include the following:

- Abnormal fatty tissue function
- Abnormal lipids (i.e., blood fat levels such as cholesterol, HDL, low-density lipoprotein [LDL], and triglycerides that are independent predictors of heart disease and stroke)

- Vascular endothelial dysfunction (i.e., poor blood vessel lining performance)
- Vascular inflammation (i.e., inflamed blood vessels)

> **DID YOU KNOW?**
> Heredity, body weight, abdominal obesity, and a low activity level can increase the risk of heart attack and stroke.

The cluster of risk factors for metabolic syndrome increases your risk of heart attack and stroke more than each of the risk factors alone would predict. In other words, the total risk stemming from metabolic syndrome is greater than the sum of the individual risk factors when one accumulates them.[2]

HOW FIT SHOULD I BE?

Lowering your risk of metabolic syndrome involves the following:

- Achieving a serum triglyceride level of 100 milligrams per deciliter or less. If you already have type 2 diabetes, a more aggressive goal is advised: 80 milligrams per deciliter for LDL or less. This reflects the substantially higher risk of heart disease in those with type 2 diabetes.
- Changing your exercise and nutrition routines to achieve an abdominal girth or waist circumference of less than 35 inches (measured around the widest part of your belly above the top of your hip bones)
- Normalizing your blood pressure to less than 120/75
- Raising your HDL (good cholesterol) to more than 50

While a healthy goal of a waist measurement under 35 inches for a woman is becoming a new standard, some experts still use the waist-to-hip ratio of 0.8 as a healthy target.

(Calculate waist-to-hip ratio by dividing measurement of the smallest part of your waist in inches by measurement of the widest part of your hips in inches to get the waist-to-hip ratio.)

The target of achieving a body mass index (BMI) under 25 is not realistic for anyone who has a muscular frame. Why? Consider the following:

- A healthy BMI for a person who is not more muscular than average is 19–25.
- A more realistic goal for muscular individuals is a waist circumference under 35 inches for women or a waist-to-hip ratio of 0.8.
- BMI is based on measurements of lean young white men more than a century ago and does not account for muscular builds or racial/ethnic diversity in body types.
- Muscle tissue weighs more than fat.
- Muscular individuals with healthy amounts of fat may have a skewed BMI in the obesity range.
- To determine your BMI, divide your body weight by the square of your height or use a BMI table available online.

STRATEGIES TO BECOME MORE FIT

What strategies are helpful to achieve a healthy weight, healthy endurance, and fitness? Successful strategies include:

- Accountability with documented goals
- Behavior modification
- Exercise that is enjoyable and fits your schedule
- Healthy nutrition that you can live with
- Measurable progress (not just weight on the scale)

WHAT TYPES OF EXERCISE ARE HELPFUL?

Research on midlife and menopausal women shows the following types of exercise may be effective:

- Dancing. It's enjoyable, social, and requires your attention.
- High-intensity interval training. It's time efficient and burns calories quickly. Check with your doctor first about your cardiac fitness for this fitness approach.
- Resistance bands. Use bands that increase difficulty over time. This is easy to do at home.
- Stair climbing. Do this five days a week with increasing duration.
- Strength training. Be sure to incorporate 8 to 10 major muscle groups.
- Tai chi. This exercise promotes balance and flexibility, and it adds mind–body focus.
- Walking regularly. Consider adding intervals—short bursts of faster walking interspersed with your normal pace after warmup.
- Yoga. This promotes balance, flexibility, and some strength.

BEING LEAN AND LONGEVITY

In perimenopause, you become predisposed to acquiring fat around your middle. This is a worrisome place to acquire it. Five pounds of weight gain may qualify as a "menopot." This small amount of fat acquired during peri- or early post menopause comes with the transition. After the ovaries stop manufacturing estradiol (i.e., the specific form of estrogen the ovary makes), the body's principal source of estrogen is from body fat. A small amount of extra body fat supplies a natural source of estrogen that helps offset hot flashes and thin bones.

> **DID YOU KNOW?**
> Being lean is associated with longevity, but keep in mind that you do not need to be thin to be healthy. If you are overweight, losing 5 to 10 percent of your current weight produces measurable medical benefits for your overall health such as lower blood pressure.

WAYS TO BECOME LEANER: WHAT DOES AND DOESN'T WORK

There are several strategies to consider; however, not all of them may give you the desired results.

LIPOSUCTION

Liposuction to remove abdominal fat will not improve insulin sensitivity or lower the risk of heart disease. It will also not lower the risk of diabetes or improve glucose control, nor will it improve lipids. It is purely cosmetic.

WEIGHT LOSS MEDICATIONS

To be a candidate for weight loss medications, your doctor will consider your BMI and whether you also have diabetes, heart disease, high lipids, or other concerning conditions.

Weight loss medication typically improves insulin sensitivity, lowers your risk of heart disease, lowers your risk of diabetes, and improves glucose control. Weight loss medications may also improve lipids. In addition to the weight loss medication, your doctor may also prescribe a medication to lower your cholesterol or other lipids if they are dangerously high.

There are a variety of weight loss medications available now by prescription. Insurance coverage is often based on body mass index and the presence of diabetes, metabolic syndrome, or heart disease. Many of these medications affect satiety, or the sense of fullness after eating. They also decrease appetite. The individual injects themselves with a small needle in the abdomen once a week. The dose of medication gradually increases over weeks or months. Some individuals maintain weight loss after stopping these medications. Others stay on medication to maintain a healthy weight. Examples of these medications include Wegovy, Ozempic, Mounjaro, Trulicity, Phentermine and Terzepatide (Zepbound).

BARIATRIC SURGERY

Weight loss surgery or bariatric surgery is also an option to consider if your BMI is over 40 or is 30-35 and you have other medical conditions that put you at risk, such as diabetes, heart disease, or metabolic syndrome. There are several surgical procedures to consider, and each has different pros and cons, risks, and benefits. To maintain weight loss benefits over time, you will need to modify how much and how often you eat as most procedures involve decreasing the size of the stomach and its capacity to process more than a small amount of food.

EXPLORING ALL YOUR OPTIONS

In the rest of this chapter, I will focus on research that you can explore prior to considering weight loss medication or weight loss surgery. Given the impact of aging as well as menopause, modifying your nutrition and exercise routines may involve the following:

- Apps such as My Fitness Pal, Weight Watchers, or NOOM provide coaching options and can be done remotely at your own pace
- Consulting with your doctor or a weight loss specialist in person or via telehealth
- Joining group exercise sessions
- Working with a nutritionist, behavior therapist, or fitness coach in person or online

THE MYSTERY OF "VITAMIN X"

The most frequent request I hear as a doctor is, "Just give me a pill to fix everything." I often refer to this panacea as "vitamin X." It is not on the market with this name, but you deserve to know about it so you can look for it. Want to know more about it? I'll let you in on the secret.

Vitamin X lowers the risk of diabetes, obesity, heart disease, and stroke. Vitamin X lowers your risk of breast cancer and other cancers. It strengthens bones and helps prevent osteoporosis and Alzheimer's disease. It also improves your sex life. Vitamin X is inexpensive. It comes in many forms. If you select the right version for you, it rarely has adverse side effects. Every woman can benefit from some type of vitamin X, regardless of her medical history, physical condition, or phase of menopause. Vitamin X also helps all women regardless of whether they have hot flashes, irregular menstrual periods, or no symptoms at all.

What is vitamin X? If you guessed it is exercise, you are correct. Research has shown that perimenopausal women who exercise up to 40 minutes a day, four times a week decrease their risk of breast cancer by 60 percent. If vitamin X could be packaged and sold as a pill, cream, or powder, it might be the only supplement most people would need.

WHY EXERCISE IS MORE IMPORTANT NOW THAN EVER

Women who do not exercise during perimenopause will have a higher risk of breast cancer, osteoporosis, obesity, diabetes, and heart disease than they would have otherwise. Why is exercise so critical at this time of life?

Women begin to lose muscle mass in their mid-thirties. From that time on, even if a woman eats the same amount and exercises the same way, she is still likely to gain weight. Muscle tissue burns more calories per hour than fat, 24 hours a day, while awake or at rest and even during sleep. Loss of muscle mass means fewer pounds of muscle are burning fewer calories all day long. As you have just read, once additional weight accumulates around the waist, the risk of diabetes, heart attack, and stroke increases dramatically.

Your body composition and metabolism both change as you progress from perimenopause to post menopause. The gradual loss of muscle mass is one of the changes that contribute to a slower metabolism. Almost all women begin to accumulate more fat around the waist and abdomen. This provides our bodies with natural reserves of the weaker estrogen (estrone) that is released from fatty tissue. The weaker estrone, synthesized from fat tissue, offsets the loss of the ovarian estrogen (estradiol).

Attaining and maintaining a lean healthy physique and a healthy level of physical activity increases the likelihood that you will enjoy many years of good quality life. Accomplishing this involves strategizing while living in a sedentary culture.

CHOOSING YOUR ACTIVITIES

"Activity" includes planned exercise and encompasses more than that. Many of you may find the thought of exercise off-putting, overwhelming, and exhausting. Exercise is the last thing on many women's to-do lists—if it even makes it on the list at all. If you are not active, you may remain healthy in your twenties and early thirties, but you are unlikely to stay healthy over age 40 without some form of regular activity.

The activity you select should be enjoyable for you and doable. Start with what you enjoy and figure out how you can do it regularly. After that, things will fall into place more readily. Once you are moving and you have considered what is appealing to you, you can begin to assess whether you are incorporating the types of activities that will maintain your physical and mental health.

> **DID YOU KNOW?**
> Exercise improves blood pressure, promotes weight loss, and removes abdominal fat, especially in women.

Exercise helps remove weight and keep it off. Thirty minutes of brisk walking most days is the minimum recommendation, but you can break this up into shorter intervals if you are pressed for time. If the aerobic or weight/resistance sessions are at least 10 minutes each, you will get more aerobic benefit. That doesn't mean you cannot add shorter spurts of activity whenever possible. Every bit counts. More exercise is even better—ideally, we would all do 60 minutes or more of daily activity—but it is better to start with a realistic goal. It's important to do at least 10 minutes of an activity at a time that requires effort, raises your heart rate, and makes you sweat. A casual stroll is good for your health, but it won't help you lose weight or build muscles as effectively.[3]

FOR WOMEN WHO DO NOT EXERCISE

If you do not exercise or get regular physical activity at least once a week, start slowly. Start small. See your doctor first and get the green light to exercise. Do not go from a parking spot closest to the front door to parking a mile away overnight. Consider any small habits that you can change daily. For example, if you take a train or bus each day, can you get off one or two stops early and walk the rest of the way? Can you take a walk during lunch? Are there stairs you can take as often as possible instead of the elevator? Can you choose to take extra flights of stairs rather than avoiding them? Can you deliver a message in person instead of emailing?

Do you like to garden? Do you like to dance? Put on the radio, Spotify, or Pandora, and dance to your heart's content. Check out exercise and dance classes on You Tube, or take a dance class. Inexpensive classes are often available in adult education programs or community centers as well as online. Go with a friend or partner or meet one there. Dancing is an excellent form of exercise, and it is good for the brain in addition to having a positive social component. It increases blood flow, and remembering the routines requires mental sharpness.

Do you like to walk? Consider wearing a pedometer, a small device attached to your waist that counts your steps. You can also use a pedometer app on your phone or smartwatch. Eventually, your goal may be to take 5,000 to 10,000 steps a day. In our sedentary society, some individuals take as few as 1,000 steps a day.

If you are not walking regularly but like to walk, consider starting with five-minute walks in the morning. Perhaps you can walk for five minutes when you go to get your mail. Then add another five minutes at lunchtime and before dinner. Then increase to a minimum of 10 minutes of cardio.

Consider cycling or walking to work or while doing errands.

FOR WOMEN WHO EXERCISE IN MODERATION

Women who are moderately active may use the strategies I have just reviewed to add to their activity level. Motivation may be an issue. You may feel you must choose an activity that does not appeal to you. You may "force" yourself to do it because it is "good" for you. Incorporating adequate amounts of activity into your schedule to enhance your mental and physical health is difficult enough without asking yourself to do things that are not enjoyable.

I have found it helpful both personally and professionally to think about the social aspect of exercise and look at individual preferences through that lens. Do you like to have time alone when you walk or garden? Do you like to let your thoughts roam or listen to music or a book on tape? Would you like to watch a show you've taped or a movie while you use an exercise bike, elliptical machine or treadmill? Free exercise sessions are available online, on TV, and YouTube.

Do you prefer company? Would you rather go for a walk with a friend or join a group class that meets at a fixed time? Do you prefer the flexibility of a gym or an exercise franchise that has "open hours" for exercising? Some of these facilities have other exercisers there to chat with if you wish, but you are not committed to a particular time/schedule each day. Sometimes seeing others exercising can be personally motivating.

FOR WOMEN WITH PHYSICAL RESTRICTIONS

If you have hip, knee, or ankle issues, consider aqua aerobics or swimming. Consider aqua jogging classes. For aqua classes, you do not need to be able to swim. You typically do not need to put your head in the water or get your hair wet. A flotation device around your waist keeps you buoyant while you move your legs to music while in the water. This alleviates stress on your joints and may appeal if you have pain or problems with your feet, ankles, knees, or hips. If you are wheelchair-bound, you may also enjoy aqua jogging. When I have attended these classes in a variety of locations and settings, I am impressed by the range of ages and body types. You do not have to have a certain size bathing suit to benefit or feel comfortable.

If you have hip, knee, ankle, or foot issues, water aerobics is another alternative. Exercises are conducted in shallow water. The water provides resistance and buoys up your body so that there is minimal stress on your joints. The classes I have seen or taken at the YMCA enroll women of all shapes, sizes, and health statuses.

When checking out classes, see if there are modifications provided to the standard routine that accommodate whatever physical restrictions or discomforts you may have. Consider Rita's and Sharon's stories.

Rita's Story
SOCIAL EXERCISER

I am a genetic counselor who is disciplined in my professional life, but I was having difficulty sticking to an exercise regimen. My cousin suggested I compile a list of friends and acquaintances that became my "walking buddies." Different friends were available during the week or on weekends. I try to make three or four walking dates a week, some planned and some spur of the moment. I no longer struggle to make myself go for a walk because I look forward to seeing my friends and enjoying their company.

Sharon's Story
SOLITARY EXERCISER

I am an introvert by nature. When I exercise, I would rather hop onto a treadmill. I borrow audiobooks from the local public library, and I only listen to them while I am on the treadmill, so it feels like "a treat." This way, I am motivated because I want to hear what happens next in the book. Occasionally, for variety, I record a favorite show and watch that instead. I seldom miss an exercise session.

WE ALL NEED THESE FOUR TYPES OF EXERCISE

As you begin to exercise more and try out different activities, keep in mind that four kinds of exercise should ultimately be a part of your routine after you warm up. A warm-up can be as simple as walking in place for two to three minutes before stretching. Warming up means getting your circulation going and your muscles limber.[4,5]

STRETCHING

Flexibility is lost with age. Stretching helps preserve flexibility and range of motion. Not only does stretching keep you flexible, but it also helps prevent injury and preserve range of motion. If you stretch regularly, it is less likely you will become stiff and limited in terms of what you can do. Stretching also enhances muscle strength by an additional 18 percent.

Stretch after you warm up. Bob Anderson's book, *Stretching*, has a variety of stretches that may help you warm up or cool down and ease the muscles you use most during the activities you plan.

Yoga naturally incorporates stretching with relaxation, and it enhances flexibility and strength. Tai chi and Pilates also incorporate stretching.

STRENGTHENING

Working with dumbbells or weights increases muscle strength and tone. Weight-bearing exercise may be done on weight machines, with free weights, or with exercise bands. It is also possible to work against your own body weight to build strength, as in doing push-ups, squats or planks.

Weight-bearing activity forces your body to work against gravity, strengthening your bones and muscles. Targeted strengthening helps preserve and replenish healthy muscle mass that is naturally lost with increasing age. Muscle conditioning helps ward off osteoporosis. It also helps keep your body trim and may decrease your waist and hip size by inches even before you lose any weight. Most important, muscle conditioning helps preserve your independence.

If you preserve your strength, you may continue to lift your own grocery or shopping bags and travel independently if you choose. Aerobic activity alone is not as important to heart health as muscle conditioning and strengthening. Rowing indoors or outdoors is becoming more popular because it strengthens the upper body while simultaneously providing aerobic benefits. Indoor rowing machines are available at health clubs and gyms. Light kayaks, rowboats, or skulls are fun if you have access to the water.

Bonus: Muscle tissue burns more calories per minute, even when you are not exercising.

> **DID YOU KNOW?**
>
> Working out with weights does not create bulky muscles. You are never too old to begin a weight-bearing exercise regimen. Supreme Court Justice Ruth Bader Ginsburg was working on her pushups with a trainer even in her 80s.

AEROBIC/CARDIOVASCULAR ACTIVITY

Raising the heart rate is sometimes referred to as "cardio" for short. You do not have to be a runner or triathlete to attain cardiac fitness. Cardiac exercise can be as simple as marching in place as fast as you can or using the stairs more at home or at work. It can consist of doing your own housework or gardening. It can be using a treadmill, a stationary bike, an elliptical machine, or a combination of these. It can be dancing. It can be jumping rope to prevent fractures from osteoporosis. (Note: Avoid jumping rope if you have already had an osteoporotic fracture.) A nontraditional sport such as fencing can be enjoyed well into your 80s. Convenience and the activity's appeal are key to entice you to do it regularly.

BALANCING

Maintaining a healthy posture and preserving your balance become increasingly important as you age. With age, your posture may deteriorate, and you lose your sense of balance. Now we know that specific types of exercise can help us regain balance. One of the simplest balance exercises is this:

1. Stand on one foot while you brush the top row of teeth.
2. Stand on your other foot while you brush the bottom row of teeth.

(Do not try this while wearing sandals or shoes with heels.)

Exercises to regain balance range from walking on rugged uneven terrain to doing Pilates to working on an exercise ball or a rubber disc placed on the floor. Improving your balance decreases your risk of falling. Fewer falls mean fewer fractures of the hip or the wrists when you reach out to break a fall. Activities that contribute to standing tall and preserving straight posture as well as balance include tai chi, yoga, and Pilates, all of which can be practiced well into the senior years.

TAI CHI

Tai chi is an ancient form of slow movements that enhance one's posture, alignment, and range of motion. You may find a class taught by a certified instructor, borrow a videotape or DVD from the library, or find an instructor on YouTube.

YOGA

Yoga combines exercises that incorporate stretching and strengthening with breathing. It originated in India thousands of years ago. Yoga develops strength, flexibility, and a steady mind. It can be as gentle or demanding as you make it.

PILATES

Pilates was developed by Joseph Pilates, a German boxer. While in England during World War II, he devised a system of pulleys and resistance exercises on bunk beds to stay in shape. These exercises were designed to work the core of the body from the ribs to the pelvic area and stabilize it. Pilates differs from muscle training in that the core of the body is stretched, strengthened, and stabilized with each movement. Alignment of the body is also emphasized. Pilates can be performed in a vigorous way on special machines or mats on the floor. A certified instructor may assist you in learning the subtleties of the technique and enhance the benefits you will derive. There are also books and YouTube videos available that provide Pilates activities at various levels of difficulty, including wall Pilates.

OPTIMAL NUTRITION

You may have already noticed your metabolism slowing down over time. You may have also noticed that your muscles are not as strong as they were, especially if you do not do weight-bearing exercise. Losing muscle mass results in fewer calories burned per hour.

> **DID YOU KNOW?**
>
> If you enter perimenopause and keep eating the same way you always have—and exercise as much as you always have—you will gain weight as you age.

Perimenopause and post menopause bring other variables to the weight/balance picture. In addition to the decrease in metabolism associated with aging—as well as the fewer calories needed as one ages—other effects related to perimenopause and post menopause are difficult to sort out.

Some researchers report that women metabolize smaller meals better than larger ones beginning in perimenopause and lasting into their postmenopausal years. Typically, perimenopausal and postmenopausal women need fewer carbohydrates than they did earlier in life. Smaller portions are helpful. The smaller portions should include whole grains (avoid white sugar or flour) and high-fiber carbohydrates that provide longer-lasting satisfaction and superior nutrition. Enjoying your carbohydrate servings early in the day is also helpful. Nutritionists also advise including a protein serving with any carbohydrate serving to improve metabolism and satiety.

Consuming more calories than the amount of energy you expend will cause weight gain. This is true even if you only overestimate your calorie needs by a modest amount. Cutting calories too drastically to lose weight will not serve you well either. Cutting calories drastically (i.e., below your body's healthy requirements) will prompt a "starvation response." When this happens, your body will conserve calories and store them as fat because it thinks you are literally starving. While this was originally an adaptive response when food was scarce in caveman times or during a famine, it is not adaptive for a postmenopausal woman. The last thing you want is to store extra fat while eating too few calories.[6]

As you lose weight, your calorie requirements decrease. A smaller body that has decreased in size has smaller energy demands. Activity can offset this so your minimal caloric requirement is not too restrictive.

Researchers are reporting that eating 80 percent of your body's requirement leads to living longer. If you are leaner and consume fewer calories (i.e., 1,800 or fewer calories a day), you may also have a lower body temperature. Lower body temperature is associated with longevity. On the other hand, excessive dieting and even anorexia are surfacing in perimenopausal and postmenopausal women. This kind of "thinness" is not healthy.

INSTEAD OF COUNTING CALORIES, MAKE EACH CALORIE COUNT

Keep in mind that all calories are not created equal. Some foods are "nutrient-dense," meaning there is a high ratio of nutrients to calories, and you get more benefit from eating them. Processed, sugary, commercially prepared foods have few nutrients but lots of calories.

Proteins, carbohydrates, and fats are all essential to health. Different fad diets will discount one while overemphasizing another, but it's important to remember that the body needs a balance of all three. Consider the following:

- Carbohydrates are used primarily for fuel but also contribute to healthy moods.
- Fats are used by every cell in the body. Healthy fats are incorporated into cell membranes.
- Protein is needed for your body to build and repair cells, tissues, organs, hormones, antibodies, hair, fingernails, and so on.

Healthy carbohydrates include whole grains that contain fiber to help digestion and elimination. Whole grains help maintain healthy levels of serotonin that are essential for good moods. Whole grains also help prevent heart disease and several types of cancer, including bowel cancer. Whole grains should be on every woman's plate.

CALORIES AND THE FOOD PYRAMID

Do not feel you must use the traditional food pyramid to govern your food choices. The government dietary guidelines represent input from special interest groups, including the dairy industry, the meat industry, and those who grow corn, to name a few. The food pyramid is not a consensus of the latest developments in medical research on nutrition. Dr. Walter Willett, an internationally respected MD (medical doctor), PhD, at Harvard School of Public Health, reviews some of the issues in his book *Eat, Drink, and Be Healthy*.

A WORD OF CAUTION ABOUT DIET BOOKS AND PROGRAMS

Diet books or programs often include content that is not regulated or monitored. Nor are the recommendations necessarily supported by research. Celebrities in the diet and exercise domain are akin to "pied pipers" mesmerizing the attention of adult women. A celebrity need only provide a charismatic book cover photo exuding sex appeal to draw women in. The implication is, "Do what I say, and you will achieve my looks and appeal for yourself!" There are also books that have intrinsic appeal but no evidence backing them up. For example, the book *Eat Right for Your Blood Type* has/had an enthusiastic following. Although it is an interesting book, the author does not cite a single research study. Published articles are needed to validate this theory. Blood type could theoretically be the key to how we should eat, but some proof is in order.

FOODS TO AVOID

In your journey to become healthier, you'll want to stay away from these foods as much as possible or avoid them altogether:

- White stuff
  "White stuff" refers to carbohydrates that offer poor nutritional value per calorie. White stuff includes white flour, white sugar, and starch with minimal fiber and vitamins. When you eat white stuff, you digest it too quickly, leaving you with a "sugar low" after the carbohydrate sugar rush suddenly leaves your bloodstream. After quickly digesting white stuff, you may feel weak and especially hungry. You

may even crave more white stuff. The nutritional value of white flour has been stripped away in preparing it. Further, white stuff has no fiber, so it can lead to constipation. White stuff is calorie-dense, so you do not have to eat a large portion to pack in many nutritionally empty calories that will only leave you begging for more.

- Sodas
  Sodas, whether they are diet, sugar-free, or regular, lead to thinner bones. Avoid colas to avoid one cause of osteoporosis.
- Alcohol
  Alcohol (i.e., beer, wine, or liquor) typically decreases inhibitions and compromises judgment about how much to eat and what to select. Alcohol is also calorie-dense. Lastly, it disrupts sleep, which disturbs the body's ability to tell when it is satisfied with the amount of food that has come in (see chapter 9 for more information).
  Consider Janelle's story.

Janelle's Story
CHANGING EATING HABITS

I am 53 and newly postmenopausal. I have been keeping a food diary for three weeks and adjusting portion sizes of protein and carbohydrates. My doctor suggested I consult a nutritionist. I used to skip breakfast, but now I have yogurt in the morning. I try to have carbohydrates more often at lunch. A month ago, I would eat a whole chicken cutlet for dinner, but I have reduced my portion size to four ounces. Now I only buy whole wheat pasta and measure out a one-cup serving. When I eat out, I request brown rice instead of white. I know I am on the right track. I am moving away from the white stuff and increasing my whole grains. This increases my fiber consumption and provides extra nutrients in my diet. I am also becoming more aware of what I eat by keeping a food diary and trying healthier portion sizes, especially for my protein and carbohydrate servings.

STRESS EATING

Janelle's story illustrates the role of keeping a food diary to learn more about your eating patterns. It is easy to forget what you are putting in your mouth. Even studies looking at nutritionists' behavior and calorie tracking show that estimating food consumption and calories hours after consuming them is inaccurate by hundreds of calories.

> DID YOU KNOW?
> The process of keeping a food diary and tracking electronically or on paper can help awareness and decrease stress eating.

Are you prone to stress eating? Consider meditating for five minutes a day, and then gradually increase that to 15 or 20 minutes a day. Meditating can be as simple as repeating a word to yourself over and over. When your mind wanders, bring it back to the word you are repeating in your head. If you have too much on your mind, it may be helpful to have a pad of paper to write down "to do's" if they disrupt your mind–body practice.

Sometimes food preferences or stronger cravings influence you to eat food with a particular texture or flavor. If you are stressed, you may succumb to the urge to eat a certain type of food. Consider healthier substitutions that satisfy you as well. For example:

- Consider fat-free pudding instead of chocolate mousse.
- Consider frozen yogurt instead of full-fat ice cream.
- Crunch on a crispy apple instead of pretzels.
- Crunch on baked potato chips instead of fried potato chips.

Alternatively, some of my patients successfully use portion control to enjoy the same food their family, friends, or housemates enjoy but in smaller servings.

Experiencing stress releases the stress hormone cortisol. Cortisol promotes storage of abdominal and core fat around the internal organs. This type of fat storage is the most hazardous. It increases the risk of heart attack, stroke, and diabetes as well as metabolic syndrome. Those who are stress eaters may find that stress reduction is a critical component of their improved nutritional plan.

Identifying whether you are a stress eater is helpful. Before eating a meal or snack, ask yourself these questions:

- Am I stimulated by appealing food? For example, did I just walk past a bakery and smell the special of the day?
- Am I hungry? Might I be thirsty instead?
- Am I bored, nervous, or stressed?

If you identify yourself as a stress eater, you've found important information. You will likely benefit from strategies to decrease stress and stress eating. Strategies may include meditation, cognitive behavioral therapy, hypnosis, and acupuncture, to name a few. Exercise is also an excellent stress reducer.

Support from others reduces stress, and it also contributes to the ability to attain and maintain a healthy weight. Support may come in different forms such as meeting with your doctor, consulting a nutritionist, online forums (e.g., My Fitness Pal, Lost It!, Weight Watchers, or NOOM), and weight loss support groups (e.g., Overeaters Anonymous). Consider Sabrina's story.

Sabrina's Story
A SPEED EATER

I am a "speed eater." I grew up in a large family where those who ate fast got more of what they wanted! Throughout school, I kept up this rapid eating pace. Plus, I always had somewhere else to go. When I am hungry, I can eat a lot of food quickly without realizing how much I have eaten. This way of eating is why I have never really developed the ability to tell when I am full. Now, at 65, I am 40 pounds overweight and having trouble with my knees. My doctor diagnosed osteoarthritis of the knees and told me that the arthritic changes in my knees were a result of the extra stress they bore from my added weight. They said the bony changes would continue to create further damage and increasing pain if I did not remove the excess weight. They recommended that I consider Weight Watchers. I was under a lot of stress at the time and was not ready to begin the Weight Watchers program. I wanted to try to modify my eating on my own. The doctor recommended a food diary where I record everything I eat—before, during, or immediately after I eat it, including the portion size. In addition, they recommended that I eat more slowly. Taking at least 20 minutes to eat a meal helps me tell when I am getting full. My doctor says it takes 20 minutes to register how full you are. During this period of ongoing stress in my life, I have continued to keep my food diary and to eat more slowly. When I am mentally ready, I will start the Weight Watchers program online.

WEIGHT LOSS DIETS

The food you eat is your diet, not the food you have to give up or restrict yourself to eating. Anything you put in your mouth constitutes your diet. Over time, the term *diet* has become synonymous with attempts to lose weight. Unfortunately, the term *diet* has been distorted to connote depriving yourself of the food you want.

To shift your thinking to focus on how to best nourish your body, consider focusing on nutrition. Long-term nutrition with healthy choices will help you enjoy a healthy body over time.

In North American culture, women are constantly enticed to become unreasonably slim or to attain an unrealistic shape. The relentless pressure and exposure to painfully thin models are beginning to ease as websites and ads begin to incorporate larger models to showcase their stylish clothing. This societal pressure and background noise make it harder to start or maintain healthy nutrition. Unrealistic expectations can be overwhelming.[6]

IS IT THE RIGHT TIME TO BEGIN?

Before starting a new nutrition plan, decide if this is a good time for you to begin. Pick a time in your life when you are likely to succeed. It is better to maintain your weight and avoid weight gain than to make a lukewarm effort and fail or binge and regain weight. If you are under extra stress due to a relative or friend's illness, unusual demands inside or outside your home, or not in a favorable mindset for weight loss, consider maintaining your current weight until you are ready to make some lifestyle changes. On the other hand, don't wait too long for the right time to begin.

One way to start gradually is to make one change a month. For example, you could commit to keeping a food diary every day. Even though you may not change your choices deliberately, keeping a daily food log has been shown to contribute to weight loss. It makes eating more conscious. By increasing awareness of what you are consuming, you have more detailed and accurate information on which to base your future food choices.

ASSESS YOUR READINESS FOR WEIGHT LOSS OR NUTRITION CHANGES

There's a process that supports success. Where are you in the stages of change?

- *Action.* How confident are you that you can make the change you plan and do it consistently?
- *Contemplation.* What are the positive or negative consequences of changing your behavior? Will it affect your family, relationships, coworkers, or housemates?
- *Maintenance.* What accountability and support can you put in place to maintain the healthy changes?[5]
- *Precontemplation.* We all have mixed feelings about change. On the one hand, you would like to lose weight and be

healthier. On the other hand, you have too much stress now to modify your routines.
- *Preparation.* What barriers do you anticipate when making the changes you plan, and what goals are realistic for you?

Maintaining a healthy weight also requires effort. Some menopause experts say that maintaining your weight in perimenopause and early post menopause is a victory. As metabolism slows during the perimenopause and future decades, weight maintenance becomes challenging. Consider Landa's story.

Landa's Story
THE LOW-FAT MAVEN

Ten years ago, I lost 30 pounds, and I have maintained my weight over that time by eating low-fat foods and monitoring my portion sizes. I eat whole-grain carbohydrates. I do eat breakfast, but I often miss lunch. I get very hungry in the evening and crave carbohydrates. My weight is good, but my nails have become more brittle, and my hair is drier. My eyesight is worse. At 75, I have chalked these changes up to my age.

Landa is a victim of the low-fat approach to losing weight. She lacks healthy fats. All individuals need some healthy fat. Fats help to digest essential vitamins and minerals. Fat-soluble vitamins include vitamins A, D, E, and K. Vitamin A is important for eyesight. Vitamin D is important for bone health. Vitamin K is important for blood clotting. Without sufficient fat, these vitamins are not adequately absorbed by the body. Taking excess amounts of these vitamins will not correct this problem if there is not adequate fat to promote their digestion and absorption. Landa's doctor found that she had a vitamin D deficiency that contributed to thin bones. They prescribed supplemental vitamin D by mouth and recommended that Landa have two teaspoons of olive oil each day or a few nuts to give her adequate amounts of healthy oils in her diet. Over time,

Landa noticed that her hair was not as dry, and her nails were less brittle several months after she added the healthy oils to her diet. She also found she was not as hungry after dinner. The oils helped her to feel more satisfied.

MEDITERRANEAN DIET

Weight reduction is the cornerstone of treatment for metabolic syndrome as well as diabetes and heart disease for those who are overweight, and the Mediterranean diet is an ideal strategy. Different versions of the Mediterranean diet vary by country and cuisine. In general, they emphasize lean protein, olive oil, nut oil, or avocado oil, as well as fresh fruits and vegetables. One version of the Mediterranean diet is presented in the *Sonoma Diet Cookbook* by Connie Guttersen. This version includes a detailed description of the program and recipes. Although the Sonoma diet is not promoted as a low-carbohydrate or low-calorie diet, it has features of both. The healthy fats in this program, including olive oil along with the fruits, vegetables, and whole grains, promote lower blood pressure, weight loss, more normal lipid profiles, and less severe insulin resistance as well as less inflammation of the blood vessels.

DASH DIET

Another program that targets metabolic syndrome is the DASH diet, which limits daily sodium intake to 2,400 milligrams and promotes a higher dairy intake compared with the Mediterranean diet. It also may improve triglycerides, diastolic blood pressure, and fasting glucose. A program with low carbohydrates and a low glycemic index will improve glucose control and blood lipids.

HOW TO EVALUATE A WEIGHT LOSS DIET

When you are considering a weight loss plan, your doctor may be able to help you answer these questions (or they will refer you to a nutritionist):

- Are there enough fats to maintain skin, hair, and nail health? Are fats healthy ones such as those from nuts, avocados, and olive oil?
- Are there enough fruits and vegetables to keep the risk of cancer and heart disease at bay?
- Are there enough healthy carbohydrates to sustain serotonin levels and maintain good humor as well as maintain healthy digestion and elimination?
- Do you have the option of eating out and still staying on the program?
- Does it promote a healthy heart and strong bones?
- How do you feel about eating the way the weight loss plan advises for the rest of your life?
- If you are diabetic, does the program meet your needs, or should you consult a nutritionist or diabetic expert as well?
- Is there a behavioral piece to the program? Are there strategies for coping with various roadblocks you may encounter, such as cravings, urges, parties, or emotional eating? Consider adding other behavioral tools, such as hypnosis or meditation to reduce stress, or even cognitive behavioral therapy to give you insights into why you may be a stress eater or an emotional eater.
- Is there a maintenance phase built in? Are you willing to commit to the maintenance program? Would it fit into your lifestyle? Committing to the weight loss plan without a maintenance plan just sets you up to regain weight. You will need to commit to long-term lifestyle modifications and new nutritional choices to allow your hard-won progress to stick to you permanently. Researchers have shown that Weight Watchers followers do not achieve larger or faster losses than followers of other nutritional programs such as Atkins or South Beach, but Weight Watchers members do keep the weight off longer if they follow the maintenance program faithfully. The NOOM weight loss program also

has a behavioral component to modify your approach to eating.
- Is there an adjustment for decreasing your food intake as your weight loss progresses? You will need fewer calories as you remove weight. Beware: if you eat too little at first, your metabolism will slow down to guard you against starvation. Your body thinks you are starving it and will hold on to the calories and store them as fat to prepare for the famine.
- What is the appeal and flavor attraction of the program that you are considering? Do you like the foods in the program and the way they are prepared? Are you open to trying the foods they suggest? Is there enough variety for you to experiment with or create healthier versions of your favorites? Flavor and appeal count. If you are not accustomed to eating vegetables and do not like them, switching to a vegetarian diet should not be your first move. Eventually, your palate may become more accustomed to enjoying the taste of vegetables, after several transitions. When you decrease the amount of white stuff you eat, you will notice fewer sugar cravings, and your tastes may shift to enjoying the nuances of various sensations other than the sweet ones. Varying textures and taste may help. Many women stick to sweet or salty and creamy or crunchy. At some point, you can expand your horizons to include sour, salty, savory, or bitter in addition to sweet. Textures can include crunchy, chewy, or creamy, as well as combinations of these.
- What is the nutritional value of the program?
- What prep work is involved for the program? For example, the South Beach diet is a heart-healthy program that also has cancer prevention features and is nutritionally sound, but substantial preparation is needed to create the dishes it advises. Are you someone who will devote the time and energy to chopping and assembling the foods ahead of time? The Sonoma diet is another program that emphasizes

Mediterranean cuisine. The food is delicious, but it helps if you like to cook and cook often. Conversely, there may be minimal or no prep work with a program such as Jenny Craig, where the meals are provided for you. To be successful, you need to be committed to the maintenance phase when you will no longer have the portion control built into the premade dinners.

As every woman knows all too well, if you eat too much, you will not lose weight. The problem that sets in during perimenopause and persists throughout post menopause is that the range between eating just a little too much (resulting in unwanted weight gain) and eating too little (with its inevitable slowing of metabolism and calorie burn) is that the range between the two narrows in peri- and post menopause. Consider Madelyn's story.

Madelyn's Story
LIKES PROTEIN AND CARBOHYDRATES

I was brought up on meat and potatoes. I grew up eating salty, soggy canned vegetables that held no appeal. I have tried low-carbohydrate diets such as Atkins in the past and found my mood plummeted without carbs. I have tried low-protein diets and found that I could not think straight and felt weak. My husband is also fond of meat and potatoes, so we always returned to that tried-and-true pattern. Recently, my doctor told me I have high blood pressure and high cholesterol. I am ready to make a change and pick healthier food choices. Even though I am 70, they said it is not too late!

My doctor recommends a low-sodium diet with more fruits and vegetables. To start, they suggest filling half my plate with non-starchy vegetables, one-quarter of the plate with carbohydrates (preferably whole grains), and one-quarter with lean meat, chicken, or fish. They referred me to a nutritionist who recommends I try to have one or two vegetarian meals each week. The nutritionist recommended a few programs with ideas about serving raw vegetables, in addition to those that include lightly steamed ones as well as frozen vegetables. Also, they provided vegetarian versions of some of my favorite recipes. I found I like low-fat moussaka, a recipe with no meat, from the American Heart Association cookbook. I also was surprised how much I enjoy vegetarian lasagna made with tofu crumbles (found in the freezer section of the supermarket) instead of ground beef as one of the fillings. Low-fat soup, another of my new discoveries, leaves me feeling full and satisfied with fewer calories and better nutrition.

COMPARING DIET PLANS

How do you feel after trying new foods or recipes? Are you satisfied? Do you feel full for hours? Do the portion sizes and recommended foods and recipes meet your metabolic needs without causing you to gain weight? Avoid restricted choices that rob you of flexibility. It is important to be able to enjoy special occasions with friends, family, and coworkers.

ATKINS DIET

Atkins emphasizes unlimited protein and fat with minimal vegetables and carbohydrates. There are minimal fruit options at first. Nutrition experts have voiced concerns about the types of fat Atkins promotes. Full-fat dairy and saturated fat products are not heart-healthy and promote cancer over time. For some Atkins devotees, adding back carbohydrates and fruits results in unwanted weight gain.

The advantage of Atkins is that it is simple to understand. You do not have to measure portion sizes or track food.

> **DID YOU KNOW?**
>
> Nutrition experts attribute the success of all diet programs, Atkins included, to calorie restriction. In the end, they say, one can eat only so much steak and full-fat dairy. Any nutrition program that restricts calories will help you lose weight if you follow it consistently.

Advantages of the Atkins Diet
- Consistently tends to produce weight loss.
- Helps retain muscle mass during weight loss.
- Minimal vegetables and almost no fruit is hard for some individuals to sustain.

Drawbacks of the Atkins Diet
- Bad moods can occur due to carbohydrate deprivation and low blood serotonin levels.
- High animal and dairy fat diets may lead to heart problems.
- High-protein, high-fat diets are associated with constipation (due to very low fiber).
- Insulin sensitivity does not improve with weight loss on a high-protein regimen.
- Ketosis may result in bad breath due to muscle breakdown.
- Extremely high-protein diets are associated with a higher risk of bone loss and osteoporosis.

MEDITERRANEAN DIET OR SONOMA DIET

Consider the following key details about the Mediterranean or Sonoma diet:

- Advises lean protein such as poultry and seafood in lesser amounts
- Emphasizes heart-healthy fats (e.g., olive oil and avocado oil) in lesser amounts
- Recommended by the American Heart Association
- Stresses healthy, high-fiber carbohydrates

SOUTH BEACH DIET

The South Beach diet, introduced by Dr. Arthur Agatston, is a healthier, more nutritionally sound, balanced low-carbohydrate program. Programs like the South Beach diet, the Core Program in Weight Watchers, NOOM weight loss program, and the Sonoma diet (Mediterranean diet) all stress healthy high-fiber carbohydrates and heart-healthy fats in lesser amounts with liberal amounts of lean protein and nonstarchy vegetables and fruits. These are all heart-healthy strategies.

DASH DIET

Consider the following key details about the DASH diet:

- Emphasizes low sodium choices
- Low in sodium, added sugars, and saturated fat
- Recommended by the American Heart Association and the American Diabetes Association
- Rich in calcium, potassium, protein, fiber, and magnesium

LOW-FAT DIETS

Three large randomized controlled trials looked at the effects of low-fat diets on weight loss in postmenopausal women. It took 4 to 12 months of treatment with a low-fat diet and fewer calories for postmenopausal women to see a 6 to 8.5 percent weight loss. In the Women's Health Initiative Dietary Modification Trial, more than 19,500 postmenopausal women followed a low-fat diet with only 20 percent fat and no restriction on calories for seven years. Their body weight went down by 1.7 percent during the first year, and they maintained a 1 percent weight loss after seven years compared to women who did not follow the low-fat regimen.[6,7]

VEGETARIAN OR VEGAN DIETS

If you are not ready to commit to a vegetarian diet or strict vegan diet with no dairy, eggs, or seafood, consider trying one or two vegetarian meals a week.

Research on vegetarian nutrition shows fewer hot flashes and night sweats than in meat eaters as well as a significant reduction in vasomotor symptoms with just a half cup of soybeans or edamame a day. In addition to weight loss, other advantages of a vegetarian diet include lower blood pressure and lower risk of diabetes and heart disease (see chapter 2).

Dr. Neal Barnard, an expert on vegetarian and vegan nutrition, founded the Physicians' Committee for Responsible Medicine (PCRM). PCRM has a free starter kit for vegetarian meals at www.PCRM.org/kickstart. In addition to this free resource, there are books, tapes, and materials for cooking and eating out and planning healthy meals. You may also find information from Dr. Barnard on YouTube.

Benefits of a vegetarian or vegan nutrition program include the following:

- Associated with excellent health, including a lower risk of bowel or colon cancer
- Associated with living longer, especially when partnered with regular exercise
- Helps you get better nutrients and feel full
- Produces healthy food for more individuals at a lower cost with less pollution and waste
- Lowers the risk of bowel/colon and breast cancer and other types of cancer[7]
- Lowers the risk of heart attack and stroke
- Promotes digestion and satiety that allows individuals to feel full longer on fewer calories
- Reverses existing heart disease

INTERMITTENT FASTING OPTIONS

- Alternate-day fasting diets are becoming popular. Here is one way it works: On the fast day, you eat 500 calories throughout the day. The next day is a feast day where you eat with no restrictions on the type or quantity of food. After six months, postmenopausal women lost twice as much weight as premenopausal women. Valuable information about intermittent fasting.
- Bone mineral density is not weakened by intermittent fasting.
- Postmenopausal women lost one-fifth of their body weight over six months.

- Postmenopausal women stuck to the fasting protocol more closely.
- Premenopausal women lost 5 percent of their body weight over six months.[8]

KEEPING A FOOD JOURNAL FOR WEIGHT LOSS

If you are on a budget or not ready to set aside the time or devote the effort to a formal program, you can use this simple, low-cost option: Keep a food diary. Record everything you eat, just before or after you eat it, on a piece of paper, your computer, or a handheld device. Merely recording your food intake makes you more conscious of what you are eating, how much, when, and where. Understanding the circumstances of when and where you eat will assist you in identifying the issues you want to address. Consider Marina's story.

> **DID YOU KNOW?**
> Studies show that recording food intake changes eating habits even if you do not consciously commit to changing them.

Marina's Story
REASONABLE FOOD IN UNREASONABLE PORTIONS

I have always made healthy eating choices, and I am quite knowledgeable about nutrition. I bake or grill chicken breasts without the skin, I buy whole-wheat bread and brown rice, and I often have fresh fruit for dessert. But I was brought up to clean my plate. Although my choices were usually healthy, my portion sizes were supersized. When I ate whole-wheat pasta, I would serve myself as much as I wanted. I knew that it was healthier than white pasta and did not force myself to gauge the serving size. Even though I walk one mile with a coworker twice a week during lunch, my waist size has gradually expanded to 38 inches, and I weigh 45 pounds more than I did in high school. I thought it might be my age (59) and just an inevitable part of meno-

pause. My doctor suggested I consider several options. They took extra time to explain the negative health consequences of the excess weight I was carrying. One option was to begin a program that includes guidelines for portion sizes. Examples include the South Beach diet, Sonoma diet, Weight Watchers, or NOOM. Another option was to eat more low-fat vegetarian meals with larger portions of less calorie dense foods.

A third option was to master healthy portion sizes on my own, measure them out, and record them in a food journal. For example, if I choose to have frozen yogurt, and a regular portion of that brand is one-half of a cup, I would measure out the half cup for my serving. If I choose to have two servings, I would measure out the second half cup. Doing that would show me I was eating a second serving. Writing down the amounts and types of foods that I eat makes me more accountable to myself.

WHAT IF I REFUSE TO DIET OR TRACK MY EATING?

Not everyone finds tracking or logging food and exercise feasible at a given time. For a different approach, consider reading *The Hunger Habit: Why We Eat When We're Not Hungry and How to Stop*. The author, Judson Brewer, MD, PhD, is a psychiatrist and neuroscientist who has done extensive research in addiction medicine. Dr. Brewer developed a tool to provide individuals with insights into their approach to eating. It is a fascinating read and an excellent adjunct to any nutrition program you choose, as well as a stand-alone resource.

CANNOT LOSE WEIGHT?

At times, you can be making your best effort to develop a healthy pattern of nutrition and exercise yet not see results. In perimenopause, this may be due to hormonal shifts affecting serotonin and sleep. It could also be due to disparate estrogen levels, the full effects of which are still not understood. Other medical conditions undermine weight loss efforts. Identifying and addressing these conditions may remove these barriers.

MEDICAL SABOTEURS

Here are a few medical conditions that can slow or prevent weight loss.

- *Thyroid disease*
  Thyroid disease may prevent weight loss despite an individual's best efforts. An underactive thyroid will slow your metabolism, preventing you from being able to burn calories at a normal rate. Correcting the thyroid imbalance with treatment will enable weight loss efforts to succeed, but it is not a rapid fix. In fact, it can take more than six to eight weeks to begin to see the difference. Although an overactive thyroid often burns more calories and leaves a woman lean, it can also stimulate appetite and promote unwanted weight gain.
- *Sleep problems*
  Sleep problems may promote obesity. Sleep apnea, insomnia, or other causes of an insufficient amount of sleep disturb the body's ability to judge satiety and control hunger and eating (see chapter 10 for more information).
- *Insulin resistance*
  Insulin resistance promotes obesity when the body does not respond normally to sugar.
- *Age*
  Age impacts weight loss associated with the natural loss of muscle mass over time Muscle burns more calories per minute than fat. Decreasing muscle mass with age decreases metabolism and calorie burn. Factor in age and activity when considering the amount of food required to be healthy and maintain normal energy levels.

- *Medications*
  Corticosteroids sabotage weight loss efforts and prompt the body to store extra fat. Some types of antidepressant medication, such as SSRIs (selective serotonin reuptake inhibitors), are also associated with unwanted weight gain.

NEW PATHS FORWARD FOR WEIGHT LOSS

Researchers are developing new medications to help with weight loss, glucose control, and insulin resistance. They are also devising new surgical techniques with lower risk and less recovery time.

Meanwhile, our understanding of attaining a healthy weight in midlife is slowly growing. One area of exploration and study is the gut microbiome. In chapter 7, I discussed the vaginal microbiome, including the types of bacteria that are supposed to live in the healthy vagina. The gut or intestines have their own microbiome or healthy population of bacteria that are supposed to live there. As researchers learn more about this population of bacteria in the gut, they also learn about how healthy gut bacteria help with digestion and maintaining a healthy weight. In a few cases, they have transferred healthy segments of the intestine containing normal healthy bacteria, placed them in a recipient with unhealthy intestinal bacteria, and found improvements in health and weight control in the recipient. Equol, an active metabolite of soy isoflavone, is a weak plant estrogen. Equol has the potential to prevent hyperglycemia, elevated lipids, obesity, and metabolic syndrome. Equol production in Japanese women is associated with less prevalence of metabolic syndrome in women ages 50–69 in a large Japanese study. The gut bacteria in some women can convert daidzcin in food to Equol. Expect more information to emerge showing how the gut bacteria play a role in the health and weight control of women in peri- and post menopause.

ASSESSING YOUR PROGRESS

Like other aspects of menopausal health, reassess your nutrition and activity patterns at least once every year. Reevaluate them sooner if your schedule changes, you lack energy to do the things you enjoy, or you have a change in your health status such as trouble with your hip, knee, or ankle that forces a change in your routine. Nutrition and activity choices impact your health significantly during menopause. Wise choices will enhance the health of your heart and your bones and add to your general sense of well-being in addition to helping you achieve or maintain a healthy body size.

In some cases, an exercise stress test will be part of an assessment of your general fitness level and cardiac health. If your doctor does not think you need one based on your medical history and exam, there are other fitness goals. If you walk 10,000 steps each day, as measured by a pedometer, you are likely to be healthy and/or physically active enough to maintain your health, but you would still need to add balance, flexibility, and a weight-bearing component.

Other guides to signal physical health include your stamina and energy level. Do you have the stamina and physical energy to do the things you enjoy on a regular basis? Does your exercise or activity pattern match your schedule? Does it meet your social preferences or needs? Have you changed from a solitary exerciser who works out or walks on her own to someone who enjoys a class or a walking companion more?

Are your exercise expectations too rigorous? Are you demanding so much of yourself that you throw up your hands in defeat? For example, do you tell yourself that you either work out at the gym every day after work or not at all? Do you have alternatives that you enjoy if the weather foils Plan A for your activity that day? Regular tweaking and a set of Plan B alternatives can save you. Also, keep in mind the variety of activities that provide benefit. If you do not feel like walking or getting on a treadmill, stepper, or elliptical machine, you may be in the mood for doing yoga or tai chi. You may feel like lifting free weights in front of the television or while you play your favorite music.

You can change the social context if you develop a preference for social versus solitary exercise. This may also change with your growing fitness level. If you are sedentary, you may begin by walking five minutes a day or climbing one minute of stairs one to three times a day. Later in your fitness journey, as you gain stamina and increase your level of fitness, you may enjoy walking or exercising with others, or you may welcome the challenge of a 5K charity walk or other sports challenge.

If your schedule becomes more demanding, you may need to change the timing or location of your activities.

The savvy way to promote physical fitness and good nutrition is to consume nutritionally healthy foods and have an active lifestyle and move frequently. As anyone who has reached the second half of her life knows, healthy eating has its rewards. One patient summed it up for me when she said, after losing 30 pounds, "I used to live to eat. Now I eat to live."

IMPORTANT TAKEAWAYS

- All women need these four types of exercise: stretching, strengthening, aerobic/cardiovascular, and balancing.
- Diabetes mellitus and metabolic syndrome both drastically increase your risk of heart disease and stroke.
- Diet is critical. Consuming more calories than the amount of energy you expend will cause weight gain even if you only overestimate your calorie needs by a modest amount.
- Exercising before, during, and after menopause lowers your risk of breast cancer, osteoporosis, obesity, diabetes, and heart disease.
- If you have tried to lose weight and cannot, it is important to talk to your doctor about whether a medical condition could be the cause.

- There are many diets to consider, and a thoughtful approach is what will help you be successful in the short and long term.

QUESTIONS FOR YOUR DOCTOR

1. Am I at risk for developing diabetes mellitus or metabolic syndrome? If so, what can I do to reduce that risk?
2. Do you have any advice on how I can get more exercise?
3. How fit should I be, and what can I do to assess my level of fitness?
4. I would like to follow a healthier diet. What would you recommend?
5. I have tried to lose weight and am having trouble. Could something else be going on?
6. Am I a candidate for weight loss surgery?
7. Am I a candidate for weight loss medication?

RESOURCES

www.GaplesInstitute.org—The Gaples Institute is an educational nonprofit with courses for clinicians and the general public as well as a general lifestyle library.

www.pcna.net—Preventive Cardiovascular Nurses Association has videos, patient resources, and patient tools and handouts.

www.pcrm.org/kickstart—provides resources on vegetarian and vegan options, including recipes, restaurant options, and updated research studies on the benefits of vegetable-based eating.

Weight Watchers (www.weightwatchers.com). This program may be followed with in-person meetings, including a meeting leader and now a personal coach. The program may also be done entirely online. There are different versions of the program. Some options require tracking eating and exercise, and others have minimal tracking. You may choose to eat more carbohydrates or more protein or follow a vegan or vegetarian approach.

APPS

- My Fitness Pal
- Lose It!
- NOOM
- Weight Watchers

BOOKS

Barnard N. *Cookbook for Reversing Diabetes.* Rodale Books; 2018.

Barnard N. *The Vegan Starter Kit: Everything You Need to Know About Plant-Based Eating.* Grand Central Publishing; 2018.

Barnard N. *Your Body in Balance: The New Science of Food, Hormones and Health.* Balance Publishing; 2020.

Brewer J. *The Hunger Habit: Why We Eat When We're Not Hungry and How to Stop.* Avery Penguin Random House Publishing; 2024.

Katzen M, Willett W. *Eat, Drink, and Weigh Less: A Flexible and Delicious Way to Shrink Your Waist Without Going Hungry.* Hyperion; 2006. Walter Willett is the most quoted published nutritionist. He and his coauthors offer practical advice that is easy to implement.

LeBrasseur NK, Chen C. *Mayo Clinic on Healthy Aging.* Mayo Clinic Press; 2024.

Lyon G. *Forever Strong. A New, Science-Based Strategy for Aging Well.* Atria Books; 2023.

Nelson M, with Wernick S. *Strong Women Stay Slim.* Bantam Books; 1998.

Sowa, A. *The Ozempic Revolution.* Harper Collins. 2025

Wansink B. *Mindless Eating: Why We Eat More Than We Think.* Bantam Books; 2006.

CHAPTER 13

CURBING YOUR RISK OF CANCER

When it comes to cancer, there are ways to lower your risk, and some of them may surprise you.

CANCER IS MORE PREVALENT NOW than ever before. Why? Women are living longer, and many cancers become more common with age. While you have more opportunities to detect and prevent cancer today than your mother or grandmother did, information about preventive steps can be confusing and overwhelming.

In this chapter, I will answer these questions:

- How does your individual and family risk profile affect whether you might develop cancer of the breast, cervix, ovary, and uterus?
- What tests do doctors use to detect and diagnose various types of cancers?
- How can you reduce your risk of developing cancer? What are some lifestyle choices and other strategies to consider?

CANCER RISK: IT CHANGES OVER TIME

Modifying your lifestyle to lower your risk of cancer improves your chances of remaining cancer-free. However, it does not guarantee you will never be diagnosed with cancer. Each woman's strategy to improve their health and reduce their risk of developing cancer is unique, and it depends on their updated family and personal histories as well as new and emerging research available for each specific type of cancer.

EARLY DETECTION FOR CANCER

Some women are surprised to hear that early detection is not yet available for all types of cancer. For example, there is still no reliable way to detect early ovarian cancer. Pelvic exams, blood tests, and pelvic ultrasounds cannot reliably diagnose it. Typically, ovarian cancer is identified after it has already spread beyond the ovary. However, genetic testing using saliva or blood can help determine whether you have a higher risk of developing ovarian cancer. If you do have a higher risk, there are options to lower your risk that we will review later in this chapter. However, other types of cancer are more easily detected. Let's dive more deeply into these four types of cancer and what you need to know:

1. Breast
2. Cervix
3. Ovary
4. Uterus

BREAST CANCER

Globally, and in the United States, breast cancer is the most commonly diagnosed cancer. In the United States, breast cancer is the second most common cause of death for women after heart disease. One out of every eight women will develop breast cancer in their lifetime, but your specific risk for developing it depends on your age. Here is an estimate of the risk of developing breast cancer for American women over a lifetime based on a study of thousands of Americans[1]:

- Birth to age 49:   2.1 percent (1 in 49 women)
- Age 50–59:   2.4 percent (1 in 42 women)
- Age 60–69:   3.5 percent (1 in 28 women)
- Age 70:   7 percent (1 in 14 women)

> **DID YOU KNOW?**
> Nine out of 10 women who get breast cancer do not have a family history of breast cancer or high-risk genes.

Regardless of whether you have a personal or family history of breast cancer, certain risk factors increase or decrease your risk. Once you are aware of these risk factors, you can decide whether to act. Some of these risk factors are potentially modifiable with lifestyle choices while others are not.

Risk Factors for Developing Breast Cancer

As with many types of cancer, there are two types of risk factors: those you can potentially change and those you can't.

Potentially Modifiable Risk Factors

Consider the following potentially modifiable risk factors to determine whether any of them apply to you:

1. Absence of full-term delivery

   Women who never delivered a full-term child have a higher risk of breast cancer. That's because there has been no break in high estrogen levels due to pregnancy.

2. Alcohol consumption

   Any woman who consistently drinks more than one beer, one mixed drink, or one glass of wine in 24 hours increases her risk of breast cancer. More specifically, if you consume 10 grams of alcohol a day consistently over time, your risk of breast cancer increases by 10 percent. Why? Processing alcohol raises estrogen levels. Even three to six drinks a week will increase your risk of breast cancer.[2,3]

3. Androgen levels

   High levels of male hormone increase your risk of breast cancer. Taking male hormone without careful monitoring may produce higher male hormone levels than a woman will normally have on her own. This will increase her risk of getting breast cancer. One reason some women take male hormone is to boost their sex drive. For more information about the pros and cons of this approach, see chapter 3 and chapter 7.

4. Diet

    A Mediterranean diet with abundant vegetables, fruit, and fish with some olive oil lowers the risk of breast cancer. Eating less animal fat lowers the risk of breast cancer, as does a vegetarian diet.[4]

5. Hormone replacement therapy

    Although estrogen alone may reduce breast cancer risk during the first five years of taking the hormone, taking estrogen and progesterone hormone replacement therapy in post menopause may increase breast density (and cancer risk) after that time. See chapter 3 for more information.

6. Older age at the time of first full-term delivery

    You have a 5 percent higher risk of breast cancer if you deliver your first child after the age of 35. Interestingly, breastfeeding for 12 months lowers your risk of breast cancer regardless of age. That's because it decreases the duration of estrogen exposure and lowers your lifetime exposure to estrogen.

7. Radiation exposure to the chest

    Radiation to the chest increases your risk of breast cancer, especially when it occurs during the teenage years (for example to treat Hodgkin's lymphoma).

8. Sedentary lifestyle

    Inactivity increases breast cancer risk even if you have a normal body mass index (BMI). This is especially true for postmenopausal women who have an innately higher risk of breast cancer.

9. Smoking

    Smoking cigarettes increases the risk of breast cancer.

10. Weight

Postmenopausal women who are overweight have a higher risk of breast cancer. More specifically, for every 5 kg (11 pounds) of weight gained during post menopause, the risk of breast cancer increases. Why? Precursors of estrogen stored in women's fat deposits (adipose tissue) convert to a weaker but active estrogen. As those fat deposits increase with weight, so does estrogen. This estrogen (estrone) then circulates in the blood and increases the risk of breast cancer.

> **DID YOU KNOW?**
> Excess body fat increases your risk of breast cancer, even if your BMI is normal and you are not overweight.

Nonmodifiable Risk Factors

Consider the following nonmodifiable risk factors to determine whether any are relevant. If they are, be sure to talk to your doctor about how you can lower your risk using the strategies discussed in this chapter.

1. Age

    Your risk of developing breast cancer increases as you age.

2. Dense breast tissue that occupies 75 percent or more of the breast

    Dense breast tissue contains glands and connective tissue. The remainder of breast tissue is fat. Having heterogeneously dense breasts (i.e., breasts with a higher percentage of glandular and supportive tissue than fat) is not as risky unless the dense breast tissue occupies 75 percent or more of the breast. If this is the case, your risk of breast cancer increases by four to five times. Physical activity is associated with lower breast density and lower risk of breast cancer. I have not seen a study that proves causation, but hopefully those studies will be in the works. Dense breast tissue contains more gland tissue. Gland tissue is where breast cancer is likely to occur. Further, denser breast tissue is white, and early cancers often appear white on a mammogram and are harder to detect early with more dense breast tissue.

3. Early menarche

If you had your first menstrual period before age 13, your risk of developing breast cancer increases. That is because estrogen has circulated throughout your body for longer compared to most women.

4. Family history and genetics

Consider the following:
- If you have one first-degree relative with breast cancer (i.e., your mother or sister), you have twice the risk of developing breast cancer yourself.
- If you have two first-degree relatives with breast cancer, you have three times the risk of developing breast cancer.
- If your first-degree relative (i.e., mother or sister) was diagnosed with breast cancer under age 30, you have three times the risk of developing breast cancer.
- If your first-degree relative was diagnosed over age 60, you have one-and-a-half times the risk of developing breast cancer.
- If you have a male relative with breast cancer, you are at an extremely elevated risk for developing breast cancer. That is because male breast cancer is rare and due to a genetic mutation that is an inheritable risk. Female relatives of a male patient with breast cancer are strongly advised to get genetic testing.

5. Height
    Women who are five foot nine and taller have a higher risk of breast cancer, although the reason is unknown.
6. Personal history of atypia, personal history of benign breast disease, or personal history of breast biopsy
    Each of these increases the risk of developing breast cancer.
7. Sex
    Women are at higher risk of developing breast cancer than men.

If you have one or more nonmodifiable risk factors for breast cancer, you do have an opportunity to focus on the lifestyle modifications I will review shortly to lower your risk of breast cancer.

Lifestyle Choices That Do Not Increase Your Risk of Breast Cancer
Contrary to widespread belief, several lifestyle choices do not increase your risk of breast cancer. These include the following:

- Caffeine consumption
- Cosmetic breast implants
- COVID-19 vaccine (Note: The vaccine may cause women to have swollen lymph nodes in their armpits for up to six weeks. As a result, consider delaying routine screening mammogram for six weeks after second vaccine.)
- Deodorant (Note: Deodorant in the armpit may show up on mammograms, so it's important to wipe it off before having a mammogram.)
- Electric blankets
- Hair dye
- History of pregnancy termination or abortion
- In vitro fertilization

Symptoms of Breast Cancer
Breast cancer is usually painless, and you may not feel a lump until it is advanced. Having said that, if you have nipple discharge, especially blood nipple discharge, or new skin changes on your breast, these findings should be evaluated promptly.

Screening for Breast Cancer

Breast cancer screening is critical for all women, regardless of their risk factors. There are many options available for screening. Your doctor can advise you on which one is best for you.

Digital Mammogram

Until recently, digital mammogram was the standard for breast cancer screening in women without a personal or family history of breast cancer. Why? The detection rate was good, and the amount of radiation to which each woman was exposed was low. However, the density of your breasts may limit the effectiveness of a digital mammogram.

> **DID YOU KNOW?**
> Ten percent of women have extremely dense breasts. For these women, traditional mammogram only detects breast cancer 60 percent of the time. On the other hand, 40 percent of women have heterogeneously dense breasts. For these women, digital mammogram finds 75 percent of breast cancers. Tomo mammo (3D mammo) increases the cancer detection rate in women with heterogeneously dense breasts.

The degree of breast tissue density refers to the prevalence of fibroglandular tissue versus fat when viewed on a mammogram. Fat shows up as black or dark gray, and fibroglandular tissue shows up as white. The white can hide cancers. Also, cancer is most likely to develop in glandular breast tissue, not fatty breast tissue.

> **DID YOU KNOW?**
> Dense breast tissue is the most common risk factor for breast cancer. It is responsible for more breast cancer diagnoses than a positive family history or inheriting a mutation or high-risk gene for breast cancer. Individuals with extremely dense breast tissue have a risk of breast cancer that is as high as

a history of a previous breast biopsy showing atypical cells. Researchers are working on innovative technology to detect breast cancer in women with dense breasts. For now, consider modifying your lifestyle to lower your risk of breast cancer and consider getting an ultrasound or MRI (magnetic resonance imaging) along with your regular mammogram.

A radiologist interprets your mammogram to determine your breast density. Breast density is not related to breast size or shape. A digital mammogram's ability to detect breast cancer improves when breasts include more fatty tissue and less dense tissue. With digital mammograms, the number of false positives or false alarms (i.e., incorrectly telling a woman she has breast cancer when she does not) is not high, and the number of false negatives or missed cancers (i.e., telling a woman she has no breast cancer when she really has it) is low unless the individual has a lot of dense breast tissue.[5]

3D Mammogram

Now that clinicians and researchers have established the importance of breast density in interpreting mammograms, the tomosynthesis (3D) mammogram has become the new standard for breast cancer screening, especially for individuals with heterogeneously dense breast tissue. With a 3D mammogram, radiologists can view extra images and view the breast tissue in three dimensions, providing greater insight into potential breast cancer that may be present. The 3D mammograms lower the risk of being called back for additional images. They also increase cancer detection in all women except those with extremely dense breasts.

Radiology departments have made adjustments so that a 3D mammogram does not use more radiation than a digital mammogram.

Thermogram

A thermogram is a test that uses an infrared camera to detect heat patterns and blood flow in body tissues. However, it is not useful as a screening or diagnostic test. It has a worse track record for finding cancers than a 2D mammogram. Even though there is no radiation, there are also no helpful results. It is too unreliable. Consider Taneeka's story.

Taneeka's Story
THERMOGRAM VERSUS MAMMOGRAM

I am a healthy 40-year-old woman. I asked my doctor for a thermogram. A friend told me that the thermogram uses heat and no radiation. Since I have no family history of breast cancer, and I want to avoid radiation, I prefer to have a thermogram. My doctor did not agree. They told me that a thermogram imaging study will not reliably detect breast cancer and that a mammogram is a better option because it finds 80 percent of breast cancers that are present.

I got another opinion and had a thermogram on my own. The next year, I went back to my original doctor. I felt a lump. It turned out to be a benign cyst, but after that I decided to pursue mammograms instead.

Breast Ultrasound

Ultrasound is an important diagnostic tool for detecting breast cancer. If your doctor identifies a palpable lump, or a radiologist sees an abnormal area on your mammogram, a breast ultrasound can provide additional clues. More specifically, it can help your doctor look more closely at the area of overlapping tissue or density and image the palpable lump to learn more about its features (i.e., whether the lump is cystic or solid).

The ultrasound uses sound waves to image breast tissue. It is an excellent adjunct to mammogram screening, but it is not a good screening tool on its own. It is not designed to find cancer when there is no lump on exam or specific mammogram finding. Breast ultrasound used with a mammogram is also better at finding certain types of breast cancer such as lobular cancer. A breast ultrasound can also help determine whether a breast biopsy is appropriate.

BREAST MAGNETIC RESONANCE IMAGING (MRI)

Breast MRI uses magnetic energy (not radiation) to image the breasts, and it can be an important test for women with a high-risk profile because it increases the chances of finding breast cancer early in women with a high risk history. Here is the flip side: as a very sensitive test, breast MRI can also produce false positives if you are not considered at elevated risk (e.g., if you do not have a personal or family history of breast cancer). If you have an elevated risk of developing breast cancer, you may be advised to have a breast MRI regardless of your breast density. However, you should also have a mammogram either at the same time or annually, unless you are under age 30. High-risk women under age 30 may have breast MRI annually to detect early breast cancers until an annual mammogram is added to their screening regimen at age 30. Consider Leona's story.

Leona's Story
A 34-YEAR-OLD WOMAN WITH A HIGH-RISK FAMILY HISTORY OF BREAST CANCER

My mother died at age 40 from breast cancer. I had genetic testing, and I have the BRCA2 cancer gene. My doctor told me to start having mammograms at age 35, which is five years before my mother was diagnosed. The doctor also advised me to have a breast MRI every 12 months. I am planning to do a mammogram once a year and a breast MRI once a year. I'm also following the recommendation to have a breast exam with my doctor every six months. In my case, the sensitivity of the MRI is an advantage because my baseline risk of breast cancer is higher than that of my friends, and the MRI is less likely to miss an early breast cancer.

Breast Cancer and the COVID-19 Vaccine

The COVID-19 vaccine does not increase your risk of breast cancer. However, it can cause swelling of the lymph nodes in the axilla (armpit) for as long as six to eight weeks. These changes can mimic the appearance of cancer. In some cases, your doctor may recommend postponing a routine screening mammogram for two months after you get a COVID vaccine to minimize false alarms. However, if you need a diagnostic study due to a lump in your breast or abnormal finding on a mammogram, this follow-up study should not be delayed. Consider Rihanna's story.

Rihanna's Story
BREAST LUMP FOLLOWING A COVID-19 VACCINE

I am a 50-year-old woman who gained 15 pounds in perimenopause during the pandemic. I have also become sedentary while working from home for the past two years. After I received my second COVID-19 vaccine, I waited six weeks and then went for my overdue screening mammogram. Three weeks later, I noticed a breast lump. I had read that the vaccine could cause breast lumps. Since my mammogram was negative and reassuring, I was not worried. When the lump was still there after another two months, I saw my doctor. The doctor was concerned and told me that a persistent lump needs to be evaluated.

I had a biopsy that showed early breast cancer. The cancerous lump was surgically removed, and then I had radiation. My doctors say my risk of recurrence is low and that I have a complete cure. I told the doctor I thought my lump was from the COVID-19 vaccine. My doctor told me the lumps from the vaccine are usually enlarged lymph nodes in the armpit and last about six weeks. I am glad I did not wait longer. If I had waited, the outcome might have been very different.

Breast Cancer and Family History

As stated earlier in this chapter, family history can profoundly affect your risk of breast cancer. It is important to understand your screening options and talk with your doctor about which options are best for you based on your unique circumstances. Consider Sasha's story.

Sasha's Story
A 40-YEAR-OLD WOMAN WITH NO FAMILY HISTORY OF BREAST CANCER

I am a healthy 40-year-old, although I am thirty pounds overweight. I have a glass of wine three times a week and walk my dog daily. I do not have a family history of breast cancer. My first child was born when I was 35 years old. My doctor said the birth of my first child after age 30 is a risk factor for breast cancer, as is my being overweight.

A 3D mammogram showed I have extremely dense breasts, and the report states the results are less accurate. I started to worry. My doctor reaffirmed that extremely dense breasts make it more challenging to identify an early breast cancer because the dense tissue can hide an early cancer. I thought having a 3D mammogram would eliminate that concern; however, for extremely dense breasts like mine, even a 3D mammogram is not as helpful. There was an area on the 3D mammogram that was even more dense than the surrounding area. It wasn't clear if it was overlapping tissue or a worrisome new finding. My doctor spoke to the radiologist, and they agreed I should have a breast ultrasound to look at the area of concern. The breast ultrasound did not show anything worrisome.

Two months later, my older sister was diagnosed with breast cancer. I called my doctor, and she said I should have a breast MRI because my new family history puts me at higher risk. My MRI showed I had early breast cancer that was so tiny that the 3D mammogram and breast ultrasound could not identify it. My sister's doctor and my doctor each advised us to have genetic testing. The testing shows we both have the PTEN gene for a higher risk of breast cancer. Our mother has no siblings, but our father's sister had breast cancer. We rarely see her and forgot to mention her in our family history. I am relieved that my cancer was caught early, and expect a good outcome.

MRI is not always a good screening test because it is so sensitive. There are many false alarms or false-positive signs of breast cancer in the general population when no risk factors are identified. Studies are underway to develop new screening options for women. However, a breast MRI is a useful tool for individuals who have an elevated risk of breast cancer in the family or who have inherited a gene or mutation for breast cancer. Consider Sage's story.

Sage's Story
A 35-YEAR-OLD WOMAN WHOSE MOTHER DIED AT AGE 40 OF BREAST CANCER

My mother died of breast cancer at age 40 after she was diagnosed at age 35. I had genetic testing and was found to have the BRCA2 gene. My doctor said I should start having mammograms at age 30. My doctor also recommended I have a breast MRI every 12 months starting at age 25. I have an MRI once a year and a mammogram once a year. I also have a clinical breast exam every six months—once with my gynecologist and once with my internal medicine doctor. For me, the extra sensitivity of the MRI is a plus because my baseline risk of breast cancer is higher than other women, and the MRI is less likely to miss an early breast cancer.

Breast Cancer and Genetic Testing

If you have a family history of breast cancer, consider having medical genetic testing and speaking to a trained genetic counselor. The genetic counselor can help you decide whether testing is right for you. They can also assist you in getting the tests covered by insurance and help you to consider the implications of potential results for you and your other family members, including any children you may have.

> **DID YOU KNOW?**
>
> Direct-to-consumer labs typically do not check for all the genes that are currently associated with breast cancer. For example, if the direct-to-consumer testing only checks for BRCA1 and BRCA2 (as is common), you may be falsely reassured that you do not carry a high-risk gene for breast cancer. In this case, you may miss the chance to have additional screening tests that would allow your doctor to identify your cancer early. In addition, if you are unaware of your true genetic risk of developing breast cancer, you may not choose lifestyle measures to lower the risk.

Sometimes a patient mentions that she does not want genetic testing because she would not act on the information. This is understandable if she thinks that testing positive for a breast cancer gene means she will be advised to have a double mastectomy. In practice, genetic testing helps doctors recommend the best testing or screening to increase your chances of finding the cancer early before it spreads. Mastectomy is not the most common outcome of a positive test for a breast cancer gene. However, if your risk of breast cancer is extremely high based on a genetic mutation found on genetic testing or your breast cancer risk is high based on your personal and family histories (or both), a mastectomy and reconstruction may serve you best.

For example, if you have an inherited gene for breast cancer such as PTEN, p53, STK11, CDH1, PALB2, BRCA1, or BRCA2, you may be better served by getting a 3D mammogram once a year, a breast MRI once a year, and a clinical breast exam twice a year. Some of my patients have one breast exam with their gynecologist and one with their internist six months apart. This higher genetic risk of breast cancer would also inform your choices for contraception and hormone replacement during pre-, peri-, and post menopause. Consider Andrea's story.

Andrea's Story
A 45-YEAR-OLD WOMAN WITH A PATERNAL UNCLE WHO HAS MALE BREAST CANCER

I am 45 years old, and my paternal uncle had breast cancer. When I told my gynecologist, they said this is a red flag and that I may have a high-risk gene for breast cancer. Ideally, my uncle should undergo genetic testing as soon as possible. If he tests positive for a genetic mutation, then I should get genetic testing as well. I asked my doctor about the benefits of genetic testing. They said the testing results would allow them to customize my breast cancer screening schedule and include an annual breast MRI. It would also help them determine whether it made sense to offer me medication like tamoxifen or raloxifen. Taking one of these medications could lower my risk of getting breast cancer by 50 percent. I also asked my doctor about breast cancer modeling that could help estimate my personal risk of breast cancer. They explained we could use one or more of the models, but each model has limitations. For example, the Gail model does not include breast density in its predictions. Other models do not include family history or personal history of breast cancer in their risk calculations. They directed me to the website www.densebreast-info.org for more information about the different models to predict the risk of breast cancer. My uncle will be undergoing the genetic tests, as advised, and we will take the next steps after we get his results.

PREPARING FOR YOUR DOCTOR'S APPOINTMENT

Before your appointment, bringing the following information is often helpful:

- Detailed account of your family history, including whether your mother or sister(s) have or had breast cancer and the age of diagnosis. It also includes whether any grandparents, aunts, or male relatives had or have breast cancer and

the age of diagnosis. Do not include aunts or uncles by marriage. Do not include stepparents or step-grandparents. Your risk is based on blood relatives.
- Follow-up studies from any abnormal mammograms
- Pathology results for any breast biopsies you have had
- Prior abnormal mammogram reports, including any reports from previous facilities. Also, obtain the technical mammogram report that includes details about breast density and other specifics.

QUESTIONS TO ASK YOUR DOCTOR

1. Given my family history of breast cancer and my personal history, what are your recommendations for breast cancer screening and lifestyle modifications?
2. Should I pursue genetic testing? You will benefit from consulting a genetic counselor on this one. You may learn that if you have a living relative with breast cancer, especially if it is a mother or sister, it is helpful to have that relative get genetic testing if they are willing to do so. If the test reveals they do not have any of the many genes for inherited breast cancer, this means they may simply have a random mutation and you may not need genetic testing. The genetic counselor can advise you. If your close relative is positive for a high-risk gene for breast cancer, they may advise you to get genetic testing to see if you have the same gene. The results of your genetic testing will influence your personal screening and testing advice. It also has implications for your children's breast cancer risk.
3. Is it helpful to consider breast cancer modeling? In addition to preparing your personal medical history and family history to review with your doctor, your doctor may offer to estimate your risk of breast cancer with a model. These models try to predict your individual risk of developing breast cancer. Examples of these types of models are the

Gail model and the Tyler-Cusick model. Your doctor will advise whether these models might be helpful for you.[5]

You have an opportunity to lower your risk of breast cancer by avoiding weight gain, a sedentary lifestyle, excess alcohol consumption, and cigarettes. You may use the information here about types of breast cancer screening, including digital mammogram, 3D mammogram, and breast MRI for higher-risk women to start a discussion with your doctors. Consider reviewing the questions to ask your doctor about assessing your risk for breast cancer based on your personal medical history, breast density on mammogram, lifestyle, and family history.

Next, I will discuss uterine cancer, where the options for detection are not well established.

UTERINE CANCER

Uterine cancer rates are rising—more women have been diagnosed with uterine cancer every year since 2010. This is problematic for women and their doctors because there is no screening test for uterine cancer!

WHAT ARE THE TYPES OF UTERINE CANCER AND WHY DO THEY MATTER?

Uterine cancers can start in the muscle wall or the endometrium (uterine lining). Cancers of the endometrium are the most common. The most common type of endometrial cancer is endometrioid cancer, a type where the endometrium or lining cells become cancerous. This type of uterine cancer has an excellent survival rate when diagnosed in its early stages. It is referred to as type 1 endometrial cancer. Type 2 endometrial cancers are more aggressive and difficult to diagnose early. Researchers recently demonstrated that type 2 endometrial cancers are more common in Black women. Better tests are needed to find and treat these cancers early.

Typically, endometrial cancer is detected in an individual who has postmenopausal bleeding. The bleeding episode does not have to be heavy, painful, or long. Even a short episode of scant bleeding may represent endometrial cancer. To evaluate postmenopausal bleeding, a pelvic ultrasound is usually done to measure the thickness of the uterus lining (endometrial thickness). However, the pelvic ultrasound alone is not enough to diagnose uterine cancer. An endometrial thickness of 4 millimeters (about 0.16 in) or greater may be a sign that there could be endometrial cancer, and a hysteroscopy (microscope exam of the uterus lining) and biopsies are advised. If an individual has two episodes of postmenopausal bleeding, the hysteroscopy and biopsies are advised regardless of the ultrasound findings.

> DID YOU KNOW?
> Endometrial cancer is harder to identify in perimenopause.

In perimenopause, signs of endometrial cancer vary from irregular bleeding, heavy bleeding, or both to fewer than five bleeding episodes a year—each pattern may signify endometrial cancer. Not only are the signs of endometrial cancer more varied and confusing in perimenopause, but testing is less helpful. The ultrasound test used in postmenopausal bleeding is not as helpful in perimenopause.

For type 2, more aggressive endometrial cancers, the lining does not reliably appear abnormal or thick on ultrasound. This makes type 2 endometrial cancer harder to identify, even in post menopause. Researchers and clinicians have not yet determined how to identify these more aggressive endometrial cancers in the early stages. Currently, there are no formal clinical guidelines for diagnosing type 2 endometrial cancer. Since type 2 endometrial cancer affects Black women disproportionately, consider requesting evaluation of any postmenopausal bleeding with a hysteroscopy and biopsies of the uterus lining as well as evaluation of heavy or prolonged or abnormal bleeding in perimenopause, even if it is long-standing.[12]

Uterine cancer can be hereditary, but in most cases, it is not. While some inherited genes increase the risk of uterine cancer, lifestyle choices are a substantial influence. The rate of uterine cancer has been rising every year for all groups of women since 2010. One reason for the increasing rate of uterine cancer in the past decade is the increasing rate of obesity and the number of overweight individuals. In the past few years, researchers have reanalyzed data through the lens of ethnicity and found that Black women/women of African descent have a higher risk of dying from endometrial cancer. Black women are less likely to be diagnosed with early-stage endometrial cancer and more commonly have higher-risk, more aggressive types of uterine cancer. The survival rate for Black women is lower. One contribution to the lower survival rate is that features of these more aggressive uterine cancers are not usually identified on ultrasounds.[13]

DID YOU KNOW?
The most common sign of uterine cancer is postmenopausal bleeding.

In pre- or perimenopausal women, bleeding patterns are less specific and may include irregular bleeding with missed periods and three months or more of no bleeding between cycles. Alternatively, an individual may notice heavy or prolonged menstrual periods. Keeping a menstrual history is crucial and may enable you and your gynecologist to identify a uterine cancer or precancer earlier than if you are unclear about your bleeding patterns.

Symptoms of Uterine Cancer

Uterine cancer may be difficult to identify by symptoms alone, especially during perimenopause. During post menopause, any bleeding or spotting, whether it is heavy or light, brown, red, or pink, is a potential sign of uterine cancer. The evaluation of postmenopausal and perimenopausal bleeding is discussed in chapter 5. In perimenopause, symptoms alone will not indicate whether there is uterine cancer. In perimenopause, an ultrasound measurement of the uterus lining thickness is also not definitive. Further evaluation for uterine cancer is advised if menstrual cycles change and arrive more frequently by five days or more. For example, instead of a bleeding episode starting every 28 days, it changes to every 22 days. Or if menstrual flow is longer or heavier or spotting between menstrual periods, further evaluation is advised, including direct visualization of the uterus lining using a hysteroscope.[7]

Risk Factors for Developing Uterine Cancer

WHAT FACTORS INCREASE THE RISK FOR DEVELOPING UTERINE CANCER?

Sedentary and obese individuals are at risk. Both sedentary and obese women have more fatty tissue, or adipose tissue. The adipose tissue produces a greater amount of the weaker estrogen, estrone, outside of ovary-produced estrogen. As the number of individuals who are overweight or obese rises, so does the number of individuals who are diagnosed with uterine cancer.

> DID YOU KNOW?
>
> Currently, in the United States, 57 percent of all uterine cancers are related to obesity. Women with a normal body mass index (BMI) have a 3 percent lifetime risk of endometrial cancer. However, for every five-unit increase in BMI, the risk of uterine cancer increases by more than 50 percent.

In fact, doctors are now diagnosing young obese women with uterine cancer. In the past, the average age of diagnosis was 63 years. Sadly, data from SEER (Surveillance, Epidemiology and End Results) shows the number of endometrial cancer cases rising in women under age 50. The SEER database goes back to 1990 and allows researchers to look at trends in cancer diagnosis by age, ethnicity, and medical history.[6]

Another risk factor for uterine cancer involves conditions associated with excess estrogen such as polycystic ovary syndrome as well as women who are overweight or obese. Women who take estrogen without progesterone or take too little progesterone are at higher risk of developing uterine cancer.

DID YOU KNOW?
Uterine cancer is becoming more common and more lethal. Rates of uterine cancer are rising at an average of 1.3 percent each year.[6]

Tamoxifen, a medication given to lower the risk of breast cancer, can also increase the risk of uterine cancer. Tamoxifen blocks estrogen effects in the breast but promotes estrogen effects in the uterus. Tamoxifen doubles the risk of uterine cancer. When used for more than five years, it quadruples the risk of uterine cancer.

Individuals with diabetes or metabolic syndrome are at higher risk for endometrial cancer. Having said that, uterine cancer may be diagnosed in individuals with no risk factors. In these cases, women may have a random genetic mutation or a high-risk gene that has not yet been identified.

DID YOU KNOW?
Bearing a child lowers the risk of uterine cancer. And women who use oral contraceptives may lower their risk of uterine cancer by 30 to 40 percent.

Screening for Uterine Cancer

Unlike the Pap test to detect early cervical cancer and the mammogram to detect early breast cancer, there is no good screening test for uterine cancer. The diagnosis rests on taking a thorough medical history, including a detailed menstrual history, a family history, and specific testing of the uterus lining. The new standard of care is that thorough testing for uterus cancer involves a direct view of the uterine lining as well as getting biopsy samples. In the past, blind biopsies were done without looking directly inside the uterus lining with a microscope. Blind biopsies missed identifying many cancers. If the gynecologist takes a blind biopsy from the left side of the uterus lining and the cancer is developing on the right, it would not be diagnosed. Direct visualization with a hysteroscopy (slender microscope introduced into the uterine lining through the cervix) reduces the chances that the cancer will be missed by the biopsy. The hysteroscopy and biopsies may be done in the office or in the operating room.

Even trained gynecologists can miss the early signs of endometrial cancer. That is because the signs may be subtle, and many individuals do not report heavy bleeding or irregular bleeding when they have experienced these bleeding patterns for years or even decades. However, in peri- or post menopause, the significance of these bleeding patterns is concerning, and they are a red flag. If your doctor does not take a thorough menstrual history, bring your menstrual history to discuss with them. Consider Cerise's and Layla's stories.

Cerise's Story
A 49-YEAR-OLD WOMAN WITH HEAVY MENSTRUAL PERIODS

I have had heavy menstrual periods for decades and was advised to consider a hysterectomy after my third child was born. I typically soak a super tampon in less than an hour for one to two days a month. At my annual exam, I told my doctor I did not have any changes in my menstrual periods. However, a few weeks later, I rebled and noticed large blood clots the diameter of a 50-cent piece.

When I started to feel lightheaded, my partner took me to the emergency room. I smoke cigarettes, so they checked a blood ferritin level in addition to a regular blood count. The hematocrit was normal at 40, but the ferritin was only 3, showing my iron reserves were severely depleted.

The gynecologist on call ordered an ultrasound to image the uterus. They said my uterus felt large on pelvic exam. The ultrasound showed my uterus lining was irregular and thick in some places. The gynecologist advised a hysteroscopy with a biopsy of the uterus lining to check for cancer and precancer.

I am so used to the heavy menstrual periods that I was not concerned until the low iron reserves prompted me to follow the gynecologist's advice. The office hysteroscopy to check my uterus lining found precancer in a polyp. I was surprised. I have had heavy menstrual periods all my life! I thought it was normal! The gynecologist explained that heavy menstrual periods are common for women in their teens and twenties when menstrual cycles may still be irregular and not associated with monthly ovulation. After age 35, heavy menstrual bleeding may be associated with cancer or precancer of the uterus lining. After age 35, it is more common to find a structural or anatomic reason for the heavy bleeding, even in perimenopause. I had a choice of a hysterectomy or a progesterone-releasing intrauterine device (IUD) in the uterus with a repeat sampling of the uterus lining in six months. I chose the progesterone-releasing IUD, and now I have short, light menstrual periods. Repeat hysteroscopy and biopsy three months later showed the precancer did not recur and was removed with the polyp.

Layla's Story
A 41-YEAR-OLD WOMAN WITH IRREGULAR, INFREQUENT MENSTRUAL PERIODS IN PERIMENOPAUSE

Early menopause runs in my family. My older sister had her final menstrual period at age 45. So, I was not surprised when I started to skip menstrual periods at age 41. My partner had a vasectomy, so I was not concerned about an unplanned pregnancy. I also was not concerned when I bled every two months. I had read irregular menstrual periods are common in perimenopause. My sister is a nurse practitioner and told me 80 percent of women have irregular menstrual periods in perimenopause. What I did not learn from the internet or my older sister is that all irregular periods do not have the same significance. Some are more worrisome than others and may signify a precancer or cancer.

I began to skip four consecutive menstrual periods at a time. I thought I would have my final menstrual period earlier than my older sister. At my annual gyn exam, the clinician asked me about the frequency and duration of my menstrual periods. They had training in menopausal medicine and were concerned about my risk of endometrial hyperplasia, which can be a form of precancer of the uterus lining. They ordered an ultrasound that showed no fibroids. They remained concerned and recommended I have a hysteroscopy with an endometrial biopsy.

The hysteroscopy revealed the lining was thickened. During the hysteroscopy, they found a polyp, biopsied it, and removed it. The biopsy of the polyp returned benign, but the surrounding tissue showed complex endometrial hyperplasia with atypia. The gynecologist explained that this is a type of early endometrial cancer, and definitive treatment includes a hysterectomy if I was not planning to have more children. I agreed to the surgery.

During surgery, my doctor found an early endometrial cancer hidden in the uterine cavity. My fallopian tubes were surgically removed to lower my risk of ovarian cancer, and my normal-appearing ovaries were left in place. After my hysterectomy, I did not get hot flashes or notice other hormonal changes.

Preparing for Your Doctor's Appointment

Be sure to ask your doctor the following questions:

- Does my bleeding pattern put me at risk for uterine cancer?
- Does my body weight put me at higher risk for uterine cancer?
- Does my degree of activity put me at higher risk for uterine cancer?

- Does my family history put me at higher risk for uterine cancer?
- Does my lifestyle put me at higher risk for uterine cancer?

Summary

Your menstrual history, lifestyle factors, and family history contribute to your risk of uterine cancer. Track and discuss any heavy or irregular bleeding you experience in perimenopause, even if it is longstanding. Talking to your doctor can help you identify your personal risk and take actionable steps to reduce that risk.

Black women should be especially vigilant. They are at higher risk for having endometrial cancer and higher risk for having more aggressive types of endometrial cancer that are hard to identify early. Persist until you have a full evaluation, including hysteroscopy and biopsies of the uterus lining if you have heavy or irregular bleeding in perimenopause or have postmenopausal bleeding. Even if ultrasound findings are not worrisome, Black women are still at higher risk for more aggressive types of uterine cancer.

CERVICAL CANCER

Unlike ovarian cancer and uterine cancer, there are well-established screening tests for cervical cancer. Pap smears were introduced in 1941 as a regular, validated screening test for cervical cancer. The number of women dying of cervical cancer has been shrinking since the 1970s due to the Pap smear. Now, with the addition of human papillomavirus (HPV) testing, there is even more effective prevention and early detection of cervical cancer. That's because HPV causes most cervical cancer cases. HPV status is now critical to identifying precancerous cells in the cervix.

Risk Factors for Developing Cervical Cancer

Unlike breast, uterine, or ovarian cancer, cervical cancer is not tied to family history. In fact, 91 percent of cervical cancers are caused by acquiring high-risk HPV DNA.[8]

Additional risk factors for cervical cancer or precancer are:

- Having a high-risk sexual partner
- Having first-time sex under age 18
- Having multiple sexual partners
- Smoking cigarettes

Penile–vaginal intercourse is not necessary to acquire cervical cancer or high-risk HPV DNA. High-risk HPV DNA can be acquired by:

- Anal sex
- External genital contact
- External or surface skin contact
- Oral sex

The risk of cervical cancer is declining due to HPV vaccines and better screening, but the risk of oral cancer, vulvar cancer, and anal cancer related to high-risk HPV DNA is rising.

Symptoms of Cervical Cancer

Cervix cancer usually has no symptoms but could involve bleeding between menstrual periods or bleeding after sex.

Screening for Cervical Cancer

The Pap test is a noninvasive test that uses a brush to swab cells off the surface of the cervix and determine if they appear normal. The Pap test has been the gold standard for cervical cancer screening for more than 70 years. Since the discovery that HPV causes more than 95 percent of cervical cancers, doctors have been incorporating HPV into Pap testing to increase accuracy. However, it is still important for a doctor to check the appearance of the cervix each year. While it is not common, it is possible to have cancer or precancer of the cervix that is not found on a Pap smear or HPV test. For example, last year, I met with a healthy woman in her late thirties with a concerning-looking spot on her cervix. Her Pap was negative for abnormal cervix cells, but she had high-risk HPV DNA. I did a microscope exam of her cervix (colposcopy) with biopsies that showed a severe precancer of her cervix. She had the abnormal cervix cells removed in the office and has done well since. Ask the clinician who performs your Pap smear if they see anything on your cervix when they examine you; do not rely on the Pap smear results alone.

While HPV testing and Pap smears have enhanced doctors' ability to detect precancer of the cervix, the topic is continually evolving. More specifically, there has been a philosophical shift in how doctors identify and treat cervical cancer. Researchers and clinicians have subsequently changed the way in which they educate patients about Pap smears and cervical cancer screening.

> **DID YOU KNOW?**
> Researchers have found that HPV is responsible for more than 91 percent of cervical cancer cases. Pap smears are still used to identify abnormal cells in your cervix, and HPV DNA testing is used to determine if you have been exposed to a high-risk type of HPV DNA that increases your risk of getting cervical cancer.

In 2019, however, new screening and detection guidelines for cervical cancer emerged after a consensus of 19 professional specialty organizations. The 2019 American Society of Colposcopy and Cervical Pathology (ASCCP) Risk-Based Management Consensus Guidelines made it clear that doctors should strive to detect cervical cancer as early as possible without overtesting for it. Overtesting refers to too many Pap smears that are not warranted or too many colposcopies with biopsies that do not yield an accurate cancer or precancer diagnosis.[8]

These new guidelines were a game changer. Before 2019, the guidelines for cervical cancer screening directed clinicians to determine testing and treatment for cervical cancer based on individual Pap smear and HPV DNA results regardless of your overall personal risk. Now, the focus has shifted away from Pap smear and HPV DNA results toward assessing an individual woman's *overall* risk of developing cervical cancer. This means worrisome results from your last Pap smear alone may not warrant screening more frequently for cervical cancer, particularly if your overall risk of developing cervical cancer is low. However, it also means your doctor could bypass normal Pap smear results to screen for cervical cancer if your overall risk is high.

One upside of the new 2019 ASCCP guidelines is that less worrisome cancer precursors no longer necessarily mandate testing. However, your part in this process is crucial. What makes this novel approach possible is knowing your Pap smear history and documenting it. Your doctor can then use this information to advise you about future screening with Pap smears and HPV testing.

What is the downside? Although the 2019 ASCCP guidelines are beneficial in many ways, they're not easy for clinicians to implement. Roughly four years before the release of the new 2019 consensus guidelines, I attended a special one-day course on abnormal Pap smears and cervical cancer screening at a major professional meeting sponsored by the American College of Obstetricians and Gynecologists. I knew the material well but wanted to refresh my memory and confirm my knowledge was cutting-edge. To my dismay, the lecturers were scrutinizing their lecture notes, reading every word as if the material was new to them.

During a break, I went to the podium and asked why the lecturers were squinting at their notes. Did they not know this material cold since they were teaching it? The lecturers told me that the recommendations were so complex that no one could remember them without notes. I did not find this reassuring! As clinicians, we are expected to implement these guidelines daily in our exam rooms without the aid of lecture notes. I am not accustomed to carrying lecture notes in my white coat pocket and referring to them when I perform Pap smears. Unfortunately, clinicians cannot follow the recommendations easily without referring to the ASCCP's detailed database available via a phone app, in print, or online. Why is that? The new recommendations are based on each individual's level of risk for developing cervical cancer. This flowchart or decision tree makes it difficult to know the guidelines by memory.

When thinking about the 2019 guidelines, consider these important highlights:

1. Bleeding

    If you have symptoms such as bleeding after sex (postcoital bleeding), abnormal uterine bleeding, or abnormal vaginal bleeding, it's important to get a Pap smear test even if you are not due for one in your regular screening schedule.

2. Follow-up visits

    If your doctor tells you to follow up in one year, do not miss your follow-up visit. Your doctor recommended it because you have a higher risk of cervical cancer or precancer and should not wait three or five years between Pap smears.

3. Important historical information

    Your doctor will need to know your history of HPV test results, as well as your most recent Pap smear and any abnormal Pap smears from the past 25 years. It will also be helpful for you to track any abnormal Pap smear results, including when your doctor performed those Pap smears and the specifics of each subsequent report. The timing and specific results of your Pap smears and HPV testing will determine the age at which you can safely stop having Pap tests, how often you need them, and what other testing you need to avoid getting cervical cancer.

4. Screening

    The best way to prevent cervical cancer is to make sure you get the screening you need based on your medical history, history of Pap results, and HPV results. What are some additional factors your doctor will consider when determining whether you need screening for cervical cancer going forward? How often you have been getting Pap smears and whether you have missed Pap smears.

5. Severe precancer of the cervix

If you have severe precancer of the cervix (i.e., severe cervical intraepithelial neoplasia [CIN 3]), you may need to get Pap smears for 25 years after your last abnormal result. This may be true even if you are over 65 years old. If you do not have a worrisome result (e.g., CIN 3), you typically stop screening Pap smears after age 65 and after your Pap test results are normal for 25 years.[8]

Surveillance Versus Screening for Cervical Cancer

The most important thing I can say is that surveillance/close monitoring is different from screening. Every woman has a different set of risks for cervical cancer. It is important to do your Pap and HPV tests according to your own personal risk. This may be different from your friend's, neighbor's, coworkers', or even your sister's risk.

You're at higher risk for cervical cancer and need surveillance or close monitoring (not just routine Pap smears or HPV DNA testing every three to five years) if you:

- Had a colposcopy with abnormal tissue results
- Had a cone biopsy
- Had a loop electrical excision procedure to remove a wedge of abnormal cancerous or precancerous tissue
- Have a history of high-risk HPV DNA or abnormal cells on your Pap smear

One of the most common questions my patients ask me is: How often do I need a Pap smear?

As a gynecologist, I often worry when I answer this question. Here's why: When I tell an individual patient my recommendation for their Pap smear and HPV screening schedule, it is based on their personal medical history and other specific information, such as whether they were exposed to diethylstilbesterol (DES) in utero, whether they had regular Pap smears, when their last Pap smear was done, if they have a history of an abnormal Pap smear, and whether they have a history of high-risk HPV DNA. DES is a high-dose steroid given to women in the 1950s to prevent miscarriages. Subsequently, it was found to cause cervical and vaginal cancers in female offspring, a higher risk of breast cancer, and higher risk of male cancers in offspring.

When patients say, "Great, I'll tell my friends, relatives, and coworkers they only need a Pap smear every five years and can stop at age 65," I tell them that may not be true. Since I don't know the medical history or results of any prior Pap smears or HPV DNA results for any of those individuals, my recommendation does not apply to them.

In general, your doctor may recommend a Pap smear every three years if you:

- Are a nonsmoker
- Have no history of abnormal Pap smears or high-risk HPV in the past
- Have not missed a regular Pap smear
- Never had a colposcopy or cone biopsy

Once you are in your thirties and up to age 65, if you meet the above criteria, your doctor may recommend a Pap smear and HPV DNA every three to five years if no Pap smears are missed and none of the Pap smears have shown abnormalities. Consider Azadeh's story.

Azadeh's Story
A 37-YEAR-OLD WOMAN WHO WANTS TO KNOW
HOW OFTEN TO HAVE PAP SMEARS

I am an engineer, and I like precise recommendations. I have a new gynecologist, and I asked them how often I should have a Pap test. They said they needed more information. They reviewed my personal medical history and learned that I had an abnormal Pap smear three years ago followed by a cone biopsy. They asked for the pathology report of the cone biopsy. I am requesting a copy to review with them.

The doctor said they will review the report to see if the cone biopsy removed something serious. They recommend I have a Pap smear every year with an HPV test every three years. If the Pap is abnormal, I should also have an HPV test at the same time.

I told them I would share this information with some of my friends who have also questioned how often they should have a Pap test. They said they didn't know how often my friends needed Pap tests because they didn't have my friends' medical histories. They also explained there is no one-size-fits-all answer and that my friends should each speak with their own doctors.

If you are at higher risk of cervical cancer due to a history of abnormal Pap smears and biopsies or because you have a history of high-risk HPV DNA on a Pap smear, you may need annual testing. Consider Carmelita's story.

Carmelita's Story
A 66-YEAR-OLD WOMAN WHO IS QUESTIONING WHETHER SHE NEEDS A PAP SMEAR TEST

None of my friends still see their gynecologists for Pap tests. I am wondering if my gynecologist is up to date on Pap guidelines. They tell me I still need Pap smears.

I was widowed at age 55 and dated a lot before remarrying three years ago. At age 59, my Pap came back abnormal, and cervical biopsies showed precancer. After that, I had a cone biopsy to remove the high-risk CIN 3 precancerous tissue in my cervix. Four years ago, at age 62, I had high-risk HPV (human papillomavirus) on my Pap. My doctor told me that based on the updated 2019 guidelines, even though I never actually had cervical cancer, the high-risk HPV DNA and CIN 3 on my Pap means I still need Pap smears annually for now. While my friends who never had an abnormal Pap may safely stop having Pap smears at age 65, with my particular history, I must continue having Pap smear screening for another 25 years! My personal need for continued Pap screening is specific to my history and is very different from the needs of my friends.

In addition to personal history of abnormal Pap smears and HPV status, age is also a factor in determining how results are addressed. Here is an example of a mother and her daughter who had the same abnormal Pap smear results but were given different treatment, follow-up, and screening recommendations.

Mother–Daughter Story

Tanya, a 48-year-old woman with an abnormal Pap smear
Lola, her 21-year-old daughter with an abnormal Pap smear

TANYA

I'm a 48-year-old widow with a new partner. I have a 21-year-old daughter, Lola, who recently had her first Pap smear that showed atypical squamous cells of uncertain significance (ASCUS) with mildly abnormal cells. The reflex HPV DNA that her doctor performed after the atypical cells were found on the Pap smear showed no high-risk HPV DNA. Lola had received two of the three recommended Gardasil shots to prevent HPV DNA. Her gynecologist told her to get her third Gardasil shot to lower the risk that she would get high-risk HPV DNA or that abnormalities in her cervix would persist or recur. Lola's doctor advised her to have a repeat Pap in twelve months, since the mild changes in her cervical cells might resolve on their own.

When I had my annual gyn exam, my Pap showed ASCUS with high-risk HPV DNA. My gynecologist advised a colposcopy. I told my gyn I already heard about ASCUS since my daughter had that Pap result recently and she just needed to have a repeat Pap in twelve months. I wanted to know why I needed more testing. My gynecologist explained that the HPV infection typically resolves on its own in young healthy women, especially if they have no high-risk HPV.

After I had the office colposcopy, a microscope exam with biopsies, I learned that the pathology report of the cervix tissue showed CIN 2 (moderate dysplasia of the cervix). My doctor said CIN 2 can resolve on its own or turn into cancer. I was advised to have a cone biopsy to remove the abnormal precancerous tissue in the cervix and then have annual Pap smears. I got a second opinion, and that gynecologist agreed with my doctor. My gynecologist also advised me to use condoms to lower the risk of getting additional exposure to high-risk HPV. So even though my daughter and I had similar results, my high-risk HPV status and my age led my gyn to give me a different recommendation for testing and follow-up than my daughter's doctor gave her.

As you can see, these are two similar stories with very different recommendations for frequency of Pap smears.

Screening Guidelines Versus Surveillance After Abnormal Pap Smear Results

Any abnormal finding changes the recommendation for routine screening with Pap smears from every three to five years to more frequent surveillance. Screening is routine checking for abnormalities with no high-risk history or prior abnormal results. Surveillance kicks in when a high-risk HPV result is found or there are abnormal cells on a Pap smear. In this case, more frequent follow-up or surveillance is in order to monitor whether the abnormality resolves or persists or worsens and becomes cancerous. Surveillance mandates more intense follow-up with more frequent Pap smear testing and regular HPV DNA testing. Depending on the specific Pap results, frequent surveillance could mean Pap smears every four months or six months for a year or two until you return to screening. The frequency of the testing is customized to the type of abnormal finding.

Women who have high-risk HPV DNA may find that their body can clear the high-risk wart virus on its own without any treatment, regardless of whether there is a cervical lesion that is being treated. All cervical lesions that are seen should be biopsied, even if the Pap smear is normal or reassuring.[9]

PREPARING FOR YOUR DOCTOR'S APPOINTMENT

To prepare for your doctor visit, take these important steps:

1. Ask your doctor for their screening recommendations based on your personal history of Pap results and any biopsy results.
2. Do not rely on recommendations from friends and family members to determine how often you should have Pap smears. This is true even if their history seems like yours. Based on updated guidelines, Pap smears are scheduled according to your individual risk of getting cervical cancer, not just according to the results of your last Pap smear.
3. Keep a record of the exact Pap report results with details, especially if the report is abnormal. Have handy the specific results of any abnormal Pap smears in the past.
4. Keep a record of the pathology report from any biopsies you had regardless of whether they were done during a colposcopy or cone biopsy, or a loop electrical excision procedure to remove abnormal tissue from the cervix.
5. Keep a record of your last Pap screening and your last HPV test.
6. Request a Pap smear if you have bleeding after sex or if you have irregular, heavy, abnormal, or unexpected uterine or vaginal bleeding.
7. Ask your doctor if they see anything unusual on your cervix when they examine you.

Be prepared to ask:

- Given my prior Pap smears, history of HPV, and smoking status, how often should I have Pap smears at my age?

- I have a history of warts on my hands. Do I need more frequent Pap smears?
- I have a history of high-risk HPV. Should I get the HPV vaccine at my age?

Summary

The Pap smear is used as a screening test at certain intervals to check for the early development of precancer when there are no risk factors. The Pap smear is also used as a surveillance test to follow up closely after an abnormal Pap smear result or a finding of high-risk HPV. Updated Pap smear guidelines focus on the individual's specific medical history and risk factors. If you have not had regular Pap smears, have had a recent high-risk HPV test, or have had an abnormal Pap smear result in the past 20 years, your screening recommendations may be different, and you may need more frequent Pap smears, falling into the category of surveillance and closer follow-up after an abnormal finding.

OVARIAN CANCER

Ovarian cancer is complex because there are several different types, and it can be hard to detect it early. Let's dive more deeply into the complexities and challenges.

Types of Ovarian Cancer

There are three main categories of ovary cancer based upon three different cell types: epithelial (surface cells), stromal cells (support cells), and germ cells (generating cells). Most ovarian cancers (95 percent) are epithelial ovarian cancer (EOC). The other 5 percent are cancers of other cell types in the ovary such as germ cell tumors. EOC may appear to start in the ovary; however, it may actually start in the fallopian tube or the peritoneum and then spread to the ovaries. EOC has several subtypes and is hard to detect early. There are no good screening tests to diagnose EOC in the general population.

Symptoms of Ovarian Cancer

Symptoms of ovarian cancer are similar to those of other medical conditions such as dehydration, constipation, and other gastrointestinal problems. These symptoms include bloating, early satiety or loss of appetite, abdominal swelling, pelvic or abdominal pain, urinary urgency or frequency, difficulty eating, nausea or loss of appetite, and prematurely feeling full when you have eaten only a little food.

In the case of EOC, it is more common to see some or all of these symptoms occur almost daily. The symptoms do not typically come and go or wax and wane. The workup includes an abdominal and pelvic exam, as well as a pelvic ultrasound. In the past, a blood test, CA125, was also ordered, but CA125 has a poor track record finding ovarian cancer early. CA125 is more helpful when used to follow the progress of ovarian cancer treatment—not detection of undiagnosed ovarian cancer.

DID YOU KNOW?

A newer blood test, OVA 1 Plus, has a better track record of finding early ovarian cancer, including all cell types, not just epithelial cell types. The OVA 1 Plus test has many components in its algorithm or formula, including VEGF (vascular endothelial growth factor), as well as CA125, to predict if an ovarian cyst is cancerous or not. Clinically, OVA 1 Plus testing is preferrable because it incorporates details of your patient history, ultrasound findings, and menopause status to more accurately forecast whether ovarian cancer is present.[10]

Risk Factors for Developing Ovarian Cancer

There are several risk factors for ovarian cancer. Let's start with the hereditary ones. The first is a positive family history of ovarian cancer, especially in a mother, sister, or blood-related aunts or grandparents. Another is a family history of BRCA1 or BRCA2 genetic mutations or Lynch syndrome mutations (e.g., MLH1, SH2, or others). When you have a family history of these types of genetic mutations, you also have a higher risk of ovary, colon, uterine, stomach, kidney, or pancreas cancer. Experts advise all women who are diagnosed with ovary cancer to get genetic testing.

> **DID YOU KNOW?**
> Having your genetic heritage determined by a commercial lab without the input of a medical expert or genetic counselor is not the same thing as having medical genetic testing. While medical genetic testing may be done with a blood test or saliva test/mouth swab, the medical testing typically checks for over 50 gene mutations for genetic cancers and is tailored to your personal medical history and family medical history as reviewed by a medical professional.

If you have a high-risk family history of ovarian cancer or a known genetic mutation (e.g., BRCA1 or BRCA2, Lynch, or another mutation), your doctor may recommend closer monitoring. (You may recall from the beginning of this chapter that there is no accurate screening for women at low risk of ovarian cancer.)

> **DID YOU KNOW?**
> Having one first-degree relative (i.e., a mother or sister) with ovarian cancer increases your own risk of developing ovarian cancer by 5 percent. The risk is 3.5 percent if there is a single second-degree relative with ovarian cancer (i.e., a grandmother or aunt) and a 7 percent increase if a woman has two affected relatives.

If you have a high-risk family history or a genetic mutation, and you would benefit from closer monitoring, until recently, your doctor would typically advise blood tests for ROMA and CA125 every six months along with a pelvic ultrasound. More about ROMA in the next paragraph. Now that the OVA 1 Plus blood test is available and is more accurate in predicting cancer of the ovary, it is likely that it will take the place of CA125 and ROMA as screening blood tests. OVA 1 Plus has the advantage of incorporating both CA125 and ROMA in its algorithm or formula. This is a welcome advance because the CA125 blood test is not sensitive enough to detect early-stage ovarian cancer. Another drawback of CA125 testing is the high rate of false positives or false alarms. For example, CA125 is often elevated with common benign conditions such as endometriosis. Unfortunately, at this time, not all insurance companies cover the OVA 1 Plus test.

> DID YOU KNOW?
>
> Individuals with genetic mutations make up 25 percent of ovarian cancer cases. These individuals are at high risk of developing ovarian cancer at a younger age, for example, in their forties as opposed to in their sixties.

The ROMA test (which stands for Risk of Ovarian Malignancy Algorithm) was cleared by the US Food and Drug Administration in 2008. ROMA tests for a serum biomarker called HE4 that is elevated in women with ovarian cancer. HE4 stands for human epididymis factor. HE4 is not elevated in endometriosis and is less often elevated with other benign conditions compared to many false CA125 elevations. Typically, blood HE4 elevations precede CA125 elevations by five to eight months. Using both ROMA and CA125 in high-risk women helps doctors identify a larger number of ovarian cancers sooner than using CA125 alone. Consider Basheva's story.

Basheva's Story
A WOMAN FROM ASHKENAZI JEWISH DESCENT
WITH A BRCA1 MUTATION

I am from an Ashkenazi Jewish family. Genetic testing shows I inherited the BRCA1 mutation. I have two aunts with ovarian cancer, both diagnosed in their late forties. When I was in my twenties, my gynecologist suggested I use a low-dose birth control pill to lower my risk of ovarian cancer by more than 50 percent. After age 37, when I had my second child, my gynecologist advised me to have both of my fallopian tubes surgically removed to lower my risk of ovarian cancer. Since I have a high-risk family history and the genetic mutation for BRCA1, I get regular pelvic ultrasound tests twice a year to check my ovaries. In the past, I also had a blood test for CA125 twice a year. Now that OVA 1 Plus is available, my doctor orders that test for me since it incorporates CA125, ROMA, my latest ultrasound findings, and my high-risk family history. I am considering having both of my ovaries surgically removed at age 45 when I am closer to menopause. As a BRCA1 carrier, I'm told my risk of ovarian cancer is 40 percent until I reach age 70.

My close childhood friend Kenisha has been supportive during my medical journey and asked her gynecologist why she was not being screened for ovarian cancer. Kenisha's family history is negative for ovary, breast, and colon cancer. Her doctor told her that her personal and family history indicates her risk for ovarian cancer is extremely low and that screening for ovarian cancer with no concerning symptoms would not be helpful. If she develops abdominal or pelvic pain, nausea, early satiety, or bloating, a full evaluation would be done to find the cause. Ovarian cancer can still occur in women with no risk factors, but it is not common at age 37. The risk of ovarian cancer for women in the general population up to age 70 is less than 1 percent.

In addition to genetic mutations, other risk factors for ovarian cancer are:

- Asbestos exposure
- Endometriosis
- Not having biological children
- Pelvic radiation

FACTORS THAT DO NOT INCREASE RISK

Consider these factors that do not increase your risk of developing ovarian cancer:

- Abortion or pregnancy termination
- Family history of breast cancer (without a genetic mutation)
- Infertility and infertility treatment

- Intrauterine device
- Talc

LOWERING YOUR RISK OF OVARIAN CANCER

As with other types of cancer, there are several ways you can lower your risk of developing ovarian cancer. These include the following:

- Breastfeeding. Breastfeeding for 12 months reduces your risk by 30 percent.
- Hysterectomy. A hysterectomy reduces your risk by 20 percent reduction if tubes and ovaries remain.
- Pregnancy/childbearing. Each pregnancy lowers your risk by 8 percent.
- Surgical removal of both fallopian tubes with or without removal of ovaries
- Tubal ligation or removal of the tubes alone (studies are underway about the removal of tubes alone)
- Use of oral contraceptives. Oral contraceptives lower the risk of ovarian cancer, even in women with BRCA1 or BRCA2, by 40 to 50 percent. If you are in this high-risk group and have a mutation for BRCA1 or BRCA2, you may expect a 60 percent reduction in ovarian cancer if you take the oral contraceptives for over six years.[11]

Now consider Olga's story.

Olga's Story
A 53-YEAR-OLD WOMAN WITH TWO CHILDREN WHO STILL HAS MENSTRUAL PERIODS

My periods are becoming irregular. I bleed every two months. The flow is not heavy, and I keep track of it. At my last annual gyn exam, the doctor said my uterus was enlarged. They recommended a pelvic ultrasound. The ultrasound showed a small fibroid and a 3.5-cm complex left ovarian cyst. I was worried since my older neighbor had ovarian cancer, and I asked if I should have the ovary surgically removed and biopsied.

The doctor explained the cyst was not very large and that my family history was reassuring. There may have been a small amount of bleeding into the cyst during a regular physiologic event. They told me the ovary makes cysts normally during ovulation and prior to the menstrual period. Complex features or divisions in the ovary can be worrisome, or these findings can be due to a physiologic or cycle cyst. If the latter is true, this means that with time, my body would absorb the cyst, and the ovary would appear normal again in eight weeks or so. I was worried and wanted to do the follow-up ultrasound sooner. The doctor said this would not give the cyst time to reabsorb. Since I had no pain, it was best to wait. I asked to have a CA125 blood test to check if there were cancerous changes in the ovary. My doctor recommended an OVA 1 Plus blood test instead and explained that the OVA 1 Plus test incorporates CA125 as part of its formula. They entered the size and features of the cyst on my ultrasound as well as my perimenopausal status. The OVA 1 Plus test came back normal and reassuring. Subsequently, the ultrasound showed complete resolution of the cyst, and I returned to having normal annual exams.

PREPARING FOR YOUR DOCTOR'S APPOINTMENT

Consider asking your doctor these questions:

- I have a family history of cancer. What should I do differently to lower my own risk of developing cancer?
- I have a personal history of cancer. Do I need different testing to detect and prevent it in the future?
- What cancer prevention strategies should I consider, and why?
- Why should I consider cancer screening tests if I have no family history of cancer?
- I already sent a sample to a commercial lab to know more about my heritage. Can I use that to predict my risk of cancer?

SUMMARY

Depending upon your family history, current state of health, pelvic ultrasound results, and genetic testing, your gynecologist can advise you what lifestyle measures or risk-reducing strategies to consider lowering your risk of ovary cancer.

IMPORTANT TAKEAWAYS

Although technology to detect cancer has come a long way, early detection is not yet available for all types of ovary cancer. While the OVA 1 Plus blood test is a significant breakthrough in the early detection of many types of ovary cancer, the best strategy also includes improving your chances of remaining cancer-free by modifying your lifestyle to lower your risk. However, you may not be able to modify your personal family history and other factors, which is why it's important to talk with your doctor and come up with a screening strategy based on your unique needs.

RESOURCES

www.acog.org—American College of Obstetricians and Gynecologists
www.cancer.net—American Society of Clinical Oncologists
Densebreastinfo.org—A summary of models to estimate breast cancer

CHAPTER 14

CONCLUSION

Going Forward

IF YOU ARE SEEKING CARE during menopause, I hope you feel more empowered to advocate for your health and more informed about what to expect before, during, and beyond menopause. While menopause is a universal biological process, you will choose how you navigate the journey. And more importantly, you're not alone.

If you are a clinician, I hope the book helps you see your patients through a new lens and while they try to address a myriad of menopausal concerns.

Each of us will experience peri- or post menopause differently depending upon our age, medical history, family history, lifestyle, and life circumstances.

Strategies that may work well for your sister, mother, friend, neighbor, or coworker may or may not work well for you.

Strategies that work well for you at one point in your menopause journey may not work well at another point in your life.

Collaborating with your doctor or clinician helps you achieve optimal health and well-being regardless of your age or stage of menopause. Whenever possible, document your health concerns, including any changes in your health, when they develop, and how they affect you. Your instincts and the information you provide your doctor about what you are experiencing mentally and physically are invaluable.

If you have done your own research, as many savvy women have, I encourage you to begin your medical visit by reviewing all your symptoms with your doctor and discussing your medical history, family history, physical examination findings, and test results. Your doctor uses their training and experience to generate a comprehensive list of different causes of your symptoms driven by the entire constellation of information you provide. This process improves your medical care and helps ensure that all relevant causes of your symptoms are considered. Your research, thoughts, and concerns are also important to discuss.

Navigating menopause can feel overwhelming at times, but women are strong and savvy, and there are more lifestyle modifications and medical options to choose from than ever before. As new research emerges in women's health and menopause, individuals and clinicians can look forward to a future filled with health and well-being. I hope the information in this book empowers you to achieve health and well-being before, during, and beyond menopause.

ACKNOWLEDGMENTS

WRITING THIS BOOK has been a rewarding and enlightening experience. I am grateful to the many people whose support and contributions made it possible.

First and foremost, my heartfelt thanks to my patients—past, present, and future—who have entrusted me with their care. Your questions, challenges, and experiences have continually shaped my understanding of not just menopause, but the full spectrum of women's health. It is a privilege to be part of your journey, and I hope this book reflects the collective wisdom gained from our conversations.

I am also grateful to my friends and colleagues at The Menopause Society, the Massachusetts Medical Society, The American College of Obstetricians and Gynecologists, and my fellow clinicians across New England. Your dedication to advancing women's health through research, education, and patient care has been invaluable. Our discussions, collaborations, and shared commitment to evidence-based medicine have played a vital role in shaping the insights within these pages.

A special thank you to my developmental editor, Lisa Eramo, for her expert guidance and thoughtful clarifying questions. She challenged me to refine complex ideas, ensuring that this book is both scientifically rigorous and accessible to all readers.

I'd also like to thank my editor, Suzanne Staszuik-Silvia, and the talented editorial and production teams who helped bring this book to life. I am grateful to Johns Hopkins University Press for believing in the importance of this work and for making it available to a wider audience.

To my friends and family—especially my husband, Paul Edelman—thank you for your unwavering encouragement, patience, and support. Your belief in this project sustained me through the many hours of research and writing.

Finally, to you, the reader—whether you or someone you care about is approaching, experiencing, or navigating life beyond menopause—I wrote this book with you in mind. My greatest hope is that *The Savvy Woman's Guide to Menopause* empowers you to make informed choices, embrace the changes ahead with confidence, and take an active role in shaping your long-term health and well-being.

REFERENCES

CHAPTER 1. SUCCESSFUL HEALTH STRATEGIES FOR WOMEN: BEFORE, DURING, AND BEYOND MENOPAUSE

1. Harlow SD, Gass M, Hall JE, et al.; STRAW+10 Collaborative Group. Executive summary of the Stages of Reproductive Aging Workshop +10: addressing the unfinished agenda of staging reproductive aging. *Climacteric.* 2012;15(2):105–114.
2. Mishra GD, Chung HF, Cano A, et al. EMAS position statement: predictors of premature and early natural menopause. *Maturitas.* 2019;123:82–88.
3. Cramer DW, et al. Family history as a predictor of early menopause. *Fertil Steril.* 1995;64:740–745.
4. Shifren J, Edelman JS, Schiff I. Hormone therapy and alternative therapies for menopause. In: *Clinical Updates in Women's Healthcare.* Vol. XIV, Number 4. American College of Obstetricians and Gynecologists; 2015.

CHAPTER 2. HANDLING HOT FLASHES WITHOUT HORMONES

1. Barnard N, et al. The Women's Study for the Alleviation of Vasomotor Symptoms (WAVS): a randomized controlled trial of a plant-based diet and whole soybeans for postmenopausal women. *Menopause.* 2021;28(10):1150–1156.
2. Carpenter JS, Burns DS, Wu J, et al. Paced respiration for vasomotor and other menopausal symptoms: a randomized, controlled trial. *J Gen Intern Med.* 2013;28(2):193–200.
3. Reed SD, LaCroix AZ, Anderson GL, et al. Lights on MsFLASH: a review of contributions. *Menopause.* 2020;27(4):473–484.
4. Green SM, et al. Cognitive behavior therapy for menopausal symptoms (CBT-Meno): a randomized controlled trial. *Menopause.* 2019;26(9):972–980.

5. Hardy C, et al. Self-help cognitive behavior therapy for working women with problematic hot flushes and night sweats (MENOS@Work): a multicenter randomized controlled trial. *Menopause.* 2018;25(5): 508–519.
6. Freeman EW, Sammel MD. Anxiety as a risk factor for menopausal hot flashes: evidence from the Penn Ovarian Aging cohort. *Menopause.* 2016;23(9):942–949.
7. Setchell KDR. 2016 Wulf H. Utian Endowed Lecture. The history and basic science development of soy isoflavones. *Menopause.* 2017;24(12): 1338–1350.
8. Hernandez G, et al. Pharmacokinetics and safety profile of single-dose administration of an estrogen receptor B-selective phytoestrogenic (phytoSERM) formulation in perimenopausal and postmenopausal women. *Menopause.* 2017;25(2):191–196.
9. Wang Y, et al. Retrospective analysis of phytoSERM for management of menopause-associated vasomotor symptoms and cognitive decline: a pilot study on pharmacogenomic effects of mitochondrial haplogroup and APOE genotype on therapeutic efficacy. *Menopause.* 2019;27(1): 57–65.
10. Reame NK. Editorial: Equalizing equol for hot flash relief? Still more questions than answers. *Menopause.* 2015;22(5):480–482.
11. Castelo-Branco C, et al. Review & metanalysis: isopropanolic black cohosh extract iCR for menopausal symptoms—an update on the evidence. *Climacteric.* 2021;24(2):109–119.
12. Zaw JJT, et al. Long-term resveratrol supplementation improves pain perception, menopausal symptoms, and overall well-being in post-menopausal women: findings from a 24-month randomized, controlled, crossover trial. *Menopause.* 2020;28(1):40–49.
13. Lensen S, et al. A core outcome set for vasomotor symptoms associated with menopause: the COMMA (Core Outcomes in Menopause) global initiative. *Menopause.* 2021;28(8):852–858.
14. Simon JA, Druckman R. Non-hormonal treatment of perimenopausal and menopausal climacteric symptoms [1A]. *Obstet Gynecol.* 2016;127:12S.
15. Ghazanfarpour M, Sadeghi R, Latifnejad Roudsari R, et al. Effects of flaxseed and Hypericum perforatum on hot flash, vaginal atrophy and estrogen-dependent cancers in menopausal women: a systematic review and meta-analysis. *Avicenna J Phytomed.* 2016;6(3):273–283.

16. Dahlgren MK, et al. A survey of medical cannabis use during perimenopause and post menopause. *Menopause*. 2022;29(9):1028–1036.
17. Leon-Ferre RA, Novotny PJ, Wolfe EG, et al. Oxybutynin vs placebo for hot flashes in women with or without breast cancer: a randomized, double-blind clinical trial (ACCRU SC-1603). *JNCI Cancer Spectr*. 2019;4(1):pkz088.
18. Santoro N, et al. Effect of the neurokinin 3 receptor antagonist fezolinetant on patient-reported outcomes in postmenopausal women with vasomotor symptoms: results of a randomized, placebo-controlled, double-blind, dose-ranging study (VESTA). *Menopause*. 2020;27(12): 1350–1356.
19. Miller VM, Kling JM, Files JA, et al. Personal perspective. What's in a name: are menopausal "hot flashes" a symptom of menopause or a manifestation of neurovascular dysregulation? *Menopause*. 2018.
20. Chien TJ, Hsu CH, Liu CY, Fang CJ. Effect of acupuncture on hot flush and menopause symptoms in breast cancer—a systematic review and meta-analysis. *PLoS One*. 2017;12(8):e0180918.
21. Carroll DG, Lisenby KM, Carter TL. Critical appraisal of paroxetine for the treatment of vasomotor symptoms. *Int J Womens Health*. 2015; 7:615–624.
22. Yoon SH, Lee JY, Lee C, Lee H, Kim SN. Gabapentin for the treatment of hot flushes in menopause: a meta-analysis. *Menopause*. 2020;27(4):485–493.

CHAPTER 3. TAKING HORMONES IN MENOPAUSE

1. The 2022 hormone therapy position statement of The North American Menopause Society. *Menopause*. 2022;29(7):767–794.
2. Mørch LS, Løkkegaard E, Andreasen AH, Krüger-Kjær S, Lidegaard Ø. Hormone therapy and ovarian cancer. *JAMA*. 2009;302(3):298–305.
3. Modified from "Facts about Menopausal Hormone Therapy," an excellent general resource that can be found at "Facts about Menopausal Hormone Therapy." www.nhlbi.nih.gov/files/docs/pht_facts.pdf. Accessed November 23, 2022.
4. National Academies of Sciences, Engineering, and Medicine. The NAMS practice pearl compounded bioidentical hormone therapy: new recommendations. December 8, 2020.
5. Beral V, Peto R, Pirie K, Reeves GK, for the Collaborative Group on Hormonal Factors in Breast Cancer. Type and timing of menopausal

hormonal therapy and breast cancer risk: individual participant meta-analysis of the worldwide epidemiological evidence. *Lancet.* 2019;394:1159–1168.

6. Bioidentical Hormone Therapy © 2023 The Menopause Society. www.menopause.org. Accessed February 25, 2023.

7. Liu Y, et al. Safety and efficacy of compounded bioidentical hormone therapy (cBHT) in perimenopausal and postmenopausal women: a systematic review and meta-analysis of randomized controlled trials. *Menopause.* 2022;29(4):465–482.

8. Gallez A, Blacher S, Maquoi E, et al. Estetrol combined to progestogen for menopause or contraception indication is neutral on breast cancer. *Cancers (Basel).* 2021;13(10):2486.

9. Pickar JH, et al. Tissue selective estrogen complex (TSEC): a review. *Menopause.* 2018;25(9):1033–1045.

10. Shifren J, Edelman JS, Schiff I. Hormone therapy and alternative therapies for menopause. *Monograph for ACOG, Clinical Updates in Women's Healthcare.* 2015;XIV(4).

11. Bhupathiraju Shilpa N, et al. Hormone therapy use and risk of chronic disease in the nurses' health study: A comparative analysis with the Women's Health Initiative. *Am J Epidemiol.* 2017;186(6):696–708.

CHAPTER 4. HEART DISEASE: THE RISK OF DOING NOTHING

1. Benjamin EJ, et al. Heart disease and stroke statistics—2018 update: a report from the American Heart Association. *Circulation.* 2018;137(12): e67–e492.

2. Honigberg MC, et al. Association of premature natural and surgical menopause with incident cardiovascular disease. *JAMA.* 2019; 322(24):2411–2421.

3. O'Kelly AC, Hitches E, Shufelt C, et al. Pregnancy and reproductive risk factors for cardiovascular disease in women. *Circ Res.* 2022; 130:652–672.

4. Kaunitz AM, Kapoor E, Faubion S. Treatment of women after bilateral salpingo-oophorectomy performed prior to natural menopause. *JAMA.* 2021;326(14):1429–1430.

5. Wang XY, et al. Menstrual cycle regularity and length across the reproductive lifespan and risk for premature mortality: prospective cohort study. *BMJ.* 2020;371:m3464.

6. Jaskanwal Deep Singh S, et al. Mental stress and its effects on vascular health. *Mayo Clin Proc.* 2022;97(5):951-990.
7. Lau ES, et al. Infertility and risk of heart failure in Women's Health Initiative. *J Am Coll Cardiol.* 2022;79(16):1594-1603.
8. Wang Y-X, et al. Pregnancy loss and risk of cardiovascular disease: the Nurses' Health Study II. *Eur Heart J.* 2022;43(3):190-199.
9. Lee JJ, et al. Age of menarche and risk of cardiovascular disease outcomes: findings from the National Heart Lung and Blood Institute-sponsored women's ischemia syndrome evaluation. *J Am Heart Assoc.* 2019;8(12):1161-1175.
10. Guan C, Zahid S, Minhas AS, et al. Polycystic ovary syndrome: a "risk-enhancing" factor for cardiovascular disease. *Fertil Steril.* 2022;117(5):924-935.
11. AHA Presidential Advisory. Call to action for cardiovascular disease in women: epidemiology, awareness, access, and delivery of equitable health care: a presidential advisory from the American Heart Association. *Circulation.* 2022;145:e1059-e1071.
12. Vaccarino V, Shah AJ, Mehta PK, et al. Brain-heart connections in stress and cardiovascular disease: implications for the cardiac patient. *Atherosclerosis.* 2021;328:74-82.
13. Margolies L, et al. Digital mammography and screening for coronary artery disease. *JACC Cardiovasc Imaging.* 2016;9(4):350-360.
14. Lau ES. Aspirin for primary prevention of cardiovascular disease in women. The Menopause Society. NAMS Practice Pearl. September 13, 2022.

CHAPTER 5. UNDERSTANDING UNEXPECTED BLEEDING

1. Orlando MS, Bradley LD. Implementation of office hysteroscopy for the evaluation and treatment of intrauterine pathology. *Obstet Gynecol.* 2022;140:499-513.
2. Goldstein SR, Lumsden MA. Abnormal uterine bleeding in perimenopause. *Climacteric.* 2017;20(5):414-420.
3. DeStephano CC, Allyse MA, Abu Dabrh AMM, et al. Pilot study of women's perspectives when abnormal uterine bleeding occurs during perimenopause. *Climacteric.* 2022;25(5):510-515.
4. Davis E, Sparzak PB. *Abnormal Uterine Bleeding.* StatPearls Publishing; 2022.

5. Munro MG, Critchley HOD, Broder MS, Fraser IS. FIGO classification system (PALM-COEIN) for causes of abnormal uterine bleeding in nongravid women of reproductive age. *Int J Gynaecol Obstet.* 2011;113:3-13.
6. Török P, Krasznai Z, Molnár S, Lampé R, Jakab A. Preoperative assessment of endometrial cancer. *Transl Cancer Res.* 2020;9(12):7746-7758.
7. Management of acute abnormal bleeding in nonpregnant reproductive-aged women. ACOG Committee Opinion. Number 557, April 2013. Reaffirmed 2020. Accessed February 20, 2023.
8. Raffone, A, Raimondo D, Neola D, et al. Diagnostic accuracy of MRI in the differential diagnosis between uterine leiomyomas and sarcomas: a systematic review and meta-analysis. *Int. J Gynaecol Obstet.* 2024; 165(1):22-33.

CHAPTER 6. COMMON CONCERNS

1. Soper D. Trichomonas under control or under controlled? *Am J Obstet Gynecol.* 2004;190(1):281-290.
2. Sobel JD. Nontrichomonal purulent vaginitis: clinical approach. *Curr Infect Dis Rep.* 2000;2(6):501-505.
3. Dwyer J, Tafuri SM, LaGrange CA. *Oxybutynin.* StatPearls Publishing; 2022.
4. He Q, Xiao K, Peng L, et al. An effective meta-analysis of magnetic stimulation therapy for urinary incontinence. *Sci Rep.* 2019;9(1):9077.
5. Gardner AN, Schkenazi SO. The short-term efficacy and safety of fractional CO2 laser therapy for vulvovaginal symptoms in menopause, breast cancer, and lichen sclerosus. *Menopause.* 2021;28(5):511-516.
6. Filippini M, Porcari I, Ruffolo AF, et al. CO2-laser therapy and genitourinary syndrome of menopause: a systematic review and meta-analysis. *J Sex Med.* 2022;19(3):452-470.
7. Paraiso MFR, Ferrando CA, Sokol ER, et al. A randomized clinical trial comparing vaginal laser therapy to vaginal estrogen therapy in women with genitourinary syndrome of menopause: the VeLVET Trial. *Menopause.* 2020;27(1):50-56.
8. Huang YC, Chang KV. *Kegel Exercises.* StatPearls Publishing; 2022.
9. Te Brummelstroete GH, Loohuis AM, Wessels NJ, Westers HC, van Summeren JJGT, Blanker MH. Scientific evidence for pelvic floor devices presented at conferences: an overview. *Neurourol Urodyn.* 2019;38(7):1958-1965.

10. Rovner ES, Wein AJ. Treatment options for stress urinary incontinence. *Rev Urol.* 2004;6(suppl 3):S29-S47.

11. Ala-Jaakkola, R, Laitila A, Ouwehand, AC, Lehtoranta, L. Role of D-mannose in urinary tract infections: a narrative review. *Nutr J.* 2022;21(1):18.

CHAPTER 7. SMOOTHER SEX

1. Basson R. Female sexual response: The role of drugs in the management of sexual dysfunction. *Obstet Gynecol.* 2001;98:350-353.

2. Basson R. Using a different model for female sexual response to address women's problematic low sexual desire. *J Sex Marital Ther.* 2001;27(5):395-403.

3. Shifren JL, et al. Sexual problems and distress in United States women: prevalence and correlates. *Obstet Gynecol.* 2008:112(5):970-978.

4. Sand M, et al. Women's endorsement of models of female sexual response: the Nurses' Sexuality Study. *J Sex Med.* 2009;6(10):2761-2771.

5. Coleman EM, et al. Arousability and sexual satisfaction in lesbian and heterosexual women. *J Sex Res.* 1983;19(1):58-73.

6. Shifren JL, et al. Transdermal testosterone treatment in women with impaired sexual function after oophorectomy. *N Engl J Med.* 2000;343(10):682-688.

7. Davis SR, et al. Global consensus position statement on the use of testosterone therapy for women. *J Clin Endocrinol Metab.* 2019;104:4660-4666.

8. International Society for the Study of Women's Sexual Health. Clinical practice guideline for the use of systemic testosterone for hypoactive sexual desire disorder in women. *Climacteric.* 2021;24(6):533-550.

9. Kingsberg SA, Faubion SS. Clinical management of hypoactive sexual desire disorder in postmenopausal women. NAMS Practice Pearl. Released May 19, 2022.

10. Kling JM, Thomas HN. Female sexual function and dysfunction. In *Sex and Gender-Based Women's Health.* Springer; 2020:127-139.

11. Collar AL, et al. Medical counseling on sexual enrichment aids. Women's preferences and medical practitioner expertise. *Obstet Gynecol.* 2022;140(3).

12. Kingsberg SA, et al. Vulvar and vaginal atrophy in postmenopausal women: findings from the REVIVE (Real Women's Views of Treatment

Options for Menopausal Vaginal ChangEs) survey. *J Sex Med.* 2013;10:1790-1799.

13. Waetjen LE, et al., for the Study of Women's Health Across the Nation (SWAN). Factors associated with developing vaginal dryness symptoms in women transitioning through menopause: a longitudinal study. *Menopause.* 2018;15(10).

14. Labrie F, Archer D, Bouchard C, et al. Intravaginal dehydroepiandrosterone (Prasterone), a physiological and highly efficient treatment of vaginal atrophy. *Menopause.* 2009;16(5):907-922.

15. Kingsberg SA, Clayton AH, Portman D, et al. Bremelanotide for the treatment of hypoactive sexual desire disorder: two randomized phase 3 trials. *Obstet Gynecol.* 2019;134(5):899-908.

16. Rapkin AJ, Satmary W. A deep dive into devices for sexual health. *Contemp OBGYN.* March/April 2024:14-18.

17. Scott EE. Early effect of fractional CO2 laser treatment in postmenopausal women with vaginal atrophy. *Laser Ther.* 2018;27(1):41-47.

18. Pather K, Dilgir S, Rane A. The ThermiVa in Genital Hiatus Treatment (TIGHT) Study. *Sex Med.* 2021;9:100427.

19. Magon N, Alinsod R. ThermiVa: the revolutionary technology for vulvovaginal rejuvenation and noninvasive management of female SUI. *J Obstet Gynaecol India.* 2016;66(4):300-302.

20. Herbenick, D Reece, M, Sanders S, Dodge B, Ghassemi A, Fortenberry JD. Prevalence and characteristics of vibrator use by women in the United States: results from a nationally representative study. 2009;5(7):1857-1866.

CHAPTER 8. COMPATIBLE CONTRACEPTION

1. Grandi G, Di Vinci P, Sgandurra A, Feliciello L, Monari F, Facchinetti F. Contraception during perimenopause: practical guidance. *Int J Womens Health.* 2022;14:913-929.

2. Steinberg J, Lynch SE. Lactic acid, citric acid, and potassium bitartrate (Phexxi) vaginal gel for contraception. *Am Fam Physician.* 2021;103(10):628-629.

3. Pinkerton JV, Levy BS, et al. The perimenopausal period and the benefits of progestin IUDs. *OBG Manag.* 2023;35(5):20-27, 45, 47, e48.

4. Fruzzetti F, Fidecicchi T, Montt Guevara MM, Simoncini T. Estetrol: a new choice for contraception. *J Clin Med.* 2021;10(23):5625.

CHAPTER 9. MOODS, MEMORY, AND MENTAL HEALTH

1. Olff M. Sex and gender differences in post-traumatic stress disorder: an update. *Eur J Psychotraumatol.* 2017;8(suppl 4):1351204.
2. Armour M, Ee CC, Hao J, Wilson TM, Yao SS, Smith CA. Acupuncture and acupressure for premenstrual syndrome. *Cochrane Database Syst Rev.* 2018;8(8):CD005290.
3. Marjoribanks J, Brown J, O'Brien PM, Wyatt K. Selective serotonin reuptake inhibitors for premenstrual syndrome. *Cochrane Database Syst Rev.* 2013;2013(6):CD001396.
4. Mahboubi M. Evening primrose (Oenothera biennis) oil in management of female ailments. *J Menopausal Med.* 2019;25(2):74–82.
5. Barnard ND, Scialli AR, Hurlock D, Bertron P. Diet and sex-hormone binding globulin, dysmenorrhea, and premenstrual symptoms. *Obstet Gynecol.* 2000;95(2):245–250.
6. Soares CN. Depression and menopause: an update on current knowledge and clinical management for this critical window. *Med Clin North Am.* 2019;103(4):651–657.
7. Kravitz HM, et al. Risk of high depressive symptoms after the final menstrual period: the Study of Women's Health Across the Nation (SWAN). *Menopause.* 2022;29(7).
8. Stute P, et al. Management of depressive symptoms in peri- and postmenopausal women: EMAS position statement. *Maturitas.* 2020;131:91–101.
9. Mills E, Montori VM, Wu P, et al. Interaction of St John's wort with conventional drugs: systematic review of clinical trials. *BMJ.* 2004;329:27.
10. Knuppel L, Linde K. Adverse effects of St. John's Wort: a systematic review. *J Clin Psychiatry* 2004;65:1470.
11. Cyranowski J. Practice considerations for behavioral therapies for depression and anxiety in midlife women. *Menopause.* 2022; 29(2):236–238.
12. Vargas AS, Luís Â, Barroso M, Gallardo E, Pereira L. Psilocybin as a new approach to treat depression and anxiety in the context of life-threatening diseases—a systematic review and meta-analysis of clinical trials. *Biomedicines.* 2020;8(9):331.
13. Lazar SW, Kerr CE, Wasserman RH, et al. Meditation experience is associated with increased cortical thickness. *Neuroreport.* 2005;16(17): 1893–1897.

14. Maki PM, Jaff NG. Brain fog in menopause: a health-care professional's guide for decision-making and counseling on cognition. *Climacteric.* 2022;25(6):570-578.

15. Hölzel BK, Carmody J, Vangel M, et al. Mindfulness practice leads to increases in regional brain gray matter density. *Psychiatry Res.* 2011;191(1):36-43.

16. Whitfield T, et al. The effect of mindfulness-based programs on cognitive function in adults: a systematic review and meta-analysis. *Neuropsychology Rev.* 2022;32(3):677-702.

17. Livingston G, et al. Dementia prevention, intervention, and care. 2020 report of the Lancet commission. *Lancet.* 2020;396(10248):413-446.

18. Oliveira D, et al. Motivation and willingness to increase physical activity for dementia risk reduction: cross-sectional UK survey with people aged 50 and over. *Aging Ment Health.* 2022;26(9):1899-1908.

19. Whitfield T, Barnhofer T, Acabchuk R, et al. The effect of mindfulness-based programs on cognitive function in adults: a systematic review and meta-analysis. *Neuropsychol Rev.* 2022;32(3):677-702.

20. Krivanedk TJ, et al. Promoting successful cognitive aging: a ten-year update. *J Alzheimers Dis.* 2021;81:871-920.

CHAPTER 10. SUCCESSFUL SLEEP

1. Mure LS. Diurnal transcriptome atlas of a primate across major neural and peripheral tissues. *Science.* 2018;6381:359.

2. Zhang Y, Ren R, Yang L, et al. Sleep in Alzheimer's disease: a systematic review and meta-analysis of polysomnographic findings. *Transl Psychiatry.* 2022;12(1):136.

3. Covassin N, Singh P, McCrady-Spitzer SK, et al. Effects of experimental sleep restriction on energy intake, energy expenditure, and visceral obesity. *J Am Coll Cardiol.* 2022;79(13):1254-1265.

4. Lim AS, Kowgier M, Yu L, Buchman AS, Bennett DA. Sleep fragmentation and the risk of incident Alzheimer's disease and cognitive decline in older persons. *Sleep.* 2013;36(7):1027-1032.

5. Attarian H, et al. Treatment of chronic insomnia disorder in menopause: evaluation of literature. *Menopause.* 2014;22(6):674-684.

6. Lam C, et al. Behavioral interventions for improving sleep outcomes in menopausal women: a systematic review and meta-analysis. *Menopause.* 2022;29(10):1210-1221.

7. Nowakowski S, Meers JM. Cognitive-behavior therapy for sleep disorders at midlife. NAMS Practice Pearl. February 16, 2021.
8. Kling J, et al. Associations of sleep and female sexual function: good sleep quality matters. *Menopause*. 2021;28(6):619-625.
9. Zolfaghari S, et al. Effects of menopause on sleep quality and sleep disorders: Canadian Longitudinal Study on Aging. *Menopause*. 2019;27(3):295-304.
10. Ohayon MM. Determining the level of sleepiness in the American population and its correlates. *J Psychiatr Res*. 2012;46(4):422-427.
11. Kim M, et al. Light at night in older age is associated with obesity, diabetes, and hypertension. *Sleep*. 2023;46(3):zsac130.
12. Akhlaghi M, Kohanmeo A. Sleep deprivation in the development of obesity, effects on appetite regulation, energy metabolism, and dietary choices [published online October 31, 2023]. *Nutr Res Rev*.
13. Edelman JS. Sleep disorders update. ACOG, Clinical Updates in Women's Healthcare. September 2015.

CHAPTER 11. BETTER BONES

1. Wright NC, et al. The recent prevalence of osteoporosis and low bone mass in the United States based on bone mineral density at the femoral neck or lumbar spine. *J Bone Miner Res*. 2014;29:2520-2526.
2. Management of osteoporosis in postmenopausal women, the 2021 position statement of The North American Menopause Society. *Menopause*. 2021;28(9):973-997.
3. ACOG Clinical Practice guideline No 2. Managing postmenopausal osteoporosis. *Obstet Gynecol*. 2022;139(1):698-717.
4. Thi V, et al. Calcium intake and bone mineral density: systematic review and meta-analysis. *BMJ*. 2015;351:h4183.
5. Camacho PM, et al. Endocrinology clinical practice guidelines for the diagnosis and treatment of postmenopausal osteoporosis—2020 update. *Endocr Pract*. 2020;26(suppl 1):1-46.
6. Cosman F, Dempster DW. Anabolic agents for postmenopausal osteoporosis: how do you choose? *Curr Osteoporos Rep*. 2021; 10(2):189-205.
7. McClung MR. Role of bone forming agents in the management of osteoporosis. *Aging Clin Exp Res*. 2021;33(4):775-791.

8. Kanis JA, et al. Algorithm for the management of patients at low, high and very high risk of osteoporotic fractures. *Osteoporos Int.* 2020;31(1):1–12.

CHAPTER 12. LIFESTYLE CHOICES FOR LIVING LONGER

1. Kapoor E, et al. Weight gain in women at midlife: a concise review of the pathophysiology and strategies for management. *Mayo Clin Proc.* 2017;92(19):1552–1558.
2. Marlatt KL, et al. Body composition and cardiometabolic health across the menopause transition. *Obesity (Silver Spring).* 2022;30:14–27.
3. Knight MG, et al. Weight regulation in menopause. *Menopause.* 2021;28(8):960–965.
4. Li R, et al. Associations of muscle mass and strength with all-cause mortality among US older adults. *Med Sci Sports Exerc.* 2018;50:458.
5. Berra K, Hughes S. Counseling patients for lifestyle change—making a 15-minute office visit work. NAMS Practice Pearl. December 29, 2014. © The Menopause Society.
6. Murawski ME, Milsom VA, Ross KM, et al. Problem solving, treatment adherence, and weight-loss outcome among women participating in lifestyle treatment for obesity. *Eat Behav.* 2009;10(3):146–151.
7. Chlebowski RT, Aragaki AK, Anderson GL, et al; Women's Health Initiative. Dietary modification and breast cancer mortality: long-term follow-up of the Women's Health Initiative randomized trial. *J Clin Oncol.* 2020;38(13):1419–1428.
8. Varady KA. Dietary strategies for weight loss in midlife women. *Menopause.* 2018;25(6):697–699.

CHAPTER 13. CURBING YOUR RISK OF CANCER

1. www.SEER.cancer.gov>statfacts>html>breast. Accessed January 8, 2023.
2. World Cancer Research Fund/American Institute for Cancer Research. Diet, nutrition, physical activity and breast cancer. Continuous update project expert report 2018. wcrf.org/diet-activity-and-cancer/cancer-types/breast-cancer/. Accessed February 1, 2023.
3. US Department of Health and Human Services, US Department of Agriculture. *2015–2020 Dietary Guidelines for Americans.* 8th ed. December 2015. https://health.gov/our-work/food-nutrition/previous-dietary-guidelines/2015. Accessed February 1, 2023.

4. Mussallem D. Lifestyle for breast cancer risk reduction. *Menopause.* 2022;29(8):979–981.
5. Dense breasts Q&A guide. www.NationalBreastCancer.org. Accessed February 1, 2023.
6. Henley SJ, et al. Annual report to the nation on the status of cancer I. National cancer statistics. *Cancer.* 2020;126:2225–2249.
7. ACOG Committee Opinion # 557. Management of acute abnormal bleeding in non- pregnant reproductive-aged women. April 2013.
8. Fontham ETH, et al. Cervical cancer screening for individuals at average risk: 2020 guideline update from the American Cancer Society. *CA Cancer J Clin.* 2020;70:321–346.
9. Mills JM, et al. Eligibility for cervical cancer screening exit: comparison of a national and safety net cohort. *Gynecol Oncol.* 2021; 162:308–314.
10. Reilly G, Bullock RG, Greenwood J, et al. Analytical validation of a deep neural network algorithm for the detection of ovarian cancer. *JCO Clin Cancer Inform.* 2022;6:e2100192.
11. Huber D, et al. Use of oral contraceptives in BRCA mutation carriers and risk for ovarian and breast cancer: a systematic review. *Arch Gynecol Obstet.* 2020;301:875–884.
12. Saccardi C, et al. New light on endometrial thickness as a risk factor of cancer; what do clinicians need to know? *Cancer Manage Res.* 2022; 14:1331–1340.
13. Clarke MA, et al. Racial and ethnic differences in hysterectomy-corrected uterine corpus cancer mortality by stage and histologic subtype. *JAMA Oncol.* 2022;6:895–203.

GLOSSARY

Adenomyosis—back-bleeding that occurs when the blood pushes backward through the uterus wall instead of out of the uterus through the cervix and into the vagina

Anemia—low iron in the blood

Arteriosclerosis—hardening of the arteries, a sign of heart disease

Atrophic vaginitis—thinning and drying of vaginal wall tissue from lack of estrogen

Atypia—nucleus of cell is not normal but not distorted enough to classify as cancer

Atypical cells of uncertain significance—ASCUS, atypical cells in cervix on Pap smear

Bacterial vaginosis—most common vaginal infection with abnormal bacteria

Bone mineral density—usually checked with a DXA to estimate risk of thin bones and fracture risk typically done in women age 60 and over

Breast artery calcification—calcium deposits in breast arteries

Candida vulvitis—yeast infection of skin outside vagina

Candida vulvovaginitis—yeast infection of vagina and outside skin (vulva)

Chlamydia—infection of the cervix that may be silent, affects fertility, contagious

Cervical intraepithelial neoplasia—degrees of precancer changes in the cervix

Cervix—outer opening of the womb/uterus where Pap smear is taken

Colposcopy—microscope exam to check for abnormal tissue (on cervix, vulva, or vagina)

Condylomata—genital warts caused by the human papillomavirus

Cone biopsy—removal of precancerous tissue in the cervix (also called LEEP cone biopsy)

Contraceptive patch—birth control in patch form

Coronary artery calcium score—estimating risk of heart disease by looking at calcium in arteries

Coronary artery disease—disease of the arteries supplying the heart

Coronary CT angiography—dye study to identify changes in coronary arteries using CT scan

Cortical bone—outer covering of bones

Cystic lump—lump that has a fluid-filled cyst or cysts in it, not solid

Cystitis—bladder infection

Cystocele—weak bladder support

Digital mammogram—mammogram using technology to convert X-rays to electronic signals like a digital camera to increase accuracy

Dilatation and curettage—a gynecologist opens the cervix and samples the uterus lining to evaluate it. Hysteroscopy is recommended at the same time to directly visualize the lining

Dual-energy X-ray absorptiometry (DXA)—low-dose painless X-ray to estimate risk of fracture and thin bones in spine and hip

Echocardiogram—sound wave test of heart function

Eclampsia—high blood pressure during pregnancy, excess protein in the urine and seizures during pregnancy or shortly after birth

Endometrial (uterine) cancer—cancer of the lining of the uterus

Endometrial biopsy—tissue sample of the uterus lining

Endometrial hyperplasia—precancer of the uterus

Endometrial polyps—soft tissue growth in the uterus lining

Endometrium—uterine lining

Endothelial dysfunction—abnormal behavior of uterus lining cells

Estradiol—estrogen produced in ovaries during reproductive years

Estrogen—general term for all types of estrogen

Estrone—a weaker estrogen made in fatty tissue—the dominant form of estrogen in postmenopausal women

Factor V Leiden—a hereditary condition with a high risk of blood clots

Female sexual dysfunction—when a woman is dissatisfied with her sexual function

Ferritin—iron reserves

Fibroids—solid muscle wall tumors

Follicular stimulating hormone—FSH, a hormone that is elevated in post menopause and shows erratic levels in perimenopause

Gastritis—inflammation of the lining of the stomach

Gastroesophageal reflux disease—stomach acid pushes back to irritate the esophagus, the food tube connecting the mouth with the stomach

Genitourinary syndrome of menopause—GSM includes vaginal thinning, dryness, and tissue thinning of the urinary system due to lack of estrogen found in post menopause and often starting in perimenopause

Gonorrhea—a sexually transmitted infection, often silent, that requires antibiotics

Heart attack—blockage or spasm of an artery that supplies oxygen to the heart

Hematocrit—measures the proportion of the red blood cells in your blood, helps assess anemia

Hip structural analysis (HSA)—a research tool to check for quality of bone

Human papillomavirus—HPV, a virus that causes warts or cancer or precancer

Hysterectomy—surgical removal of the uterus

Hysteroscope—slender microscope to visualize the uterus lining

Hysteroscopy—microscopic exam of the uterus lining

Intrauterine device (IUD)—device placed in the uterus lining to prevent pregnancy; if medicated with progesterone, it may also control bleeding and prevent endometrial cancer

Isoflavones—component of soy that can act like a weak estrogen or a weak antiestrogen

Laparoscope—microscope introduced through the navel

Lichen sclerosis—a chronic skin condition of the vulva skin outside the vagina typically producing white lesions, may be painful or silent

Lichen simplex chronicus—thick scaley dry patchy areas, may occur on the vulva and result from chronic itching/scratching

Loop electrical excision procedure—use radiofrequency or laser to remove abnormal cervix tissue

Mammogram—low-dose X-ray screening exam to detect breast cancer before it is visible/palpable

Melanoma—skin cancer with irregular border and discoloration

Metabolic syndrome (syndrome X)—an individual with three of the five conditions listed has a high risk of heart disease and diabetes (excess fat at waist, high blood pressure, high triglycerides, low HDL cholesterol, and high fasting glucose)

Oophorectomy—removal of one or both ovaries

Osteoblasts—bone-building cells

Osteoclasts—bone-dissolving cells

Osteopenia—now called low bone mass, with bone thinning and a modest increase in fracture risk

Osteoporosis—critical loss of bone strength in hip or spine with a high risk for a fracture

Pelvic inflammatory disease—infection with inflammation of tubes, ovaries, and uterus

Peritoneum—inner lining of abdomen

Pessary—a ring or other device placed in the vagina to hold up the tissue

Polycystic ovary syndrome—ovaries produce excess male sex hormone and may also produce excess ovarian cysts, can lead to insulin resistance and weight gain

Polyps—soft fleshy tissue growths may occur in bowel, vagina, or uterus lining

Posttraumatic stress disorder—long-term symptoms affecting mental health after life-threatening events

Preeclampsia—high blood pressure and excess protein in the urine during pregnancy

Premature ovarian insufficiency—POI, ovaries stop functioning normally before age 40

Premenstrual syndrome—mood changes, bloating, breast tenderness, or anxiety that may occur two days or two weeks before a menstrual period and typically resolve when menses start

Rectocele—support wall above the rectum is weak, allowing the rectum to bulge into the vagina, a type of prolapse

Sarcopenia—muscle loss as part of the aging process

Sonohysterogram—test that uses sound waves and sterile salt water injected into the uterus lining to view the uterus lining indirectly using ultrasound

Stages of Reproductive Aging Workshop (STRAW) framework—a study that looks at phases of menopause in many women over time

Stroke—also called CVA, cerebral vascular accident, caused by abnormal blood vessels in the brain that are compromised by a blockage that reduces blood supply or a brain bleed

Synthetic mammogram—using a three-dimensional tomo mammo to reconstruct two-dimensional mammo images without using additional radiation

Thermogram—images the breasts using a photograph that shows differences in temperature. Research has not shown that this is an effective screening method

Therapeutic ultrasound—using highly focused ultrasound as a treatment modality for fibroids

Tomosynthesis—uses X-rays to take pictures of the inside of the breast, then a computer reconstructs three-dimensional images used to screen for early breast cancer

Trabecular bone—spongy porous bone in center of vertebrae and long bones

Trichomonas—sexually transmitted vaginal infection caused by a protozoon that typically causes irritation and an odor

Tubal ligation—cutting, tying, or cauterizing the tubes to prevent pregnancy

Ultrasound—sound wave test to image internal organs

Urethra—narrow tube that allows the urine to exit the bladder above the top of the vagina

Uterine artery embolization—technique that decreases blood flow to the uterus from its outer blood supply

Uterine (endometrial) cancer—cancer of the lining of the uterus

Vaginal ring—vaginal rings may contain medication such as NuvaRing, a ring for birth control, or Estring, a ring to supply low-dose estrogen to the vagina, or FemRing that supplies estrogen to the vagina as well as the rest of the body

Vaginal stenosis—narrowing of the vaginal opening

Vasectomy—a male sterilization procedure usually performed as an outpatient under local

Vulva—outer lips of the vagina

INDEX

Abaloparatide, 382
abdominal fat, 21, 392, 393, 396, 400
abortion, 123, 257, 442, 476
Activella, 88, 94
Actonel, 377, 378
acupuncture, 58, 328
adenomyosis, 138, 139, 143, 153–56; endometrial ablation for, 156, 164–66, 169; Lupron for, 168–69
adipose tissue, 21, 157, 158, 321, 440, 456. *See also* body fat; obesity/overweight
aerobic exercise, 408–9
age: at first menstrual period, 6; at menopause, 5–8
aging: and bone thinning, 351; and depression, 291–92; and heart disease, 8, 121–22; and memory loss, 307–8; and sleep issues, 324; societal views, 2–3, 35, 272; Stages of Reproductive Aging Workshop (STRAW) framework, 5; and weight gain, 400, 410–11, 430
agnus-castus, 289

alcohol intake, 414; and breast cancer risk, 438; and hormone therapy (HT), 79; and hot flashes, 43; during pregnancy, 251; and sexual experience, 229; and sleep quality, 340
Alendronate, 375, 376, 382–83, 385
allergies: bee stings, 56; medications, 96, 196; peanuts, 82, 100, 243; pets, 342
Alzheimer's disease, 309; and estrogen, 315–16; and mindfulness meditation, 311–14; prevention, 310–11; and sleep, 321; testing for, 316. *See also* dementia
Andriol, 240
androgen levels, 438–39
anemia, 138–40; blood tests for, 148, 150; and osteoporosis, 354; and prolonged bleeding, 137, 150, 163, 171–72
Annovera, 265
annual checkups, 76, 101, 446, 468
anorexia, 354, 357, 359, 374

antibiotics: for bacterial vaginosis, 191–92; for Bartholin gland cyst, 218; sexual effects, 213–14; for sexually transmitted infections, 195; for urinary tract infection, 178–79; yeast infection after, 190
antidepressants, 59–60, 300–301; drug holiday from, 214–15; and osteoporosis risk, 355; and sex drive, 214–15. *See also* selective serotonin reuptake inhibitors (SSRIs)
anti-estrogen medications, 355; Lupron, 168–69, 355
antihistamines, 214
anti-Müllerian hormone (AMH), 5
anxiety: counseling/therapy, 301–2, 312; and heart disease risk, 124; and mental health, 290–92, 296; and PMS/PMDD, 285, 287, 288; and progesterone, 275; and serotonin, 275; and sex, 207, 213, 215, 237; and stress response, 279
appearance, 234, 272
appetite, changes in, 283, 287, 295, 400, 430, 473
aqua jogging, 406
aromatase inhibitors, 95
arteriosclerosis, 116. *See also* cardiovascular disease (CVD)
Ashkenazi Jews, 475
aspirin: as blood thinner, 173; for CVD prevention, 129–31; and vitamin E, 57
assisted living, 314–15
Atenolol, 214, 296
Atkins diet, 421, 423, 424–25
atrophic vaginitis, 188, 189

back-bleeding, 138, 139, 143, 153–56. *See also* adenomyosis
bacterial infections, 191–92
bacterial vaginosis, 189, 191, 192, 193
balance exercises, 409; and fall risk, 371. *See also* falls
Balneol, 199
bariatric surgery, 401
Barnard, Neal, 41–42, 427
barrier contraceptive methods, 254–57
Bartholin gland cysts, 218
Basson, Rosemary, 204–5
Bazedoxifene, 102
Be Kool Strips®, 45
belly fat, 21, 392, 393, 396, 399
Benzocaine, 196, 256
Best Friends (Josselson), 280
beta-blockers, 214, 296
bilateral oophorectomy, 27
bioidentical hormones, 93–99
birth control. *See* contraception
bisphosphonates, 375, 376–80; benefits of, 377–78; side effects, 378–79
black cohosh, 54–55
Black women: and abnormal bleeding, 175; age at menopause, 6; and uterine cancer, 175, 453, 454–55, 461
bladder: anatomical support for, 176, 180, 184–85, 187, 201; Botox for, 182; cystocele, 185, 216; infection of, 177–79; irritants, 220; medication side effects, 184; overactive, 62; training of, 220. *See also* incontinence, urinary
bleeding, abnormal, 133–73; adenomyosis, 153–56; after intercourse, 143; and anemia,

138–40; anti-estrogen injections, 168–69; blood thinners, 173; causes of, 141–43, 152–53; cycle length, 143–47; diagnostic tests, 148–52; endometrial ablation, 164–68; endometrial hyperplasia, 156–59; endometrium, dyssynchronous, 162–63; fibroids, 161–62; hormone treatments for, 169; hysterectomy, 171–72; iron supplementation, 138–40; lifelong heavy periods, 137; medical procedures, 163–64; menstrual tracking apps, 135; myomectomy, 170; PALM COEIN evaluation, 136; polyps, 159–61; postmenopausal bleeding, 147–48; severity of, 137–38; spotting, 140; tranexamic acid, 172; uterine artery embolization (UAE), 170–71
bleeding, menstrual: and adenomyososis, 154, 168–69; blood loss, severity of, 137–38, 139–41; cycle length, evaluation of, 143–44; cycles and patterns, 19, 22, 134–35, 141, 145–46, 250; and endometrial ablation, 166, 168; heavy periods, 137; during perimenopause, 10, 22–23, 24, 113; and thyroid function, 149
bloating, 20, 88, 138, 154, 162, 283, 289, 473
blood clots: and estrogen therapy, 70, 80, 85, 89, 228–29, 267; and heart attack, 117; and medications for hot flashes, 59; and metabolic syndrome, 395; and oral contraceptives, 260–61; and stroke, 116; tranexemic acid, 172
blood clotting disorders, 262

blood pressure, high, 115–16; and exercise, 397, 403; and heart disease risk, 125–26; and hot flashes, 38, 41; lowering without medication, 117, 280, 369, 371; and metabolic syndrome, 395–96; and oral contraceptives, 261; and polycystic ovarian syndrome, 113; in pregnancy, 123; and sleep apnea, 330; and smoking, 108; and vascular dementia, 309. See also stroke
blood pressure medication, 61, 214; and depression, 296; and hot flashes, 59, 61; and sleep quality, 325
blood tests: for abnormal bleeding, 148–49, 150; CA125, 473, 474–75; follicle-stimulating hormone (FSH), 23–24; thyroid hormone, 39–40, 282, 296
blood thinners, 56, 57–58, 173
bloody nipple discharge, 442
BMD (bone mineral density), 358, 360, 365, 376, 380
body fat, 21, 109, 114, 321, 336–37, 392–93, 397, 399, 403, 440. See also adipose tissue; obesity/overweight
body mass index (BMI), 6, 109–10; and cancer risk, 439
bone health, 345–87; anabolic medications, 382–84; bone formation, 350–51; bone quality, 386; bone thinning/loss, 345–46, 351–53; calcium supplementation, 367–70; dual-energy X-ray absorptiometry (DXA) test, 358–65; fracture risk and treatment options, 374–76; fracture

508   Index

bone health (cont.)
  risk assessment tool (FRAX), 364–66; importance of, 346, 347–48; measurement of, 358–66; medication for, 372–81; ongoing reassessment, 384–85; promotion of, 367; selective estrogen receptor modulators (SERMs), 381–82; vitamin D, 370–71. See also osteoporosis
bone mineral density (BMD), 358, 360, 365, 376, 380
Boniva, 376, 378, 385
Botox injections, 182
brain: brain fog, 304–5; brain-heart connection, 114. See also cognitive decline
BRCA1/BRCA2 mutations, 111, 450, 473–76
breast artery calcification (BAC), 131
breast cancer, 437–53; alcohol intake and risk, 82; aromatase inhibitors, 95; breast biopsy, 60, 442, 444, 445; breast cancer modeling, 452–53; breast magnetic resonance imaging (MRI), 446–49; COVID-19 vaccine, 446–47; dense breast tissue and cancer risk, 440–41, 443–44; digital mammogram, 443–44; doctor-patient partnership, 451–53; family history, 447–48; genetic testing, 449–51, 452; and hormone therapy (HT), 72, 77, 92, 228; and oral contraceptive use, 262; questions to ask doctor, 452–53; risk factors, 72, 76, 438–42; screening, 443–45; survivors, and sex, 245–46; symptoms, 442; thermogram, 444–45; 3D mammogram, 444; ultrasound, 445
breastfeeding, 124–25
breasts: breast cyst, 445; breast disease, benign, 75, 442; breast exams, 76, 89, 446, 449, 450; breast tenderness, 10, 20, 94, 283, 284; nipple discharge, 442
breathing: disordered, in sleep apnea, 329–31; and meditation, 312; paced respiration for hot flashes, 41; relaxation for anxiety, 290, 296
bremelanotide, 244
Brewer, Judson, 429
bulimia, 354, 357, 359, 374
Bupropion, 211, 215, 300

CA125 ovarian testing, 473, 474–76, 478
caffeine, 288; and cancer risk, 442; and hot flashes, 43–44; and osteoporosis, 354; and sleep quality, 339–40
calcium: and bone thinning, 346; food sources, 363, 368–69; for PMS, 288; and risk of osteoporosis, 354, 356; supplementation, 358, 362, 367–70; and vitamin D, 371
calorie requirements, 410–11. See also diet/nutrition
cancer: bleeding as symptom, 137, 142, 143, 147, 152–53; chemotherapy, 355; and depression, 296; detection, early, 149–50, 194, 437; exercise and cancer risk, 402; fibroids and cancer risk, 161–62; hormones and cancer risk, 49, 60; polyps as precancerous, 159–61;

Index   509

risk factors, 14–15, 436; soy and cancer risk, 47–48. *See also* specific cancers
cancer antigen-125 (CA125) testing, 473, 474–76, 478
candida vaginitis/vulvovaginitis, 190, 197
cannabis, 58; and sleep quality, 340
carbohydrates: cravings, 419; healthy carbs, 412, 421, 423; metabolism, 336, 394, 410; and mood, 412; and sleep, 339; "white stuff," 413
carcinoid cancer, 81
cardiovascular disease (CVD), 105–32; aspirin for prevention, 129–31; definitions and measurement, 115–17; diagnosis of, 131; gender differences, 118–21; and hormone therapy (HT), 77; lactation as protection against, 124–25; medication for, 126–27; prevention, 107; risk, reducing, 124–31; risk assessment, 106, 128–29; risk factors, 14, 108–14, 121–24; stress as risk factor, 114–15
cardiovascular exercise, 408–9
Catapress, 61
Caya (diaphragm), 256
CBT (cognitive behavioral therapy). *See* cognitive behavioral therapy (CBT)
celiac sprue disease, 354
central sleep apnea (CSA), 329
cervical cancer, 194, 461–72; American Society of Colposcopy and Cervical Pathology guidelines, 463–66; doctor's visits, 471–72; risk factors, 461–62; screening for (Pap smear), 462–66; surveillance vs. screening, 466–70; symptoms, 462; vaccine for, 194, 462. *See also* Pap smears
cervical cap, 257
cervical dysplasia/precancer, 194, 470
chasteberry, 289
chemotherapy, 355
chlamydia, 143, 150, 193, 194–95, 255, 260
cholesterol levels, 7, 10, 13–14, 110; and estrogen supplementation, 261; HDL cholesterol, 395, 396, 397; and heart disease risk, 125, 126; LDL cholesterol, 110, 114, 396, 397; and metabolic syndrome, 395–96; during perimenopause, 114; and polycystic ovarian syndrome, 113; reducing, 117; and testosterone supplementation, 239, 240
Cialis, 209–10, 242
Citrucel, 220
Climara, 84
clitoral changes, 96, 197–98, 208, 209, 238, 240
Clonidine, 61
CO_2 lasers, 188–89, 245
coffee. *See* caffeine
cognitive behavioral therapy (CBT), 42–43, 246, 288, 301–2; for anxiety, 290–91; for insomnia, 325–26; for urinary issues, 181
cognitive decline, 305–7; and sleep, 321. *See also* dementia
collagen: and stress urinary incontinence, 179–80, 184–85; and uterine prolapse, 187, 216; and vaginal scarring, 245
colorectal cancer, 15, 68, 74, 321, 369, 371, 427

colposcopy, 462
CombiPatch, 88–89, 100
compounded bioidentical hormone therapy (cBHT), 95–99; customization, 99–101; safety vs. risks, 98–99
computed tomography angiography, 131
condoms: female, 254–55; male, 255–56
constipation, 186, 220–21, 414, 425
contact dermatitis, 196–97
contraception, 249–68; barrier methods, 254; cervical cap, 257; Depo Provera, 260; diaphragms, 256–57; estetrol, 267; female condoms, 254–55; female sterilization, 265–66; IUDs, 259–60; male condoms, 255–56; male sterilization, 266–67; "morning after" pill, 257–58; on-demand birth control, 253–54; oral contraceptives, 260–63; "rhythm" method, 252; skin patches, 264; spermicide, 253; vaginal rings, 265; "withdrawal" method, 252–53
controlled positive airway pressure (CPAP), 331
coronary artery disease, 116. See also cardiovascular disease (CVD)
coronary heart disease (CHD), 8. See also cardiovascular disease (CVD)
cortical bone, 350, 363, 386
corticosteroids: and bone thinning, 359; and weight gain, 430
cortisol: and sleep, 336; and stress, 279, 311–12, 415
counseling, 301–2. See also cognitive behavioral therapy (CBT)
COVID-19 vaccine, 251, 442, 446–47

CPAP (controlled positive airway pressure), 331
cranberry juice/supplements, 177
C-reactive protein, 129
CSA (central sleep apnea), 329–30
cultural contexts, 291–92
Cymbalta, 300
cystitis, 177, 183. See also bladder
cystocele, 185, 216–17

daidzein, 47–48
dairy products, 362, 368, 420, 424
D&C (dilatation and curettage), 151, 159
DASH diet, 420, 426
Data Registry on Experiences of Aging, Menopause and Sexuality (DREAMS), 334
deep vein thrombosis (DVT), 382
dehydration, 340. See also hydration
Dehydroepiandrosterone (DHEA), 241–42, 245
dementia, 309; and estrogen, 315–16; and mindfulness meditation, 311–14; prevention, 310–11; testing for, 316; vascular dementia, 309. See also Alzheimer's disease
Denosumab, 375, 376, 380–81, 383
deodorant, 199, 442
Depakote, 355
Depo Provera, 260, 354
depression, 114, 291–304; counseling/psychotherapy, 301–2; and estrogen, 275, 303; exercise as treatment, 303; factors affecting, 296; Geriatric Depression Scale, 296–97; in perimenopause, 270–71, 293–94; prescription medications, 300–301; psilocybin as treatment, 303–4; risk factors,

293; screening/assessment of, 295–97; and social isolation, 295; St. John's wort, 299–300; treatment options, 297–99
dermatitis, contact, 196–97
DES (diethylstilbestrol) exposure, 466–67
Desipramine, 215
desquamative inflammatory vaginitis (DIV), 193
DHEA (dehydroepiandrosterone), 241–42, 245
diabetes, 14–15, 393–94; and cardiovascular disease (CVD) risk, 110; osteoporosis risk, 354; and sex, 219
diaphragm, contraceptive, 256–57
Diethylstilbestrol (DES) exposure, 466–67
diet/nutrition, fats, dietary: and cancer risk, 439; fiber intake, 220–21; foods to avoid, 413–14; high-fat diets, 108; high-fiber, 220–21, 289; hot flashes, impact on, 34–35, 41–42, 47–50, 64; optimal nutrition, 410–12; PMS, 283; processed foods, 108; vegan diets, 41–42, 288–89. See also cholesterol levels
diets for weight loss, 126, 417–20; Atkins diet, 424–25; calorie counting, 412; cautions concerning, 413; DASH diet, 420, 426; evaluation of, 420–23; food journals, 428–29; foods to avoid, 413–14; high-protein, 356; intermittent fasting, 427–28; low-fat, 426; Mediterranean Diet, 420, 425; Sonoma diet, 422, 425; South Beach diet, 422, 425–26;
vegetarian/vegan, 426–27. See also weight reduction
digital mammography, 443–44, 453
Dilantin, 355
dilatation and curettage (D&C), 151, 159
diuretics, 214, 289
Divigel, 84
D-mannose, 178
doctor-patient team, 12–16, 28–29, 451–53, 478
doctor visits, 30–31, 451–52, 460–61, 471–72, 478; annual checkups, 76, 101, 446, 468
dong quai, 56, 173
douching, 200
dual-energy X-ray absorptiometry (DXA) test, 348, 358–65; advantages of, 363–64; limitations of, 364–65; ongoing reassessment, 384–85; T scores and clinical diagnosis, 359–63; Z scores, 365
Duavee (bazedoxifene), 102
Duloxetine, 300
DVT (deep vein thrombosis), 382
DXA. See Dual-energy X-ray absorptiometry (DXA) test
dyslipidemia, 395. See also cholesterol levels

early menopause: and cardiovascular disease (CVD) risk, 111–12; and hormone therapy (HT), 83–84
Eat, Drink, and Be Healthy (Willett), 413
eating disorders, 354, 357, 359, 374
eczema, 196, 218
Effexor, 59–60, 300
EKG (electrocardiogram), 118, 120

electrical stimulation for urge incontinence, 181
electrocardiogram (EKG), 118, 120
EMBR cooling device, 45
"empty nesters," 236, 272–73
Emsella™ chair, 183–84
endometrial ablation, 164–69; types of, 166–68
endometrial biopsy, 149, 150, 151, 154, 156, 158, 159, 165, 172
endometrial cancer. *See* uterine cancer
endometrial hyperplasia, 143, 156–59; diagnosis, 159; risk factors, 157–58; types of, 157
endometriosis, 138, 475, 476. *See also* adenomyosis
epinephrine, 279
Equelle, 48–49
Equol, 431
erectile dysfunction, 209–10
Escitalopram, 300
Estetrol, 102, 267
Estraderm, 84
Estradiol, 20, 84; gel, 84
EstraTest, 240
Estring vaginal ring, 89, 227–28
estrogen levels, 3–4, 18–19; and bone thinning, 375; and cognition, 315–16; fluctuations, 19–20; and osteoporosis, 15; and sleep, 334; types of estrogen, 20; and weight gain, 392
estrogen therapy: for bone health, 381; depression, as treatment for, 303; estrogen alone, 87–88; estrogen-related options, 101–2; low-dose vaginal cream, 226; for low sexual desire, 242; oral, decreasing effectiveness of, 89–90; oral, for low sexual desire, 243; safety guidelines for, 81–82; and serotonin, 274–75; stopping, 91–92; systemic, contraindications, 80; vaginal, 181, 211
Estromineral Serena, 326
Estrone, 21
ethnicity: and cancer risk, 455; and osteoporosis risk, 357; and timing of menopause, 6
Evamist, 84
evening primrose oil, 288
Evenity, 376, 382
Evista, 381–82
exercise: choosing activities, 403–6; and constipation, 220; and CVD risk, 125–26; and dementia prevention, 310; and hot flashes, 34–35, 50; inactive lifestyles and cardiovascular disease (CVD) risk, 109; and insomnia, 326, 328; and osteoporosis risk, 356; and overall health, 401–2; for physical restrictions, 405; and sexual experience, 230; and sleep quality, 339; strength training, 408; and timing of menopause, 7; as treatment for depression, 303; types of, 407–10; weight-bearing and bone health, 371
exercise stress test, 120, 127, 432

falls: and balance exercises, 371, 409; fall risk, 324, 353, 367, 371; and osteoporotic fracture, 349
family history: Alzheimer's disease, 309; bleeding, abnormal, 134, 145; breast cancer, 262, 386–87, 438, 441, 443, 446–47, 449–50; and

cancer risk, 441, 447; clotting disorders, 262; depression, 296; diabetes, 110, 219; heart disease, 109, 128–29; osteoporosis, 355, 359, 364, 366, 374; ovarian cancer, 473–74; psychosis, 304. *See also* medical history
fasting, intermittent, 427–28
fats, dietary: healthy fats, 411, 419; low-fat diets, 127, 288–89, 419, 424, 426; omega-3 fatty acids, 57; processed foods, 108; and weight loss, 126
FDA. *See* U.S. Food and Drug Administration (FDA)
female condom, 254–55
female sexual dysfunction (FSD), 205–6
Femring, 80, 89
ferritin test, 148, 151, 161, 167, 173, 458
fertility, 21–22, 272
fiber in diet: and calcium absorption, 368; and constipation, 186, 220–21; and estrogen levels, 289; and hot flashes, 47
fibroids, 143, 161–62
"fight or flight" response, 277. *See also* stress
fitness, 397–98. *See also* exercise
flaxseed, 51, 56–57
flexibility: mental, 304, 310, 312; physical, 399, 405, 407, 410
Flibanserin, 243–44
fluid intake, 340
Fluoxetine, 300
folate, 251
follicles (ovarian), 5, 18, 19, 25, 27
follicle-stimulating hormone (FSH), 5; blood tests for, 23–24

food journal/diary, 414, 428–29
food pyramid, 412–13
Forteo, 376, 382
Fosamax, 370, 375, 376, 383
fractures: fracture risk and treatment options, 374–76; fragility fractures, 346; hip, 347–48, 366, 379; osteoporotic, 15, 347–50; risk for, 361–62, 363, 364–66, 374–76; spinal, 352, 357, 376, 387; wrist, 409
Framingham Heart Study, 6–7
FRAX tool (fracture risk assessment) tool, 364–66
friendship, 280–81; and social exercising, 406
FSH (follicle-stimulating hormone), 5, 23–24

Gabapentin, 61–62, 245
Gardasil, 469
garlic, 57
gastric bypass surgery, 354
gastroesophageal reflux disease (GERD), 339
gender-based medical research, 2
genetic patterns and timing of menopause, 7
genetic testing, 449–50, 452
genistein, 47–48
genital herpes, 193
genital warts, 193–94, 256
genitourinary syndrome of menopause (GSM), 189
GERD (gastroesophageal reflux disease), 339
Geriatric Depression Scale (GDS), 296–97
ghrelin, 337
ginger, 57

ginkgo, 173
ginseng, 173
glucocorticoids, 355
gonorrhea, 143, 193, 195, 255, 260
grief, 297, 302. *See also* depression
growth hormone, 337
gut microbiome, 431; and soy supplements, 48
Guttersen, Connie, 420
gynecological examination, 148, 154, 155, 195, 211, 224

hardening of the arteries, 116. *See also* cardiovascular disease (CVD)
HDL cholesterol, 395, 396, 397. *See also* cholesterol levels
health history, 48, 68, 213
hearing loss, 311
heart attack, 117; gender differences, 118–21; risk of, 121–22. *See also* cardiovascular disease (CVD)
heart disease. *See* cardiovascular disease (CVD)
heart health, 6–7
heavy bleeding, 137, 152; and anemia, 138–39; bleeding, abnormal; and endometrial ablation, 164; and fibroids, 162. *See also* adenomyosis
Hematocrit (HCT), 148
Hemoglobin (Hgb), 148
hemorrhoids, 199, 200
Heparin, 355
herbal remedies, 54–55, 56, 173, 289, 299–300, 328
herpes, genital, 193
hidden threats to health, 14–15, 105
high blood pressure. *See* blood pressure, high
high-risk pregnancy, 112–13

high sensitivity C-reactive protein (hsCRP), 129
hip fracture, 347–48, 366, 379
hip structural analysis (HSA), 501
HIV/AIDS, 194
hormones: changing levels, 18–20; and mood, 273–75; in post menopause, 21. *See also* estrogen therapy; progesterone
hormone therapy (HT), 66–104; after hysterectomy, 84–85; and alcohol, 79; author's recommendations, 69; bioidentical hormones, 93–99; breast cancer, risk of, 72, 77, 439; combination therapy, 88–89; compounded bioidentical hormone therapy (cBHT), 95–101; decision-making, 66–69, 101, 276; and early menopause, 83–84; estrogen, safety guidelines for, 81–82; estrogen, stopping, 91–92; estrogen alone, 87–88; estrogen-related options, 101–2; heart disease, risk of, 77; hormone-releasing IUDs, 259; menopausal hormone therapy (MHT), history of, 67–68; new developments, 102–3; oral contraceptives, 86–87; oral estrogen, decreasing effectiveness, 89–90; ovarian cancer, risk of, 79; precautions, 82–83; progesterone alone, 88; stroke, risk of, 71; systemic estrogen, contraindications, 80; for vaginal dryness, 224–29; vaginal estrogen, 86; Women's Health Initiative (WHI), 69–74
hot flashes, 31–64; alcohol and, 43; antidepressants, 59–60; beginning after age 60, 80–81; blood

Index 515

pressure medication, 61; and caffeine, 43–44; cognitive behavioral therapy (CBT), 42–43; diet, impact of, 34–35; exercise, impact of, 34–35, 50; hot weather, tips for keeping cool, 44–45; lifestyle modifications, 41–42; medicine, new class of, 63; natural remedies, 50–58; nerve adjustment medication, 61–62; nonmenopausal causes, 38, 81; overactive bladder medicine, 62; paced respiration, 41; physical changes during, 34; prescription medications, 58–59; reframing attitudes, 35–36; stress reduction, 42; temperature control devices, 45–46; and thyroid disease, 38–40; treatment decisions, 37; triggers for, 41; variations in, 37–38
HTA (hydrothermal ablation), 165, 166–67
human papilloma virus (HPV), 193–94, 461–62; DNA testing, 466–67, 470; Pap smears, 462–66; vaccine, 194, 462
Hunger Habit, The (Brewer), 429
HyaloGyn, 223
hydration, 177, 181, 186, 235, 340
hydrothermal ablation (HTA), 165, 166–67
hyperthyroidism, 39; osteoporosis risk, 354. *See also* thyroid disease
hypnosis, 326
hypothyroidism, 39. *See also* thyroid disease
hysterectomy, 27–28; for abnormal bleeding, 171–72; and hormone therapy (HT), 84–85

hysteroscopy, 149–50, 151, 152, 164–65, 454, 458

Ibandronate, 376, 378
incontinence, urinary, 179–84; mixed incontinence, 182; stress incontinence, 179–80; treatment options, 183–84; urge incontinence, 62, 181, 182
independent living, 297
infections: sexually transmitted disease, 193–95; urinary tract, 177–79; vaginal, 189, 219
infertility, 112, 476
inflammatory bowel disease, 354
inhibin, 24–25
insomnia, 322–29; cognitive behavioral therapy for, 325–26; primary vs. secondary, 324; and sleep deprivation, 329. *See also* sleep problems
insulin, 336–37, 394. *See also* diabetes
insulin resistance, 321, 330, 394, 396, 420, 430
insulin sensitivity, 400, 425
intellectual stimulation, 279, 291, 294, 310
intermittent fasting, 427–28
internet research, 101, 142
interpersonal psychotherapy (IPT), 301–2
intrauterine device (IUD), 83–84, 254, 259–60, 459, 477; for endometrial hyperplasia, 156; levonorgestrel, for abnormal bleeding, 169; Mirena, 100
iron (ferritin) levels, 148, 151, 161, 167, 173, 458
iron supplements, 138–39, 167

irritability, 20, 37, 270, 275, 287, 323
irritable bowel syndrome, 221, 282
isoflavones, 47, 49–50, 56, 326
itching, vulvovaginal, 187–88, 189, 190, 192, 196–97, 201, 218–19
IUD. *See* intrauterine device (IUD)

Jenny Craig program, 423
Josselson, Ruthellen, 280

Kampo, 328
Kaplan, Helen Singer, 204
kegel exercises, 180; for cystocele, 185; Emsella™ chair, 183–84; for incontinence, 185–86; and painful sex, 212
kidney disease, 355
KNDy neurons, 63
Konsyl, 220
KULKUF cooling device, 45–46
K-Y Long-Lasting Vaginal Moisturizer, 223

lactation, 124–25
lactose intolerance, 362, 368, 369
latex allergy, 255
laxatives, 220–21. *See also* constipation
LCDs (liquid crystal displays), 342
LDL cholesterol, 110, 114, 396, 397. *See also* cholesterol levels
leanness, 399
Lensen, Sarah, 52–53
leptin, 337
Levonorgestrel Intrauterine Device, 169
Lexapro, 59–60, 300
LGBTQ populations, 205
Lichen sclerosis (LS), 197–98, 218–19
Lichen simplex chronicus, 197

Lidocaine, topical, 245
life expectancy, 5, 11–12
lifestyle choices, 390–434; exercise, 401–10; foods to avoid, 413–14; leanness and longevity, 399; metabolic syndrome (syndrome X), lowering risk, 397–98; nutrition, optimal, 410–12; stress eating, 415–16; weight loss, 400–401; weight loss diets, 417–28
lipid levels, 114; dyslipidemia, 395. *See also* cholesterol levels
liposuction, 400
liquid crystal displays (LCDs), 342
lithium, 355
loop electrical excision procedure, 466, 471
low bone mass (osteopenia), 348–49
low-fat diets, 426
lubricants, 223; and condom use, 255
Lupron, 168–69, 355
Lynch syndrome mutations, 473–74

magnesium intake, 289
magnetic resonance imaging (MRI): breast, 446–49; cardiac, 131
Maki, Pauline, 304–5
mammography: breast artery calcification (BAC), 131; digital, 443–44, 453; false alarms, 75–76
MARA (water vapor ablation), 165, 166–67
marijuana. *See* cannabis
massage, 327
medical history, 23, 28–29, 38, 101, 143, 145, 148, 357–58. *See also* family history
meditation, 290–91
Mediterranean Diet, 420, 425; and breast cancer risk, 439

Medroxyprogesterone acetate (Depo Provera), 260
melatonin, 320–21, 326–27, 334
memory: memory loss, 307–9; memory testing, 316. *See also* Alzheimer's disease; dementia
menarche, 113; and cancer risk, 441
Menest, 94
menopause, definitions, 4
MENOPOD cooling device, 46
menstrual calendar, 135, 139, 143, 168
menstrual cycles: cycle length, 143–47; irregular periods, 145–47; patterns, 134–36; during perimenopause, 22–23; shortened, in perimenopause, 113
menstrual history, 136, 455, 457, 458, 461
mental decline. *See* cognitive decline
mental exercise, 310
mental health, changes in, 269–73. *See also* depression; mood
metabolic syndrome (syndrome X), 394, 394–97; lowering risk, 397–98
Metronidazole (Flagyl), 192
microbiome, gut, 431
migraine headaches, 261
Miller, Jean Baker, 281
Million Women Study, 100–101
mindfulness-based therapy, 246
mindfulness meditation, 311–14, 327
Minerva ablation technique, 165, 167
Mirena IUD, 100, 156
Mirtazapine, 215
mood: anxiety, 290–91; changes in, 269–73; connection and friendship, 279–81; depression, 291–304; and hormones, 273–76; premenstrual dysphoric disorder (PMDD), 287–88; premenstrual syndrome (PMS), 281–86
"morning after" pill, 257–58
Mounjuaro, 400
MRI. *See* magnetic resonance imaging (MRI)
multiple sclerosis, 296
multitasking, 305, 306–7
multivitamins, 57
muscle mass loss, 391, 402, 410, 425, 430
myocardial infarction (MI). *See* heart attack
myomectomy, 170

naps, 341
National Health and Nutrition Examination Survey (NHANES), 347
National Osteoporosis Foundation, 346, 359, 389
natural remedies: cranberry juice/supplements, 177; herbal, 54–55, 56, 173, 289, 299–300, 328; for hot flashes, 50–58; paced respiration, 41; for PMS/PMDD, 288–89; yoga, 407. *See also* bioidentical hormones
Nelson, Miriam, 371
nerve adjustment medication, 61–62
NEST (native estrogen with selective action in tissues), 102–3
neurontin, 61–62
niacin, 38
night sweats, 36. *See also* hot flashes
nipple discharge, 442. *See also* breasts
nonrapid eye movement (NREM) sleep, 332

NOOM weight loss app, 126, 421, 425
nortriptyline, 215
NREM (nonrapid eye movement) sleep, 332
Nurses' Health Study II, 111
nutrition. *See* diet/nutrition
NuvaRing, 265

obesity/overweight, 109–10; and abnormal bleeding, 175; and cancer risk, 440; and uterine cancer, 456. *See also* diets for weight loss; weight reduction
obstructive sleep apnea (OSA), 330
odor: in urine, 178; vaginal, 189, 191, 192, 195
omega-3 fatty acids, 57
oophorectomy, 27, 85, 111
oral contraceptives, 27, 260–63; for abnormal bleeding, 169; contrasted with hormone therapy (HT), 86–87; interaction of, with natural remedies, 52, 55; for PMS/PMDD, 284, 289; risk of early menopause, 27
orgasm, 204–5, 206, 210, 213, 233, 244–45; sexual side effects of medications, 214, 215
Ortho Evra, 264
Ospemifene (Osphena), 211, 223, 228–29, 245
osteoarthritis, 54, 383, 416
osteonecrosis, 378–79
osteopenia (low bone mass), 347, 348–49
osteoporosis: bone thinning/loss, 351–53; fracture risk and treatment options, 374–76; osteoporotic fractures, 349–50; risk factors, 15, 353–57; statistics, 346–47. *See also* bone health
osteoporosis medications, 372–84; anabolic medications, 382–84; bisphosphonates, 376–77; bisphosphonates, efficacy of, 377–78; bisphosphonates, side effects, 378–80; denosumab (Prolia), 380–81; hormone therapy, 381–82
OVA Plus blood test, 474–76
ovarian cancer, 472–78; doctor's appointments, 478; and hormone therapy (HT), 79; risk factors, 266, 473–76; risk factors, lowering, 477; symptoms of, 473; types of, 472
ovarian cysts, 85, 149, 217–18
ovaries, 18–19
overactive bladder medicine, 62
ovulation, 18–19, 25, 217, 252
Oxybutynin, 62, 181
oxytocin, 279–81
Ozempic, 400

paced respiration, 41
pain: chest pain, 116, 119; nerve pain, 61–62; and ovarian cysts, 217–18; perception of, 54; during sex, 10, 26, 86, 189, 196, 197, 206, 212–13, 214, 219–20, 230–32; and sexually transmitted diseases, 193, 194–95; and uterine cancer, 153; vulvar, 245; while urinating, 177, 178, 197
PALM COEIN evaluation tool, 136
Pap smears, 150, 152–53, 194, 462–66; timing of, 466–70
parathyroid hormone (PTH), 382
Parkinson's disease, 296
Paroxetine, 300
patient-doctor team, 12–16, 28–29, 451–53, 478

Paxil, 59–60, 300
PCE (Pooled Cohort Equations) risk estimator, 128
pelvic examination, 148, 154, 155, 195, 211, 224
pelvic floor physical therapy, 213
pelvic inflammatory disease (PID), 259, 260, 502
pelvic ultrasound, 437, 454, 473, 474
Per Diem, 220
perimenopause: definitions, 4; depression, 293–94; duration of, 20, 23–25; and fertility, 21–22; fluctuating hormone levels, 19–20; menstrual bleeding during, 22–23; mood and mental health, 270–71; pregnancy during, 251–52; sleep patterns, 336–37
pessaries, 180
pets, 342
Phentermine, 400
Phexxi, 253–54
pH levels, 190; vaginal, 200, 253
physical activity. *See* exercise
Physicians' Committee for Responsible Medicine (PCRM), 427
phytoestrogens, 47
Phytofemale Complex, 327
PhytoSERM, 49
PID (pelvic inflammatory disease), 259, 260, 502
Pilates, 410
Plan B (morning after pill), 257–58
plant-based hormones, 88–89, 94; skin patches, 84
PMDD. *See* premenstrual dysphoric disorder (PMDD)
PMS. *See* premenstrual syndrome (PMS)
polycystic ovarian syndrome, 113

polyps, 143, 159–61
positron emission tomography, 131
post menopause, 11; bleeding, 147–48; definitions, 4; depression, 294; diagnosis of, 25–26; hormone levels, 21; mood and mental health, 271; sleep patterns, 336–37
posttraumatic stress disorder (PTSD), 278
posture, 409
Prasterone, 211, 223, 225–26
pregnancy: high-risk, 112–13; during perimenopause, 251–52; unplanned, 250
Premarin, 69–70, 74–75
premature menopause, 7–8, 26
premature ovarian insufficiency (POI), 111–12, 114
premenopause, definitions, 4
premenstrual dysphoric disorder (PMDD), 287–88; natural treatments, 288–89; prescription treatments, 289–90
premenstrual syndrome (PMS), 281–86; diary of symptoms, 284; natural treatments, 288–89; prescription treatments, 289–90; symptoms, 283; and thyroid disease, 282, 284–85
Prempro, 88, 108; in WHI study, 69–70, 75, 77
preventive care, 2, 12, 15, 29, 393–97; cardiovascular disease (CVD), 75, 106–7, 129–31; cervical cancer, 194, 165; dementia, 310–15; urinary tract infection (UTI), 177–78; vaginal health, 198–99
primary care provider. *See* doctor-patient team

primary ovarian insufficiency (POI), 6
progesterone, 18; fluctuating levels, 20; for insomnia, 327; for low sexual desire, 242–43; and mood, 275; progesterone therapy, 88; and sleep, 335
prolapse, uterine/vaginal, 187, 216–17
Prolia, 375, 376, 380–81
Prometrium, 60, 82, 94, 100, 243; for insomnia, 327
Propranolol, 296
protein, 411–12; balanced with carbohydrate, 411, 414, 423; high-protein diets, 356, 424–25
proton pump inhibitors, 355
Provera, 74, 76, 88, 243
Prozac, 59–60, 300
psilocybin, 303–4
psoriasis, 196, 197, 218
psychotherapy, 301–2. *See also* cognitive behavioral therapy (CBT)
puberty, 18
Pycnogenol, 327

radiation exposure and cancer risk, 439
radiofrequency (ThermiVA), 216–17
Raloxifene, 375, 381–82
rapid eye movement (REM) sleep, 332
Reclast, 376, 377, 378
rectocele, 186–87, 216–17
red clover, 56
Relizen, 55–56
Remifemin, 55
REM sleep, 340
REON POCKET cooling device, 46
RepHresh, 223
Replens, 223

restless leg syndrome, 335, 342
resveratrol, 54
retirement, 297
Revaree, 223
rheumatoid arthritis, 355
rhythm contraceptive method, 252
Risedronate, 377, 378
role overload, 292–93
role transitions/disputes, 302
ROMA (Risk for Ovarian Malignancy Algorithm) screening, 474–76
Romosozumab, 376, 382

salivary hormone levels, 24
sarcopenia, 392
screening tests: blood tests, 474–75; for cervical cancer, 461, 466; direct-to-consumer, 450; for uterine cancer, 453, 457–58. *See also* mammography; Pap smears
seasonal affective disorder (SAD), 292
sedentary lifestyles, 109, 356; and cancer risk, 439; exercise program, starting, 403–4; and uterine cancer, 456
seizure medications, 355
selective estrogen receptor modulators (SERMs), 101–2, 381–82
selective norepinephrine reuptake inhibitors (SNRIs), 291, 300
selective serotonin reuptake inhibitors (SSRIs), 215, 290, 291, 300–301; and osteoporosis risk, 355; and weight gain, 430
S-Equol, 48–49
serotonin, 300–301; and estrogen, 274–75; and sleep, 334

Index 521

serotonin-norepinephrine reuptake inhibitors, 215
sex, 203–46; arousal difficulties, 211–12; breast cancer survivors, 245–46; and cervical cancer risk, 461–62; female sexual dysfunction (FSD), 205–6; interest/lack of interest, 232–38; lack of desire for, 208–9, 210–11; lifestyle factors affecting, 229–30; linear vs. cyclical models, 204–5; lubricants, use of, 211; male erectile dysfunction, 209–10; medical conditions affecting, 215–29; medications affecting, 213–15; medications for low sex drive, 238–44; motivation for, 237; orgasm difficulties, 213; pain during, 212–13, 217–18; physical changes affecting, 207; pleasure, 237–38; positions for, 210; scheduling, 233; seeking medical care for, 230–32; sexual aids, 244–45; and sleep quality, 334; social context of, 207; vaginal dryness, 211
sex drive, 18, 205, 208, 232, 233–38; and alcohol, 229; and exercise, 230; medication, effect of, 211, 214–15; medication to treat low sex drive, 238–43; and thyroid problems, 219
sex hormone binding globulin (SHBG), 90, 243
sexually transmitted infections, 143, 193–95; and barrier contraception, 254
Sexy Years, The (Somers), 98
Sheehy, Gail, 35
Shifren, Jan, 239–40
Silent Passage (Sheehy), 35

sitz baths, 199, 200
skin issues, vulvar, 187–89, 196–98
skin patches, contraceptive, 264
sleep, 320–43; importance of, 320–21, 333; and menopause, 334–35; nonrapid eye movement (NREM) sleep, 332; phases of, 332–33; pre-sleep rituals, 341; rapid eye movement (REM) sleep, 332; scheduling, 342; and sex, 334; sleep environment, 342; sleep improvement, 338–41; sleep patterns, 336–37; snoring, 330, 335, 337; and weight control, 336–37
sleep apnea, 329–31
sleep deprivation, 329, 333
sleep hygiene, 338–41
sleep problems: diagnosis of, 321–22; doctor, discussions with, 332; insomnia, 322–29; and weight gain, 430
sleep restriction therapy (SRT), 327–28
smoking, 7, 27; and cancer risk, 439; and cardiovascular disease (CVD) risk, 108, 126; and osteoporosis risk, 356; and sleep quality, 340
snoring, 330, 335, 337
soap pH levels, 190
social history, 213
social interactions, 310
social isolation, 295. *See also* friendship
societal views on menopause, 2–4
soda intake: and bladder issues, 181, 220; and bone health, 356–57, 367, 372, 379, 414; caffeine, 288, 340
Somers, Suzanne, 98
sonohysterogram imaging, 149

Sonoma diet, 425
Sonoma Diet Cookbook (Guttersen), 420
South Beach diet, 126, 425–26
soy foods, 41–42, 47–50
spermicide, 253; and diaphragms, 256
spotting, 135, 140, 147; menstrual calendar, recording, 144–45; from polyps, 159–61
SSRIs (selective serotonin reuptake inhibitors). See selective serotonin reuptake inhibitors (SSRIs)
stages of menopause, 16–18
Stages of Reproductive Aging Workshop (STRAW), 5
starvation response, 411, 422
statins, 14, 299
sterilization: female, 265–66; male, 266–67
steroid medications: and bone health, 358; corticosteroids, 359, 431
STIs. See sexually transmitted infections
St. John's wort, 52, 173, 299–300
St. Louis University Mental Status exam (SLUMS), 316
strength training, 408
stress: anxiety, 290–91; and cardiovascular disease (CVD) risk, 114–15; gender differences, 276–79; oxytocin, 279–81; posttraumatic stress disorder, 278; and sexual experience, 230; stress eating, 415–16; stress hypothesis and dementia, 311; stress reduction, 42; vulnerability to, 302
stretching, 407

stroke: and hormone therapy (HT), 71, 74–75; and oral contraceptives, 260–61; overview of, 116; PCE risk estimator, 128–29; risk of, 70, 106–9, 121–22; risk of, lowering, 125–26; TIA (transient ischemic attack), 315. See also blood pressure, high; cardiovascular disease (CVD)
Strong Women Stay Young (Nelson), 371
sun exposure and vitamin D, 371
sun sensitivity: with dong quai, 56; with estrogen, 82; with St. John's wort, 299
supplements: for hot flashes, 50–58; research concerning, 52–53; soy, 48–50. See also natural remedies
surgical menopause, 27
Surveillance, Epidemiology and End Results (SEER), 456
swab tests, 150
SWAN (Study of Women Across the Nation), 114
swimming, 370, 406
syndrome X (metabolic syndrome). See metabolic syndrome (syndrome X)

tai chi, 409
talc, ovarian cancer and, 477
tamoxifen, 102, 381, 457
temperature control devices, 45–46
Teriparatide, 376, 382
Terzepatide, 400
testosterone, 18, 238–41; for low sexual desire, 210; testosterone pellets, 96
ThermiVA technology, 186–87, 188, 216–17, 245–46

3D mammogram, 444
thyroid disease, 143; and hot flashes, 38-40; hyperthyroidism, 39; hypothyroidism, 39; and mood, 273-74; and PMS, 282, 284-85; and sex, 219; and weight gain, 430
thyroid test, 148-49
TIA (transient ischemic attack), 315
timing of menopause, 5-8
tissue-selective estrogen complex (TSEC), 102
toxoplasmosis, 251
trabecular bone, 350, 363-64
tranexamic acid, 172
transient ischemic attack (TIA), 315
transvaginal ultrasound, 159
Triamcinolone, 196
trichomonas, 185
tricyclic antidepressants, 215, 245
Tri-Est, 99
triglycerides, 110
Trulicity, 400
tryptophan, 282, 339
tubal ligation, 265-66
Tums, 368
twins and premature menopause, 7-8
Twirla, 264

UAE (uterine artery embolization), 170-71
ultrasound tests, 149; breast, diagnostic, 145; transvaginal, 159
urethrocele, 179
urge urinary incontinence (UUI), 62
urinary problems, 176-87; incontinence, 62, 179-84; medication that cause, 184; and sex, 219; weakened internal support, 184-87
urinary tract infection (UTI), 177-79
urologists, 182, 201

U.S. Food and Drug Administration (FDA), 51, 88, 93, 95-98, 100
U.S. Preventive Services Task Force, 295
uterine artery embolization (UAE), 170-71
uterine cancer, 143, 153, 453-61; diagnosis, 145; doctor's appointments, 460-61; endometrial cancer, 453-54; and endometrial hyperplasia, 142; risk factors, 456-57; screening for, 457-60; symptoms, 455-56; types of, 453-55
uterine prolapse, 187, 216-17
UTI (urinary tract infection), 177-79

vaccines: COVID-19, 442, 446-47; HPV, 462, 471
Vagifem, 225
vagina: douching, 200; vaginal health, promotion of, 198-99; vaginal symptoms, 189
vaginal dilators, 213
vaginal dryness, 188, 211, 221-23; hormones for, 224-29; laser treatment for, 189, 217, 245; vaginal moisturizers, 223
vaginal estrogen, 86, 94-95, 211
vaginal infection, 189, 219
vaginal moisturizer, 211, 213
vaginal ring, 227-28, 265
vaginal ultrasound, 149, 159
Vagisil, 192
valerian root, 328
vascular dementia, 309
vasectomy, 266-67
vasomotor symptoms, 33; and cardiovascular disease (CVD) risk, 113-14. See also hot flashes; night sweats

vegetarian/vegan diets, 34, 41–42, 47, 126, 288–89, 426–27, 439
Venlafaxine, 300
vertebral spine fractures, 357, 376, 387
Viagra, 209–10, 242
vibrators, 244–45
victimization of women, 292
Vitamin A, 357, 419
Vitamin B$_6$, 57, 289
Vitamin D, 289, 356, 370–71, 419
Vitamin E, 57–58, 419
Vitamin K, 419
Vitamin X. *See* exercise
vitex, 289
Vivelle, 84
vulvar cancer, 198, 462
vulvar changes, 196, 218–19. *See also* Lichen sclerosis (LS)
vulvar problems, 187–89; itching, 190–91; pain, 245
vulvovaginitis, 190

waist circumference, 109, 393, 397
waist-to-hip ratio, 109
walking, 50, 230, 328, 371, 399, 403–4, 406, 409, 432
warts, 193–94, 256
wart virus. *See* human papilloma virus (HPV)
water, exercise in, 406
water intake, 177, 181, 186, 235, 340
Wegovy, 400
weight: and sleep, 336–37; underweight and osteoporosis risk, 354
weight gain, 14, 391–93; foods to avoid, 413–14; misleading claims, 413; nutrition, optimal, 410–12;
stress eating, 415–16; weight loss diets, 417–20; weight loss diets, evaluation/comparison, 420–28. *See also* obesity/overweight
weight lifting, 408
weight reduction: assessment of progress, 432–33; challenges, 430–31; and CVD risk, 126; food journal/diary, 428–29; maintenance phases, 421; medications, 400; options, 401; portion sizes, 428–29; readiness for, 418–20; research/future trends, 431. *See also* diets for weight loss; obesity/overweight
Weight Watchers, 126, 421, 425
Wellbutrin, 300
WHI (Women's Health Initiative), 69–74, 108
WHIMS (Women's Health Initiative Memory Study), 315–16
WHO (World Health Organization), 365–66, 395
wild yam cream, 54
Willett, Walter, 412
WISDOM (Women's International Study of Long Duration Oestrogen after Menopause), 315–16
withdrawal contraceptive method, 252–53
women's experiences of menopause, 9–10
Women's Health Initiative (WHI), 69–74, 108
Women's Health Initiative Memory Study (WHIMS), 315–16
Women's International Study of Long Duration Oestrogen after Menopause (WISDOM), 315–16

World Health Organization (WHO), 365–66, 395
wrist fracture, 409

Xulane patch, 264

Yaz, 289
yeast infections, 189, 190; after antibiotics, 213–14; contrasted with bacterial, 191, 192; and diabetes, 219; and vulvar changes, 196, 201
yoga, 328, 410; and libido, 211
youth-centered culture, 35
Yuvafem, 225

Zoledronate, 377, 378
zoledronic acid, 376

Browse more books from HOPKINS PRESS

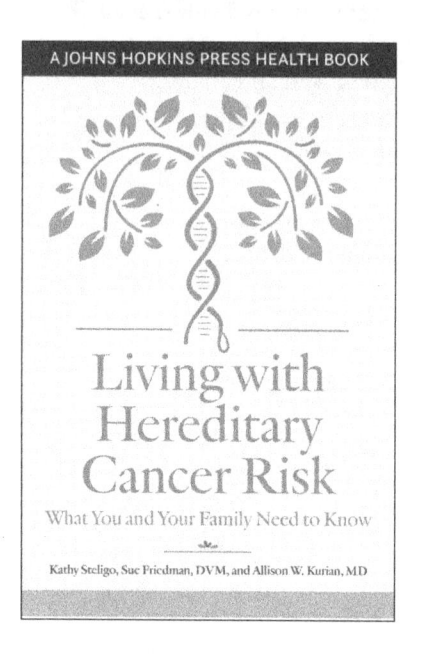

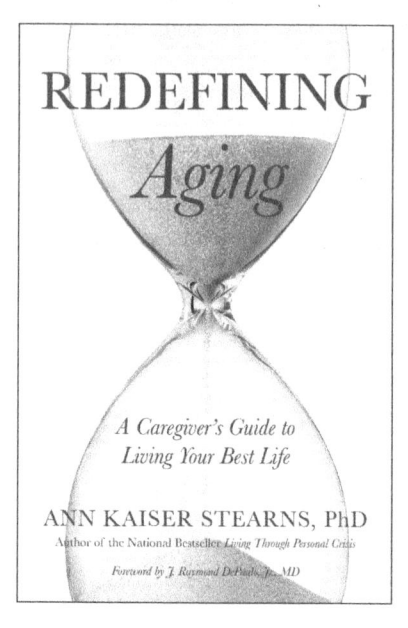

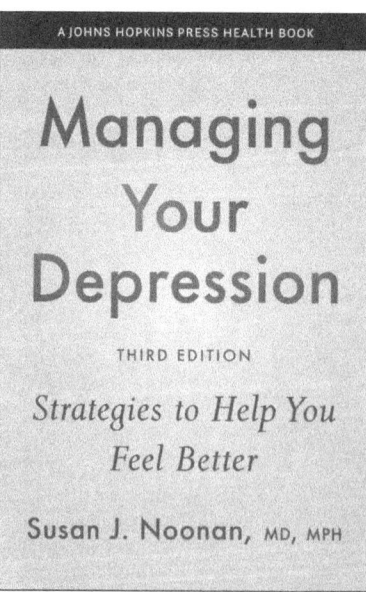

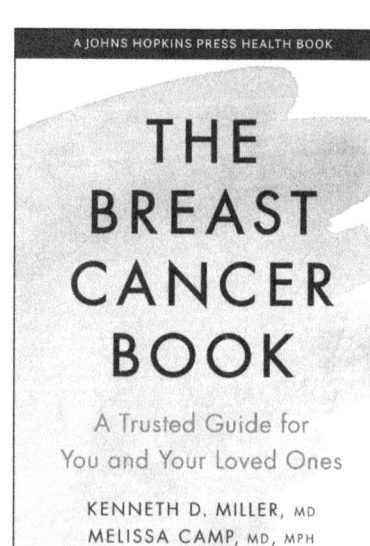

Living with Hereditary Cancer Risk
A JOHNS HOPKINS PRESS HEALTH BOOK

What You and Your Family Need to Know

Kathy Steligo, Sue Friedman, DVM, and Allison W. Kurian, MD

REDEFINING Aging
A Caregiver's Guide to Living Your Best Life

ANN KAISER STEARNS, PhD
Author of the National Bestseller *Living Through Personal Crisis*

Foreword by J. Raymond DePaulo, Jr., MD

Managing Your Depression
A JOHNS HOPKINS PRESS HEALTH BOOK

THIRD EDITION

Strategies to Help You Feel Better

Susan J. Noonan, MD, MPH

THE BREAST CANCER BOOK
A JOHNS HOPKINS PRESS HEALTH BOOK

A Trusted Guide for You and Your Loved Ones

KENNETH D. MILLER, MD
MELISSA CAMP, MD, MPH
WITH Kathy Steligo

JOHNS HOPKINS UNIVERSITY PRESS | PRESS.JHU.EDU